METHODS IN MOLECULAR BIOLOGY

Series Editor
John M. Walker
School of Life and Medical Sciences
University of Hertfordshire
Hatfield, Hertfordshire, AL10 9AB, UK

For further volumes:
http://www.springer.com/series/7651

Clostridium difficile

Methods and Protocols

Second Edition

Edited by

Adam P. Roberts and Peter Mullany

Department of Microbial Diseases, UCL Eastman Dental Institute, University College London, London, UK

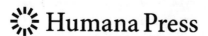 Humana Press

Editors
Adam P. Roberts
Department of Microbial Diseases
UCL Eastman Dental Institute
University College London
London, UK

Peter Mullany
Department of Microbial Diseases
UCL Eastman Dental Institute
University College London
London, UK

ISSN 1064-3745   ISSN 1940-6029   (electronic)
Methods in Molecular Biology
ISBN 978-1-4939-8176-2   ISBN 978-1-4939-6361-4   (eBook)
DOI 10.1007/978-1-4939-6361-4

Printed on acid-free paper

This Humana Press imprint is published by Springer Nature
The registered company is Springer Science+Business Media LLC New York

Preface

This is an update of the highly successful book first published in 2010 describing the available methods for the study of the important human pathogen *Clostridium difficile*. This book is required as the methods available to study the organism have moved forward at an impressive rate. Here, leading authors in the field describe methods used in their laboratories for investigating the physiology of the pathogen, which is vital if we are to thoroughly understand the diseases it causes. Excitingly, the experimental techniques used to investigate potential new treatments, including vaccine development, bacteriophage and phage product therapy, and fecal transplantation, are detailed as are the techniques used to analyze the various different mechanisms of horizontal gene transfer that have been observed for *C. difficile* and which account for its highly variable genome. This book now provides a comprehensive catalogue of molecular tools and techniques which will be current for a good while and illustrates the maturing techniques now available for the study of this once intractable pathogen.

London, UK   *Adam P. Roberts*
London, UK   *Peter Mullany*

Contents

Contributors

ELAINE ALLAN • *Department of Microbial Diseases, UCL Eastman Dental Institute, University College London, London, UK*

ROBERT E. ASHLEY • *Department of Medicine, The Pennsylvania State University College of Medicine, Hershey, PA, USA; Department of Microbiology & Immunology, The Pennsylvania State University College of Medicine, Hershey, PA, USA*

JENNIFER M. AUCHTUNG • *Alkek Center for Metagenomics and Microbiome Research, Department of Molecular Virology and Microbiology, Baylor College of Medicine, Houston, TX, USA*

FABRIZIO BARBANTI • *Department of Infectious, Parasitic and Immune-Mediated Diseases, Istituto Superiore di Sanità, Rome, Italy*

JAMEEL BATAH • *Unité Bactéries Pathogènes et Santé (UBaPS), Faculté de Pharmacie, Université Paris-Sud, Université Paris-Saclay, Châtenay-Malabry, France*

ROBERT A. BRITTON • *Alkek Center for Metagenomics and Microbiome Research, Department of Molecular Virology and Microbiology, Baylor College of Medicine, Houston, TX, USA*

MICHAEL S.M. BROUWER • *Department of Bacteriology and Epidemiology, Central Veterinary Institute of Wageningen UR, Lelystad, The Netherlands*

CAROLINA PIÇARRA CASSONA • *Instituto de Tecnologia Química e Biológica António Xavier, Universidade Nova de Lisboa, Oeiras, Portugal*

CAROLINE H. CHILTON • *Healthcare Associated Infection Research Group, (Leeds Institute for Biomedical and Clinical Sciences), University of Leeds, Old Medical School, Leeds General Infirmary, Leeds, West Yorkshire, UK*

ANNE COLLIGNON • *Unité Bactéries Pathogènes et Santé (UBaPS), Université Paris-Sud, Université Paris-Saclay, Châtenay-Malabry, France*

GRACE S. CROWTHER • *Healthcare Associated Infection Research Group, (Leeds Institute for Biomedical and Clinical Sciences), Old Medical School, Leeds General Infirmary, University of Leeds, Leeds, West Yorkshire, UK*

CÉCILE DENÈVE-LARRAZET • *Unité Bactéries Pathogènes et Santé (UBaPS), Université Paris-Sud, Université Paris-Saclay, Châtenay-Malabry, France*

ADRIANNE N. EDWARDS • *Department of Microbiology and Immunology, Emory University School of Medicine, Atlanta, GA, USA*

MUHAMMAD EHSAAN • *Clostridia Research Group, BBSRC/EPSRC Synthetic Biology Research Centre (SBRC), School of Life Sciences, Centre for Biomolecular Sciences, University of Nottingham, Nottingham, UK*

CRAIG D. ELLERMEIER • *Department of Microbiology, University of Iowa, Iowa City, IA, USA*

KYLIE FARRELL • *Alkek Center for Metagenomics and Microbiome Research, Department of Molecular Virology and Microbiology, Baylor College of Medicine, Houston, TX, USA*

KELLY A. FIMLAID • *Department of Microbiology and Molecular Genetics, University of Vermont, Burlington, VT, USA; Program in Cellular, Molecular & Biomedical Sciences, University of Vermont, Burlington, VT, USA*

LOUIS-CHARLES FORTIER • *Département de Microbiologie et d'infectiologie, Faculté de Médecine et des Sciences de la Santé, Université de Sherbrooke, Sherbrooke, QC, Canada*

DALE N. GERDING • *Research Service, Hines VA Hospital, Infectious Diseases, Loyola University Medical Center, Chicago, IL, USA*

SHAN GOH • *Department of Pathology and Pathogen Biology, The Royal Veterinary College, Hatfield, Hertfordshire, UK*

SHA HA • *Vaccine Analytical Department, Merck Research Laboratories, Merck and Co., West point, PA, USA*

SUSAN HAFENSTEIN • *Department of Medicine, The Pennsylvania State University College of Medicine, Hershey, PA, USA; Department of Microbiology & Immunology, The Pennsylvania State University College of Medicine, Hershey, PA, USA*

JOHN P. HEGARTY • *Department of Surgery, Division of Colorectal Surgery, The Pennsylvania State University College of Medicine, Hershey, PA, USA*

JON H. HEINRICHS • *Merck Research Laboratories, Merck & Co., Inc., Kenilworth, NJ, USA; Sanofi Pasteur, Swiftwater, PA, USA*

ADRIANO O. HENRIQUES • *Instituto de Tecnologia Química e Biológica António Xavier, Universidade Nova de Lisboa, Oeiras, Portugal*

SANDRA JANEZIC • *National Laboratory for Health, Environment and Food (NLZOH), Maribor, Slovenia; Faculty of Medicine, University of Maribor, Maribor, Slovenia*

PRISCILLA JOHANESEN • *Infection and Immunity Program, Monash Biomedicine Discovery Institute and Department of Microbiology, Monash University, Victoria, Australia*

STUART JOHNSON • *Research Service, Hines VA Hospital, Infectious Diseases, Loyola University Medical Center, Chicago, IL, USA*

IMAD KANSAU • *Unité Bactéries Pathogènes et Santé (UBaPS), Faculté de Pharmacie, Université Paris-Sud, Université Paris-Saclay, Châtenay-Malabry, France*

ADAM KRISTOPEIT • *Merck Research Laboratories, Merck & Co., Inc., Kenilworth, NJ, USA*

SARAH A. KUEHNE • *Clostridia Research Group, BBSRC/EPSRC Synthetic Biology Research Centre (SBRC), School of Life Sciences, Centre for Biomolecular Sciences, University of Nottingham, Nottingham, UK; Nottingham Digestive Disease Centre, NIHR Biomedical Research Unit, The University of Nottingham, University Park, Nottingham, UK*

CATHERINE LANCASTER • *Vaccine Analytical Department, Merck Research Laboratories, Merck & Co., Inc., West Point, PA, USA*

CHRISTINE H. LEE • *Department of Pathology & Molecular Medicine, St. Joseph's Healthcare Hamilton, McMaster University, Hamilton, ON, Canada*

DENA LYRAS • *Infection and Immunity Program, Monash Biomedicine Discovery Institute and Department of Microbiology, Monash University, Victoria, Australia*

SHONNA M. MCBRIDE • *Department of Microbiology and Immunology, Emory University School of Medicine, Atlanta, GA, USA*

NIGEL P. MINTON • *Clostridia Research Group, BBSRC/EPSRC Synthetic Biology Research Centre (SBRC), School of Life Sciences, Centre for Biomolecular Sciences, University of Nottingham, Nottingham, UK; Nottingham Digestive Disease Centre, NIHR Biomedical Research Unit, The University of Nottingham, University Park, Nottingham, UK*

PETER MULLANY • *Department of Microbial Diseases, UCL Eastman Dental Institute, University College London, London, UK*

ROLAND MYERS • *Department of Neural and Behavioral Sciences, The Pennsylvania State University College of Medicine, Hershey, PA, USA*

PAOLA PANNIZZO • *Merck and Co., West point, PA, USA; Johnson & Johnson, Spring House, PA, USA*

SÉVERINE PÉCHINÉ • *Unité Bactéries Pathogènes et Santé (UBaPS), Université Paris-Sud, Université Paris-Saclay, Châtenay-Malabry, France*

FÁTIMA PEREIRA • *Instituto de Tecnologia Química e Biológica António Xavier, Universidade Nova de Lisboa, Oeiras, Portugal; Division of Microbial Ecology, Department of Microbiology and Ecosystem Science, University of Vienna, Vienna, Austria*

ELIZABETH PEREZ • *Department of Medicine, Gastrointestinal Diseases Research Unit, Kingston General Hospital, Queen's University, Kingston, ON, Canada*

ELAINE O. PETROF • *Department of Medicine, Gastrointestinal Diseases Research Unit, Kingston General Hospital, Queen's University, Kingston, ON, Canada*

KEYAN PISHDADIAN • *Department of Microbiology and Molecular Genetics, University of Vermont, Burlington, VT, USA*

MARK D. PRESTON • *National Institute for Biological Standards and Control, South Mimms, UK*

ERIC M. RANSOM • *Department of Microbiology, University of Iowa, Iowa City, IA, USA; Johne's Testing Center, School of Veterinary Medicine, Madison, WI, USA*

ADAM P. ROBERTS • *Department of Microbial Diseases, UCL Eastman Dental Institute, University College London, London, UK*

CATHERINE D. ROBINSON • *Alkek Center for Metagenomics and Microbiome Research, Department of Molecular Virology and Microbiology, Baylor College of Medicine, Houston, TX, USA; Institute for Molecular Biology, University of Oregon, Eugene, OR, USA*

RICHARD R. RUSTANDI • *Vaccine Analytical Department, Merck Research Laboratories, Merck & Co., Inc., West Point, PA, USA*

SUSAN P. SAMBOL • *Research Service, Hines VA Hospital, Infectious Diseases, Loyola University Medical Center, Chicago, IL, USA*

WILLIAM SANGSTER • *Department of Surgery, Division of Colorectal Surgery, The Pennsylvania State University College of Medicine, Hershey, PA, USA*

OGNJEN SEKULOVIĆ • *Département de Microbiologie et d'infectiologie, Faculté de Médecine et des Sciences de la Santé, Université de Sherbrooke, Sherbrooke, QC, Canada*

MÓNICA SERRANO • *Instituto de Tecnologia Química e Biológica António Xavier, Universidade Nova de Lisboa, Oeiras, Portugal*

AIMEE SHEN • *Department of Microbiology and Molecular Genetics, University of Vermont, Burlington, VT, USA*

PATRIZIA SPIGAGLIA • *Department of Infectious, Parasitic and Immune-Mediated Diseases, Istituto Superiore di Sanità, Rome, Italy*

DAVID B. STEWART SR. • *Department of Surgery, Division of Colorectal Surgery, The Pennsylvania State University College of Medicine, Hershey, PA, USA*

RICHARD A. STABLER • *Faculty of Infectious & Tropical Diseases, London School of Hygiene and Tropical Medicine, London, UK*

DAVID S. THIRIOT • *Merck Research Laboratories, Merck & Co., Inc., Kenilworth, NJ, USA*

FENG WANG • *Merck Research Laboratories, Merck & Co., Inc., Kenilworth, NJ, USA*

FRANÇOIS WASELS • *Department of Infectious, Parasitic and Immune-Mediated Diseases, Istituto Superiore di Sanità, Rome, Italy*

DAVID S. WEISS • *Department of Microbiology, University of Iowa, Iowa City, IA, USA*

MARK H. WILCOX • *Healthcare Associated Infection Research Group, (Leeds Institute for Biomedical and Clinical Sciences), Old Medical School, Leeds General Infirmary, University of Leeds, Leeds, West Yorkshire, UK; Leeds Teaching Hospitals NHS Trust, Old Medical School, Leeds General Infirmary, Leeds, West Yorkshire, UK*

Chapter 1

Restriction Endonuclease Analysis Typing of *Clostridium difficile* Isolates

Susan P. Sambol, Stuart Johnson, and Dale N. Gerding

Abstract

Restriction endonuclease analysis (REA) typing using *Hin*dIII enzyme is a highly discriminatory, reproducible, and consistent method of genetic typing of *Clostridium difficile* (CD) isolates. REA typing analyzes CD whole cellular DNA on two levels of discrimination: REA Group designation and REA Type designation, which distinguishes specific subtypes within the REA Group. This methodology has enabled the tracking of epidemiologically significant CD strains over time and in some cases has allowed documentation of the evolution of previously rare REA Group strains that have subsequently become epidemic. The chapter details the methods used to isolate and purify CD colonies from stool samples, to obtain intact, full-length whole cellular DNA from CD isolates by use of guanidine-EDTA solution, and to analyze the *Hin*dIII-digested DNA after electrophoretic separation on agarose gels.

Key words *Clostridium difficile*, whole cellular DNA, REA, Agarose gel electrophoresis, *Hin*dIII, Guanidine thiocyanate, Phenol-chloroform

1 Introduction

Restriction endonuclease analysis (REA) was one of the first genotypic methods used for typing *Clostridium difficile* [1]. Subsequent genotypic methods have involved refinements of electrophoretic separation of DNA banding patterns, PCR amplification of specific genomic regions, and sequencing of specific genes or whole genomes. While these subsequent typing methods have specific advantages, our laboratory has retained *Hin*dIII REA typing of *C. difficile* for several reasons [2]. REA typing allows for two levels of discrimination: REA Group designation refers to a level which correlates with PCR ribotyping [6], and REA Type designation, which distinguishes subtypes within each REA group, further enabling epidemiological data refinement. In addition, our REA typing system includes a database of more than 600 distinct REA types from thousands of *C. difficile* isolates, many of which date back to the 1980s, thus providing a valuable epidemiological resource for the emergence of epidemic and non-epidemic CD strains over time.

Adam P. Roberts and Peter Mullany (eds.), *Clostridium difficile: Methods and Protocols*, Methods in Molecular Biology, vol. 1476, DOI 10.1007/978-1-4939-6361-4_1, © Springer Science+Business Media New York 2016

Identification of isolates to the REA group level (*see* analysis below) has been helpful in tracking important strain groups and their association with specific outbreak settings, populations at risk, and antibiotic associations. For example, multiple US hospital *C. difficile* infection (CDI) outbreaks in the early 1990s associated with clindamycin use were linked to an epidemic strain group identified as REA group J [3]. The current epidemic strains responsible for outbreaks of severe disease in North America and Europe over the last decade were identified as REA group BI [4]. Group BI strains were also identified in our 10-year survey of CD isolates in one tertiary care hospital in the 1980s [5]. Unlike Group BI strains recovered during the current epidemic since 2000, these historic BI isolates were not associated with outbreaks and were susceptible to fluoroquinolones. The BI group designation corresponds to the following strain designations by other genotypic methods: PCR ribotype 027 and the North America pulse-field gel electrophoresis pattern 1 (NAP1) [6]. In addition to REA group designations, specific REA banding patterns (REA types) can be distinguished within the REA groups and allow for more detailed epidemiologic studies of transmission and acquisition. With the exception of whole-genome sequencing, REA typing is more discriminating than most other typing systems for *C. difficile* [7] and comparable in discrimination ability to multilocus variable-number tandem-repeat analysis, MLVA [6]. We describe the methodology and interpretation of *Hin*dIII REA results with inclusion of examples of REA group and typing patterns.

2   Materials

Use molecular biology-grade DNase-, RNase-, and protease-free water or 18 MΩ purified water, and molecular biology-grade reagents for solutions unless otherwise noted, i.e., double-distilled water for electrophoresis components.

2.1 Selective Media Components

1. Taurocholate-cefoxitin-cycloserine fructose agar (TCCFA) plates: Weigh out 5.0 g dibasic sodium phosphate, etc..., 1.0 g monobasic potassium phosphate, 2.0 g sodium chloride, 0.12 g magnesium sulfate, 6.0 g fructose, 1.0 g taurocholic acid (sodium salt), 50.0 g proteose peptone (Difco), 800 ml H_2O. Add 2.5 ml Neutral Red solution (0.33%, Life Technologies), and then bring volume up to 1000 ml with mixing.

   Aliquot media into two 500 ml autoclave-safe (Pyrex) bottles, each containing 8.3 g of Bacto agar (*see* **Note 1**). Autoclave on liquid cycle for 30 min, and then cool to 50 °C in water bath. When cooled, add to *each* 500 ml bottle 2.5 ml stock (50 mg/ml) cycloserine, and 2.5 ml stock (1.6 mg/ml) cefoxitin, cap bottle tightly, and then mix by gently inverting 5–6 times (*see* **Note 2**).

Pour media into sterile, disposable 100 mm petri dishes at 22–25 ml per plate. Let harden, then bag, and store at 4 °C. Prior to use, pre-reduce in anaerobe chamber overnight.

2. Stock cycloserine for TCCFA plates, 50 mg/ml: Add 5.0 g of d-cycloserine (Sigma) to 90.0 ml molecular biology-grade water, mix by inversion or by shaking, and add water to final volume of 100.0 ml. Aliquot into sterile tubes at 10.0 ml per tube, and store at –20 °C.

3. Stock cefoxitin for TCCFA plates, 1.6 mg/ml: Weigh out 0.160 g of cefoxitin (Sigma), dissolve in 90.0 ml molecular biology-grade water, mix by inversion or by shaking, and add water to reach final volume of 100.0 ml. Aliquot into sterile tubes at 10 ml per tube, and store at –20 °C.

2.2 Nonselective Media Components

1. Trypticase soy broth (TSB): Weigh out 30.0 g of trypticase soy broth powder (BBL), and dissolve in 1000 ml final volume of molecular biology-grade water. Aliquot into two 500 ml heat-resistant (Pyrex) bottles, cap bottles loosely, and autoclave on liquid cycle for 30 min. Let cool, cap tightly, and store at 4 °C. Pre-reduce in anaerobe chamber overnight before use.

2. Columbia anaerobic sheep blood agar plates (BBL/Fisher): Pre-reduce in anaerobe chamber overnight before use.

2.3 DNA Isolation Reagents

1. Tris–EDTA solution (TE), pH 7.6: Add 10 ml of 1 M Tris base, pH 7.6 and 2 ml of 0.5 M EDTA, pH 8.0 to a 1000 ml graduated cylinder containing 800 ml molecular biology-grade water. Bring final volume up to 1000 ml with molecular biology-grade water, and then aliquot into ten 100 ml glass bottles. Autoclave on liquid cycle for 30 min, and store at room temperature.

2. 50 mg/ml Lysozyme (Sigma): Weigh out 0.1 g of lysozyme into sterile 4 ml tube, and take into anaerobe chamber. Add 2 ml of pre-reduced sterile TE (pH 7.6), and solubilize lysozyme by pipetting up and down.

3. Guanidine-EDTA-Sarkosyl solution (GES): Weigh out 30.0 g of guanidine thiocyanate into a sterile 50 ml tube, and add 10.0 ml of 0.5 M EDTA (pH 8.0) and 7.0 ml of molecular biology-grade water. Mix at 37 °C with shaking until dissolved, and then cool to room temperature (*see* **Note 3**). Add 2.5 ml of 10% Sarkosyl (*n*-lauroyl sarcosine), and bring final volume up to 50 ml with molecular biology-grade water. Filter through a 0.45 μm syringe filter, and store in the dark or in foil-covered tube at room temperature.

4. 7.5 M Ammonium acetate: Weigh out 28.9 g of ammonium acetate into sterile 50 ml tube, add molecular biology-grade water to a volume of 40 ml, warm solution to room temperature by placing in 37 °C water bath for 10 min, and mix by inversion

(*see* **Note 4**). When completely dissolved, add more molecular biology-grade water to final volume of 50 ml. Store at 4 °C.

5. Phenol-chloroform-isoamyl alcohol (25:24:1): Life Technologies (*see* **Note 5**).

6. Isopropanol (Sigma): Store at –20 °C.

7. 75% Ethanol (EtOH): Place 12.5 ml of molecular biology-grade water in a sterile 50 ml tube, add absolute ethanol to final volume of 50 ml, mix by inversion, and store at –20 °C.

2.4 HindIII Restriction Enzyme Solution

1. *Hin*dIII enzyme set (Promega/Fisher): For each digestion reaction sample, combine 2.0 μl of sterile molecular biology-grade water, 3.0 μl of 10× restriction buffer (Buffer E), 3.0 μl of 1:10 dilution of bovine serum albumin (acetylated, Promega/Fisher, included with kit), 2.0 μl *Hin*dIII restriction enzyme (10 U/μl), and 0.25 μl RNace-IT RNase cocktail 2 mg/ml (Agilent) (*see* **Notes 6** and **7**).

We generally multiply the amount of each reagent in the reaction solution by the total number of samples plus two extra; in other words, if we have 12 samples, we multiply the amount of each reagent by 14, to compensate for any pipetting inaccuracies when adding the reaction solution to each tube.

2.5 Horizontal Agarose Gel Electrophoresis Components

1. TAE electrophoresis buffer (10× Tris–acetate–EDTA solution): Weigh 48.45 g of Tris base, 16.4 g of sodium acetate, and 6.8 g of EDTA, and combine in 1000 ml flask containing 800 ml of double-distilled water. Mix until dissolved, and then adjust pH to 7.9 using glacial acetic acid. Bring volume up to 1000 ml, and store in glass bottle at room temperature. Dilute 1:10 in double-distilled water for running buffer and gel buffer (*see* **Note 8**).

2. 0.7% Agarose gel (*see* **Note 8**): Weigh 1.4 g of SeaKem GTG agarose (Lonza, Rockland ME, USA), add to 200 ml of 1× TAE electrophoresis buffer in heat-proof (Pyrex) bottle, and melt agarose by heating in microwave for 2 min on high setting. Swirl to mix, and heat for 1 additional minute in microwave or until all agarose particles have dissolved. Cool agarose solution by placing bottle under cold running water and swirling to mix every 30 s, and bring to approximately 50–60 °C (hot but not burning to touch).

3. 6× Loading buffer III (LB III): Place 3.0 ml of sterile glycerol in a sterile 15 ml tube. Add 1.0 ml of 2.5% bromophenol blue and 1.0 ml of 2.5% xylene cyanol to glycerol in tube, bring final volume to 10.0 ml with molecular biology-grade water, and mix thoroughly by inversion. Aliquot into 1.5 ml Eppendorf tubes at 1 ml per tube, and store long term at –20 °C, and then at 4 °C just before use [8].

4. Ethidium bromide solution, 10 mg/ml (Sigma).

3 Methods

3.1 Clostridium difficile (CD) Recovery and Purification from Stool Specimens by Sequential Selective (TCCFA) and Non selective (Anaerobic Sheep's Blood Agar) Plate Culture

1. Using a sterile cotton swab, inoculate a small portion of stool onto one quadrant of a pre-reduced TCCFA selective plate, and then streak for isolation using a sterile bacterial loop. Incubate at 36 °C in anaerobe chamber (anaerobic atmosphere = 90 % nitrogen, 5 % hydrogen, 5 % carbon dioxide) for 48 h. Choose distinct colonies with typical CD morphology (yellowish, "dry"-looking colonies with characteristic "fried-egg" appearance) for subculture onto nonselective media (*see* **Note 9**).

2. Inoculate one or more distinct CD colonies from TCCFA plate onto one quadrant of a pre-reduced anaerobic sheep's blood agar plate (BAP), and streak for isolation using a sterile bacterial loop. Incubate at 36 °C in anaerobe chamber for 48–72 h (*see* **Note 10**).

3.2 Isolation of Whole Cellular CD DNA

1. For each sample to be typed, inoculate a single large (2–4 mm) purified CD colony from BAP into 20 ml of pre-reduced trypticase soy broth (TSB) in a 50 ml sterile disposable tube (*see* **Note 11**). Incubate for 18–20 h at 36 °C in anaerobe chamber; no agitation of broth culture is required.

2. Cap tubes tightly, and then remove from chamber. Spin down cells at 3000 rpm ($2500 \times g$) in a tabletop centrifuge for 15 min.

3. Return tubes to anaerobe chamber, decant supernatant from each tube, and gently resuspend cell pellet in 1 ml of sterile pre-reduced TE, pH 7.6. Transfer to labeled 1.5 ml microcentrifuge tubes, and cap tightly.

4. Centrifuge for 4 min in a clinical microfuge (6-position) set up in anaerobe chamber, decant supernatant, and blot tube on clean paper towels. Add 100 µl of 50 mg/ml lysozyme to each tube and thoroughly resuspend cell pellet by pipetting up and down multiple times. Cap microfuge tubes, remove from anaerobe chamber, and place in 37 °C water bath for 15 min.

5. Add 500 µl of GES to each tube, and mix gently by inverting tube 4–7 times (*see* **Note 12**). Incubate in the dark (inside cabinet) for 15–20 min at room temperature.

6. Add 250 µl of chilled 7.5 M ammonium acetate to each tube, and mix gently by inverting tube 4–7 times. Incubate on ice for 10 min.

7. Under fume hood, add (using sterile glass pipet) approximately 700 µl of phenol-chloroform-isoamyl alcohol to each tube until nearly full. Cap tightly, place tubes in tube rack, and mix by inversion for 2 min, approximately two inversions per second. Place tubes in refrigerated microcentrifuge (3–4 °C) to separate phases by spinning at $22,000 \times g$ for 7 min. Carefully remove tubes from microcentrifuge and place in fume hood. Gently draw off the upper (aqueous) phase using either poly-

propylene transfer pipet or 1000 µl pipette, taking care to avoid interface, and place aqueous phase in sterile, labeled 1.5 ml microcentrifuge tube (*see* **Note 13**).

8. Add chilled isopropanol (approximately 400–500 µl, 0.5× volume of aqueous layer) to tubes until nearly full. Cap tightly and mix by inversion for 2 min, approximately two inversions per second. Place tubes in –20 °C freezer and allow DNA to precipitate for 20 min.

9. Transfer tubes to refrigerated microcentrifuge (3–4 °C) and spin at 22,000×*g* for 15 min. A small, 1–2 mm, whitish DNA pellet should form on bottom, "outer" portion of microcentrifuge tube (*see* **Note 14**). Decant supernatant and add 0.75 ml of chilled 75 % ethanol to tube. Mix gently by inversion, then place in refrigerated microcentrifuge (3–4 °C), and spin at 22,000×*g* for 3 min. Decant or gently draw off ethanol, taking care to leave DNA pellet in tube. This is Wash #1.

10. Repeat ethanol washes three more times for a total of four washes, keeping 75 % ethanol on ice to maintain low-temperature washes. After the fourth wash, carefully draw off all remaining fluid from DNA pellet, using small pipet tip to draw off last drop. Invert tubes on clean paper towels and allow to air-dry for 5–10 min, until all microdroplets of fluid have dissipated from tube.

11. Resuspend each DNA pellet in 20.0 µl sterile TE, pH 7.6, using a wide-bore sterile polypropylene pipette tip and pipetting up and down repeatedly until pellet appears fully dissolved in TE. DNA may be used immediately in *Hin*dIII restriction (our usual method), or stored at 4 °C for several days before *Hin*dIII restriction, or at –20 °C if used in future PCR or sequencing reactions (*see* **Note 15**).

3.3 HindIII Restriction of Purified Whole Cellular C. difficile DNA

Add 10.0 µl of *Hin*dIII restriction enzyme solution to tube containing 20.0 µl of purified CD DNA (*see* **Note 16**). Place tubes in 37 °C water bath for 2 h to attain complete digestion with *Hin*dIII. Remove tubes from water bath, and dry outside of each tube with lab tissue or paper towel. At this point, *Hin*dIII-digested DNA can be stored at 4 °C for the next 3–5 days.

Just before loading the gel, add 6.0 µl of loading buffer III (LBIII) [8] to inside of each tube and spin briefly (8 s) in tabletop microfuge to bring LBIII down to digested DNA. DNA is now ready to be loaded onto agarose gels.

3.4 Horizontal Agarose Gel Electrophoresis of HindIII-Restricted CD DNA

1× TAE electrophoresis buffer is the only buffer that will facilitate even separation of the *Hin*dIII-restricted CD DNA fragments, so a custom electrophoresis chamber is essential to hold the large amount of running buffer (approximately 1500–1600 ml) needed to run the gels overnight at low voltage without exhausting the buffer. We use custom-made horizontal electrophoresis chambers

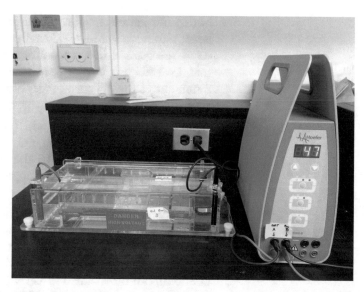

Fig. 1 REA gel electrophoresis system. DanKar horizontal agarose gel electrophoresis system with gel in casting stand (dams removed) in large electrophoresis chamber holding 1500 ml of 1× TAE electrophoresis running buffer (*see* **Note 18**)

and casting stands manufactured by DanKar Corporation (Woburn, MA). The electrophoresis chamber holds 1500 ml of running buffer, while the gel-casting stand holds a 200 ml agarose gel (Fig. 1). The sample well comb has only seven wells: one for the DNA size standard and six for the *Hin*dIII-restricted DNA samples. Each well holds approximately 100 μl volume, although the restricted DNA is only 36 μl with loading buffer.

1. Set up gel casting stand, making sure that it is completely clean (no residual agarose). Slide dams into grooves at both ends of the stand, and then test for leaks by placing water inside, tipping and looking for water leaking from beneath dams. Reset dams if necessary. Using a bubble level, make sure that the casting stand is on a level surface. Weigh out 1.4 g of SeaKem GTG agarose, and place in Pyrex bottle with 200 ml of 1× TAE electrophoresis buffer (*see* **Note 17**). Cap loosely, microwave on High for 2 min, and swirl bottle to resuspend agarose particles. Microwave on High for 1 additional minute, and then swirl carefully (solution is hot!) to make sure that all agarose is dissolved. Cool melted agarose to approximately 50 °C by rotating bottle under cold running water. Pour into gel casting stand and place seven-well comb in slot at one end of gel casting stand; allow gel to solidify at room temperature for 30 min.

2. Make 1× TAE running buffer by adding 160 ml of stock 10× TAE to 1000 ml of double-distilled H₂O in 2 L graduated cylinder; bring final volume up to 1600 ml with double-distilled H₂O. Mix by inversion, and then pour into DanKar

horizontal gel electrophoresis apparatus, taking care to avoid large bubbles. Remove dams from casting stand and place 0.7% agarose gel in electrophoresis apparatus and make sure that 1× TAE just covers the surface of the gel to a depth of 2 mm above the gel surface (*see* **Note 18**).

3. Add Lambda *Hin*dIII marker to Lane 1 to act as DNA size standard, and then carefully add *Hin*dIII-digested DNA samples (with LBIII) to each remaining well. Wait for 5 min after loading for DNA to settle to the bottom of each well, then connect electrodes to power supply, and set power supply to run at 48 V constant voltage.

4. Let run overnight for 16 h. Disconnect from power supply, and then carefully lift gel from electrophoresis apparatus using casting stand; place stand with gel in ethidium bromide (EtBr) staining solution (100 μl of 10 mg/ml stock ethidium bromide in 500 ml double-distilled H$_2$O). Rock gently to evenly distribute EtBr solution above and below gel in casting stand, and let stain for 30 min. Wearing gloves, remove gel in casting stand from EtBr solution (*see* **Note 19**) and place in basin containing approximately 1 L of double-distilled H$_2$O; let destain for 5–6 h.

5. Remove gel from destain solution, place on UV transilluminator, turn on power, and take photograph of gel using classic Polaroid or computerized gel documentation setup. We recommend taking multiple photos at different exposures to maximize readability of every lane on the gel. Save photos in organized notebooks for comparison to REA reference types.

3.5 Visual Analysis of Restriction Patterns on REA Gel Photographs

REA gel patterns consist of 70–80 distinct bands with a possible size range from 30 kb down to less than 1 kb. The largest bands toward the top of the gel are the most distinct, while on the low end of the gel, the bands are subject to blurring.

The *Hin*dIII-restricted DNA band patterns are analyzed visually by doing a millimeter-by-millimeter comparison of the bands in the top 60 mm of the gel (ranging from approximately 30 to 2 kb in length) to either (1) a known or reference REA type or (2) other isolate band patterns.

The DNA pattern is ordered using a similarity index, in which the percentage of matching bands is the basis for naming the REA group or type. If two DNA patterns show a 90% or greater similarity index (less than 10% or seven bands difference throughout the entire pattern), those two isolates are placed in the same REA group (*see* **Note 20**). REA groups have a letter nomenclature (for example, REA Group Y, Group BI) assigned in chronological order of their date of discovery and documentation, i.e., A through Z, followed by AA-AZ, BA-BZ, etc. Therefore, the order of the REA Group letter designation does not imply a relationship between consecutive REA groups; that is, REA Group A types are not similar in pattern to REA Group B types.

If two DNA patterns are identical (100% similarity index), they share the same REA type, which is the REA group followed by a number designation (for example, REA type DH7). Even a single band difference between two DNA patterns separates the isolates into two different REA types within the same REA group.

4 Notes

1. Make sure that all salts and proteose peptone are thoroughly dissolved before adjusting final volume and aliquoting into bottles containing Bacto agar. Before autoclaving, swirl contents of bottles to lightly mix the Bacto agar in a suspension. The agar will not dissolve until the media reaches autoclave temperatures. Loosely cap the bottles so that the bottles will not crack but also prevent overflow during the autoclave cycle.

2. Gentle inversion of the bottle is the best way to get the melted agar into solution while preventing the formation of foaming bubbles. Bubbles should be minimized while pouring media into plates. Excess bubbles can be moved to the edges of the plates using sterile pipet tips.

3. The reagents in GES form an endothermic reaction when mixed with water, causing the solution to become cold. This slows the dissolving of the salts, thus necessitating exposing the solution to heat in the form of a shaking incubator or 37 °C water bath to expedite the dissolving of the guanidine salt.

4. Like GES, ammonium acetate salt undergoes an endothermic reaction when added to water. Gentle heating of the tube for a limited time in a 37 °C water bath expedites the dissolving of the ammonium salt.

5. Chloroform is a carcinogen, so the phenol-chloroform extractions must be performed under a fume hood that has passed inspection. The phenol-chloroform extraction is an essential step in DNA isolation for REA and cannot be replaced by spin column purification methods. Approximately 90–95% of the DNA yield of long DNA (25 kb or longer) is lost in standard column purification methods.

   In addition, be aware that the quality of the phenol-chloroform solution is the main culprit in REA gels that fail to produce readable patterns. If gel patterns are "blown," either failing to cut, or degrading into unreadable smears, the quickest way to resolve the problem is to order a new bottle of phenol-chloroform-isoamyl alcohol.

6. The *Hind*III reaction mix should be made immediately prior to use. The small volume of the reaction solution (10 μl per sample), which will be added to 20 μl of resuspended DNA, means that the reaction buffer is in high concentration (3.3×)

until it is added to the target DNA. We have found this to be detrimental to the *Hin*dIII enzyme activity if the concentrated reaction buffer is left too long in contact with the *Hin*dIII enzyme before dilution with the target DNA.

7. RNase enzyme is a critical part of REA typing, because the DNA isolation method also isolates a large amount of RNA. The RNA will form a large white "cloud" of nucleic acid in the bottom half of the gel which will obscure the DNA pattern if it is not neutralized by the RNase enzyme.

8. 1× Tris-acetate-EDTA buffer is the only electrophoresis buffer that allows the 70 or more bands of *Hin*dIII-restricted *C. difficile* DNA to separate evenly through the length of the gel. Substituting a more robust buffer, such as TBE, will cause the *Hin*dIII-restricted bands to compress at the upper end of the gel and spread out wide at the bottom, which will make the REA pattern difficult to read.

9. It is essential to use only purified CD colonies grown on a nonselective plate such as anaerobic sheep's blood agar for DNA isolation. Picking colonies directly from a differentiating medium (such as a TCCFA plate) for inoculation into TSB broth may allow contaminants, suppressed but not killed on the TCCFA plate, to be grown along with the target CD strain. This mixed culture will interfere with REA typing.

10. Make certain that the purified anaerobic blood agar plate (BAP) culture contains only CD colonies with typical morphology. The presence of tiny white or purple, shiny, or hemolytic colonies indicates that contaminants are present in the culture, and the CD colonies must be purified again on TCCFA plates.

11. DNA isolation is a long and involved protocol in this method, so an experienced technician generally isolates DNA from a maximum of 12 samples in one day. Beginners usually start with only four samples, incrementally increasing the number of samples as they become more proficient in the technique.

12. Once the CD cells are lysed (after the lysozyme incubation), the DNA in solution must be handled gently to avoid shearing the long sequences. Vortexing is to be avoided, as is any vigorous agitation of the tube. The GES and ammonium acetate solutions are to be mixed with the DNA by gentle inversion.

13. Phenol-chloroform is both toxic and carcinogenic, so the organic layer must be decanted into glass bottles while in fume hood and discarded following hazardous chemical waste protocols. Chloroform melts brittle plastics such as polystyrene, so pipets, tips, and tubes that are used with phenol-chloroform must be either borosilicate glass or polypropylene.

14. It is essential that the DNA is kept cold throughout precipitate formation, centrifugation, and ethanol washes. Warming the solutions above 9 °C may cause the DNA to resolubilize, thus resulting in the loss of the DNA pellet. Note that in most cases, the precipitated DNA is visible as a small 1–2 mm pellet on the bottom of the microcentrifuge tube. However, from time to time, the DNA is pure enough to form an "invisible" pellet. If the technician is fairly certain that the pellet was not lost through decanting or through overheating, he or she should treat the washes, decanting, and resuspension steps as if the DNA were present on the bottom portion of the microfuge tube. For this reason, he or she should take care that the microfuge tube remains in the same orientation (usually cap hinge outward) in the microcentrifuge rotor, so that the "invisible" DNA pellet location can be inferred from the positions of visible pellets in the other samples.

15. The purified DNA is handled carefully to avoid shearing the large (>30 kb) sequences needed for REA pattern analysis. For this reason, we use wide-bore tips to resuspend the DNA pellet, and we do not freeze DNA that is earmarked for REA typing, storing it at 4 °C in TE buffer, pH 7.6, to avoid degradation of the solubilized DNA by nucleases and by possible acidic pH. However, if the intention is to use the purified DNA for further PCR studies or for sequencing, we resuspend the DNA pellet in 20–50 μl of molecular biology-grade water and store the solubilized DNA at –20 °C.

16. The average amount of double-stranded DNA isolated from a single reaction (overnight 20 ml TSB culture) is 80–100 μg. The entire amount of DNA is digested with HindIII and loaded onto a single lane on the agarose gel.

17. The agarose gel concentration is 0.7 %, significantly lower than the usual 1 % agarose concentration used in other protocols. The low concentration of agarose is essential for the separation of the large restriction fragments generated in the REA protocol. However, it also creates a relatively soft gel that breaks into pieces if handled roughly; therefore the gel is handled by keeping the casting gel stand supporting the gel during electrophoresis and through the EtBr staining step and destaining wash, until the gel is carefully slid onto the UV transilluminator for photo documentation of the restriction patterns.

18. Do not use an excess of 1× TAE running buffer. Overloading the apparatus so that the running buffer is deep above the gel only increases the temperature above the gel surface as the buffer exhausts during the run. This can cause melting of a thin layer of agarose on the surface of the gel, which in turn will cause blurring of the restriction patterns. In Fig. 1, observe the shallow level of TAE (approx 2 mm) above the surface of the horizontal agarose gel.

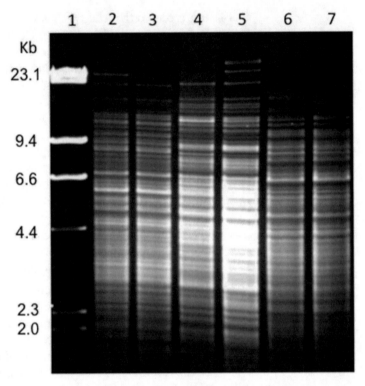

Fig. 2 REA gel photograph of three REA groups/six REA types. *Lane 1*: Lambda HindIII DNA marker. *Lane 2*: REA type DH1. *Lane 3*: REA type DH7. *Lane 4*: REA type BI6. *Lane 5*: REA type BI9. *Lane 6*: REA type M3. *Lane 7*: REA type M23. DH group and BI group are epidemic REA groups implicated in CDI in multiple countries. M group is a nontoxigenic REA group. This photograph shows that there are no distinguishing bands to differentiate toxigenic from nontoxigenic isolates using REA typing (*see* **Note 20**)

19. Ethidium bromide is a toxic, mutagenic chemical that should not be discarded down the sink. We recommend storing the EtBr stain solution in a large container and treating the waste by charcoal filtration before discarding the water down the sink, and placing the filter (as well as the photographed gel) into biohazard waste. We use the EtBr Destaining Tea Bags protocol (MoBio, Carlsbad, CA).

20. The key area of the restriction pattern to examine when grouping DNA isolates is the area that spans 12–2 kb. There are frequent variations in DNA band pattern above 12 kb that differentiate between REA types; however, we expect the patterns within an REA group to be nearly identical between 12 and 2 kb.

References

1. Kuijper EJ, Oudbier JH, Stuifbergen WNHM, Jansz A, Zanen HC (1987) Application of whole-cell DNA restriction endonuclease profiles to the epidemiology of *Clostridium difficile*-induced diarrhea. J Clin Microbiol 25:751–753

2. Clabots CR, Johnson S, Bettin KM et al (1993) Development of a rapid and efficient restriction endonuclease analysis typing system for *Clostridium difficile* and correlation with other typing schemes. J Clin Microbiol 31:1870–1875

3. Johnson S, Samore MH, Farrow KA et al (1999) Epidemics of diarrhea caused by a clindamycin-resistant strain of *Clostridium difficile* in four hospitals. N Engl J Med 341:1645–1651

4. McDonald LC, Killgore GE, Thompson A et al (2005) An epidemic, toxin gene-variant strain of *Clostridium difficile*. N Engl J Med 353:2433–2441

5. Belmares J, Johnson S, Parada JP et al (2009) Molecular epidemiology of *Clostridium difficile* over the course of 10 years in a tertiary care hospital. Clin Infect Dis 49:1141–1147

6. Killgore G, Thompson A, Johnson S et al (2008) Comparison of seven techniques for typing international epidemic strains of *Clostridium difficile*: restriction endonuclease analysis, pulsed-field gel electrophoresis, PCR-ribotyping, multilocus sequence typing, multilocus variable-number tandem-repeat analysis, amplified fragment length polymorphism, and surface layer protein A gene sequence typing. J Clin Microbiol 46:431–437

7. Manzo CE, Merrigan MM, Johnson S et al (2014) International typing study of *Clostridium difficile*. Anaerobe 28:4–7

8. Sambrook J, Russell DW (2001) Molecular cloning: a laboratory manual, 3rsth edn. Cold Spring Harbor Laboratory Press, Cold Spring Harbor, NY, A1.19

Chapter 2

Direct PCR-Ribotyping of *Clostridium difficile*

Sandra Janezic

Abstract

PCR-ribotyping, a method based on heterogeneity of ribosomal intergenic spacer region, is the preferred method for genotyping of *Clostridium difficile*. Standardly used procedure for PCR-ribotyping is culturing of *C. difficile* from fecal samples and subsequent typing. In this chapter, we describe a modified PCR-ribotyping method for direct detection of PCR-ribotypes directly in total stool DNA extract, without prior need to isolate *C. difficile*.

Key words Direct typing, PCR-ribotyping, Total stool DNA, *Clostridium difficile*

1 Introduction

Clostridium difficile infections (CDI) are a substantial burden to the health care system. Since the emergence of epidemic *C. difficile* strain of PCR-ribotype 027 that caused the first outbreaks in 2003 in Canada [1, 2] and has thereafter spread across North America and Europe [3, 4], outbreaks of CDI, which are mainly attributed, but not limited to the epidemic 027 strain, have been commonly present in hospital settings [5–10]. It is therefore important to identify epidemic strains as quickly as possible. Standard routine is to culture *C. difficile* from fecal samples and subsequent genotyping. For *C. difficile* different typing methods were developed and were reviewed by several authors [11–13]. The most commonly used method in Europe, and which has also been recently adopted in the USA, is PCR-ribotyping [14, 15]. The method is based on the amplification of intergenic spacer region (ISR) between 16S and 23S rRNA genes. The ISRs differ in length (200–600 bp) and in combination with variable number of alleles of the ribosomal operon present in different *C. difficile* strains PCR amplification of ISRs with only a single primer pair result in a banding pattern, specific for a given PCR-ribotype.

PCR-ribotyping approach was first described by Gürtler [16]. The method was then modified by O'Neill et al. [17] and was as

Adam P. Roberts and Peter Mullany (eds.), *Clostridium difficile: Methods and Protocols*, Methods in Molecular Biology, vol. 1476, DOI 10.1007/978-1-4939-6361-4_2, © Springer Science+Business Media New York 2016

such adopted in Anaerobe Reference Unit, Cardiff, UK, for a routine typing of *C. difficile* [18]. Soon after, Bidet et al. [19] designed new primers which are located closer to ISR, yielding smaller amplicon sizes (Fig. 1). Both primer sets give comparable banding patterns and are routinely used in different laboratories.

We have recently described a new primer set that enables PCR-ribotyping of *C. difficile* directly in total stool DNA, therefore avoiding the need to culture isolates. New primers were designed to anneal partially within the 16S (forward primer) and 23S (reverse primer) rRNA genes and partially within conserved regions at 5′ and 3′ of ISR (Fig. 1), resulting in specificity for *C. difficile* (Fig. 2) [20, 21]. These primers give comparable results to primers described by Bidet et al. Only difference is in amplicon lengths (relative difference in fragment lengths of 24 bp), thus hindering direct comparison of profiles generated by different primer pairs.

Direct PCR-ribotyping is a rapid method and it gives information on *C. difficile* PCR-ribotype within a day, in contrast to conventional PCR-ribotyping of cultured isolates where results are available after 2–3 days, and can be convenient typing method in situations when only total stool DNA is available.

This chapter describes material and methods used for detection of *C. difficile* PCR-ribotypes directly in total stool DNA extracts.

2   Materials

2.1   Total Stool DNA Extraction

1. Commercial kit for total stool DNA extraction, such as QIAamp DNA Stool Mini kit (Qiagen) (*see* **Note 1**).

2.2   PCR Amplification

1. Primers for amplification of 16S-23S rDNA intergenic spacer region, ISR (5′–3′):

   (a) 16S RT: GCTGGATCACCTCCTTTCTAAG (annealing on 16S rRNA gene and 5′end of ISR).

   (b) 23S RT: TGACCAGTTAAAAAGGTTTGATAGATT (annealing on 3′end of ISR and 23S rRNA gene).

2. Taq DNA polymerase with MgCl$_2$ (Roche) and amplification buffer.

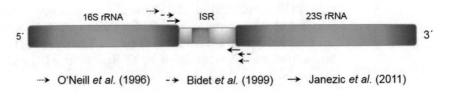

Fig. 1 Schematic representation of localizations of PCR-ribotyping primers within the *C. difficile rrn* operon

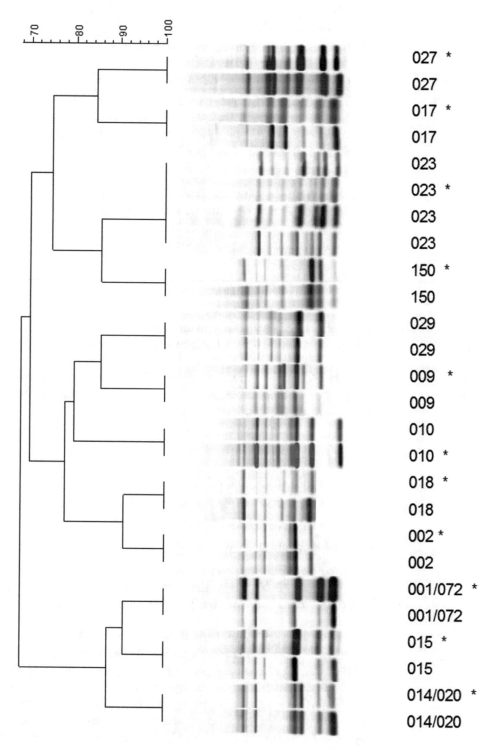

Fig. 2 Comparison of PCR-ribotyping patterns obtained from total stool DNA (marked with *) and reference strains using primers and protocol described in Janezic et al. [20] and in this chapter

3. dNTPs (Roche); working solution of 20 mM dNTPs mix (5 mM each dNTP).

4. Bovine serum albumin, BSA (10 mg/ml).

2.3 Agarose Gel Electrophoresis

1. Certified™ Low range Ultra Agarose (Bio-Rad) (*see* **Note 2**).

2. TAE buffer (50×): 2.0 M Tris-acetate, and 50 mM EDTA. Adjust pH to 7.0. For working solution (1×) dilute 20 ml of 50× TAE with 980 ml of distilled water. Cool the buffer to 4–8 °C before use (*see* **Note 3**).

3. Loading dye.

4. DNA staining solution: Ethidium bromide (EtBr) in distilled water with final concentration of 0.2 μg/ml.

2.4 Analysis of Banding Patterns

1. BioNumerics software (Applied Maths) (*see* **Note 4**).

3 Method

3.1 Isolation of Total Stool DNA

For isolation of total DNA from feces, use a commercial kit and follow the manufacturer's recommendation (*see* **Note 1**).

3.2 PCR Amplification

Prepare PCR master mix according to Table 1 and aliquot 45 μl of master mix in PCR tubes. Add 5 μl of DNA and run a PCR with the following amplification conditions:

- initial denaturation at 95 °C for 5 min,
- 35 cycles of:

    1 min at 95 °C for denaturation,

    1 min at 57 °C for annealing, and

    1 min at 72 °C for elongation,

- final elongation at 72 °C for 10 min.

After amplification, concentrate the PCR products by heating for 45 min at 75 °C. To let the water evaporate, open the caps on centrifuge tubes and leave the lid of thermocycler open.

3.3 Agarose Gel Electrophoresis

For separation of amplified ISRs prepare a 3% agarose gel (Certified™ Low Range ultra agarose; Bio-Rad; *see* **Note 2**) in 1× TAE buffer. In microwave oven melt the agarose with occasional gently mixing with magnetic stirrer; do not allow bubbles to form (*see* **Note 5**). If agarose starts to overboil, pause the microwave oven and let it to calm down and then continue with heating; repeat as many times as needed. Cool the agarose to 50–60 °C (in water bath with occasional gentle mixing on magnetic stirrer). Carefully (again avoiding bubbles) pour the agarose and let it to

Table 1 PCR mastermix composition

Reagent	Volume (µl)
PCR-grade water	36.0
10× PCR buffer (Roche)[a]	5.0
dNTPs (20 mM mix)	2.0
Primer 16S RT (50 µM)	1.0
Primer 23S RT (50 µM)	1.0
BSA (10 mg/ml)	0.5
DNA polymerase (5 U/µl)	0.25
DNA	5.0

[a]Final concentration of $MgCl_2$ in reaction mixture should be 1.5 mM

solidify for 30–45 min and run the electrophoresis at 2.5 V/cm for 4 h (*see* **Note 3**).

Load 20 µl of concentrated PCR product. It is important to include also a reference DNA standard in multiple positions in each gel (e.g., lanes 1, 7, 13, and 20 of a 20-lane gel) for normalization of a gel picture and accurate comparison of banding patterns.

To visualize DNA fragments, stain the gel in ethidium bromide (*see* **Note 6**) for 20–30 min and then de-stain in distilled water for 20–30 min. Capture the image with gel documentation system.

3.4 Analysis of Banding Patterns and Determination of PCR-Ribotypes

PCR-ribotypes can be determined by comparison of banding patterns with reference PCR-ribotypes using appropriate software (e.g., BioNumerics software; *see* **Note 4**) with in-house-built comparison library or, although not advisable and time consuming, manually by running reference strains of interest in the same gel. Isolates having identical banding patterns are considered to belong to the same PCR-ribotype. If two isolates differ in only a single band, they belong to different PCR-ribotypes.

4 Notes

1. Other commercial kits can be used for isolation of total stool DNA. A pre-step with mechanical disruption with the SeptiFast Lyse Kit on MagNA Lyser instrument (Roche) or equivalent can be included to improve the lysis of *C. difficile* cell wall.

2. Other agaroses, suitable for resolution of small PCR fragments, can be used.

3. Always use a fresh 1× TAE. A cold 1× TAE buffer should be poured to electrophoresis chamber just before loading the gel to avoid excessive heating of the buffer during electrophoresis, which can cause DNA degradation.

4. BioNumerics software (Applied Maths, Belgium) is most commonly used for analysis of banding profiles and setting up databases and reference libraries. However, other analysis software can be used as well.

5. A 3% agarose suspension is very thick, so the stirring should be gentle (100–150 rpm). If using microwave oven for melting the agarose use only stirrers covered with plastic.

6. Ethidium bromide is a potential mutagen and must be handled with care; use only appropriate gloves and dispose the staining solution and gel appropriately.

References

1. Loo VG, Poirier L, Miller MA et al (2005) A predominantly clonal multi-institutional outbreak of Clostridium difficile-associated diarrhea with high morbidity and mortality. N Engl J Med 353:2442–2449. doi:10.1056/NEJMoa051639

2. Pépin J, Valiquette L, Alary M-E et al (2004) Clostridium difficile-associated diarrhea in a region of Quebec from 1991 to 2003: a changing pattern of disease severity. Can Med Assoc J 171:466–472. doi:10.1503/cmaj.1041104

3. McDonald LC, Killgore GE, Thompson A et al (2005) An epidemic, toxin gene–variant strain of Clostridium difficile. N Engl J Med 353:2433–2441. doi:10.1056/NEJMoa051590

4. Kuijper EJ, Barbut F, Brazier JS et al (2008) Update of Clostridium difficile infection due to PCR ribotype 027 in Europe, 2008. Euro Surveill 13(31). pii: 18942

5. Baldan R, Trovato A, Bianchini V et al (2015) A successful epidemic genotype: Clostridium difficile PCR ribotype 018. J Clin Microbiol 53:2575–2580. doi:10.1128/JCM.00533-15

6. Borgmann S, Kist M, Jakobiak T, et al. (2008) Increased number of Clostridium difficile infections and prevalence of Clostridium difficile PCR ribotype 001 in southern Germany. Euro Surveill 13. pii 19057

7. Eyre DW, Tracey L, Elliott B et al (2015) Emergence and spread of predominantly community-onset Clostridium difficile PCR ribotype 244 infection in Australia, 2010 to 2012. Euro Surveill 20:21059

8. Goorhuis A, Bakker D, Corver J et al (2008) Emergence of Clostridium difficile infection due to a new hypervirulent strain, polymerase chain reaction ribotype 078. Clin Infect Dis 47:1162–1170. doi:10.1086/592257

9. Nyc O, Krutova M, Liskova A et al (2015) The emergence of Clostridium difficile PCR-ribotype 001 in Slovakia. Eur J Clin Microbiol Infect Dis 34:1701–1708. doi:10.1007/s10096-015-2407-9

10. Nyč O, Pituch H, Matějková J et al (2011) Clostridium difficile PCR ribotype 176 in the Czech Republic and Poland. Lancet 377:1407. doi:10.1016/S0140-6736(11)60575-8

11. Knetsch CW, Lawley TD, Hensgens MP et al (2013) Current application and future perspectives of molecular typing methods to study Clostridium difficile infections. Euro Surveill 18:20381

12. Killgore G, Thompson A, Johnson S et al (2008) Comparison of seven techniques for typing international epidemic strains of Clostridium difficile: restriction endonuclease analysis, pulsed-field gel electrophoresis, PCR-ribotyping, multilocus sequence typing, multilocus variable-number tandem-repeat analysis, amplified fragment length polymorphism, and surface layer protein A gene sequence typing. J Clin Microbiol 46:431–437. doi:10.1128/JCM.01484-07

13. Huber CA, Foster NF, Riley TV, Paterson DL (2013) Challenges for standardization of Clostridium difficile typing methods. J Clin Microbiol 51:2810–2814. doi:10.1128/JCM.00143-13

14. Janezic S, Rupnik M (2010) Molecular typing methods for Clostridium difficile: pulsed-field gel electrophoresis and PCR ribotyping. Methods Mol Biol Clifton NJ 646:55–65. doi:10.1007/978-1-60327-365-7_4

15. Waslawski S, Lo ES, Ewing SA et al (2013) *Clostridium difficile* ribotype diversity at six health care institutions in the United States. J Clin Microbiol 51:1938–1941. doi:10.1128/JCM.00056-13

16. Gürtler V (1993) Typing of *Clostridium difficile* strains by PCR-amplification of variable length 16S-23S rDNA spacer regions. J Gen Microbiol 139:3089–3097

17. O'Neill GL, Ogunsola FT, Brazier JS, Duerden BI (1996) Modification of a PCR ribotyping method for application as a routine typing scheme for *Clostridium difficile*. Anaerobe 2:205–209. doi:10.1006/anae.1996.0028

18. Stubbs SLJ, Brazier JS, O'Neill GL, Duerden BI (1999) PCR targeted to the 16S-23S rRNA gene intergenic spacer region of *Clostridium difficile* and construction of a library consisting of 116 different PCR ribotypes. J Clin Microbiol 37:461–463

19. Bidet P, Barbut F, Lalande V et al (1999) Development of a new PCR-ribotyping method for *Clostridium difficile* based on ribosomal RNA gene sequencing. FEMS Microbiol Lett 175:261–266

20. Janezic S, Štrumbelj I, Rupnik M (2011) Use of modified PCR ribotyping for direct detection of *Clostridium difficile* ribotypes in stool samples. J Clin Microbiol 49:3024–3025. doi:10.1128/JCM.01013-11

21. Janezic S, Indra A, Rattei T et al (2014) Recombination drives evolution of the *Clostridium difficile* 16S-23S rRNA intergenic spacer region. PLoS ONE 9:e106545. doi:10.1371/journal.pone.0106545

Chapter 3

From FASTQ to Function: In Silico Methods for Processing Next-Generation Sequencing Data

Mark D. Preston and Richard A. Stabler

Abstract

This chapter presents a method to process *C. difficile* whole-genome next-generation sequencing data straight from the sequencer. Quality control processing and de novo assembly of these data enable downstream analyses such as gene annotation and in silico multi-locus strain-type identification.

Key words Read trimming, De novo assembly, Gene annotation, MLST

1 Introduction

The first *C. difficile* genome was published in 2006 [1] after significant effort by a team of sequencers at the Wellcome Trust Sanger Centre but, with the increasing availability and quality of whole-genome sequencing equipment, the possible applications for "in-house" genomic analysis are growing for the bench scientist. This chapter shows one route to take, from the large data files generated by the sequencing hardware, transforming it and extracting biologically relevant information.

This chapter covers the processing of the raw data coming out of a sequencer by gathering sequencing reads into long genomic sequences (contigs) reflecting those found in the original sample; comparing these sequences to an existing reference; annotating these sequences; and identifying multi-locus sequencing-type (MLST) data in silico.

2 Materials

This chapter presumes that the scientist has access to a Linux machine and has working knowledge of the Linux operating system (*see* **Note 1**). Linux commands are indicated with a "$" and

Adam P. Roberts and Peter Mullany (eds.), *Clostridium difficile: Methods and Protocols*, Methods in Molecular Biology, vol. 1476, DOI 10.1007/978-1-4939-6361-4_3, © Springer Science+Business Media New York 2016

written in "Courier new" font; the "\" at the end of command lines is a textual indicator to not press return but to keep on typing and without typing the "\".

2.1 Software

First the computer system must be set up with the required software (*see* References for software sources and **Note 2**). This chapter uses the following software which must be installed prior to use:

1. fastqc [2]	Analyzes fastq data for quality, adapter sequences, etc.
2. trimmomatic [3]	Removes low-quality reads from fastq data
3. velvet [4]	De novo assembles sequences (contigs) from reads in fastq data
4. abacas [5]	Orders contigs by aligning them against a reference genome
5. prokka [6]	Transfer gene, RNA, *etc.* annotation from one species to a sample
6. BLAST+ [7]	Compares sequences and identifies the identical sections
7. act [8]	Genome comparison tool
8. mlst [9]	Sequence typing tool

These programs rely on other bioinformatic software to also be installed (for example mummer, bioperl) and further details can be on the homepage for each piece of software (*see* **Note 3**).

2.2 Preparing the System

Secondly it is advisable to create a directory structure that reflects the data, thus making it easier to locate and identify files. The following command sets up the directories; some tools will create their own directories (*see* **Note 4**):

```
$ mkdir -p reference fastq trim abacas
```

2.3 Worked Example Data

In this chapter publically available *C. difficile* sequence data will be used as an example but alternative data can be used. Download the reference annotation (.embl) and reference sequence files (.fasta) (*see* **Notes 5** and **6**):

```
$ wget "http://www.ebi.ac.uk/Tools/dbfetch/ \dbfetch?db=
    embl&id=AM180355&style=raw"
-O reference/630.embl
$ wget "http://www.ebi.ac.uk/Tools/dbfetch/ \dbfetch?db=
    ena_sequence&id=AM180355&format=fasta&style=raw" \
-O reference/630.fasta
```

Download paired-end data taken from an Illumina MiSeq-sequenced *C. difficile* sample [10] (*see* **Note 6**):

```
$ curl "ftp://ftp.sra.ebi.ac.uk/vol1/fastq/ERR788/
    ERR788977/ \ERR788977_1.fastq.gz" > fastq/sample_1.
    fastq.gz
$ curl "ftp://ftp.sra.ebi.ac.uk/vol1/fastq/ERR788/
    ERR788977/ \ERR788977_2.fastq.gz" > fastq/sample_2.
    fastq.gz
```

The Illumina MiSeq was run in "paired-end" mode to generate sequence data from both ends of genomic fragments. These fragments are ~1 kbp in length and up to 301 bp are able to be sequenced from both the start and the end of the fragment. These are known as the forward and reverse reads denoted by _1 and _2 in the file name, respectively. Together they are known as paired-end reads.

3   Methods

3.1   QC the Data

Before processing the raw data it is advisable to test its quality and remove low-quality calls. The fastqc program [2] analyzes the files taken from the sequencer. Run fastqc in interactive mode:

```
$ fastqc
```

Open (ctrl-O) the forward reads (in the file fastq/sample_1.fastq.gz). Amongst other data it shows the average base quality per cycle/position, on a logarithmic scale ($10 = 1$ error in 10, $20 = 1$ error in 100, $30 = 1$ error in 1000, and $40 = 1$ error in $10,000$). The quality of the called bases (sometimes referred to as positions or cycles) drops off (Fig. 1) and becomes more variable along the

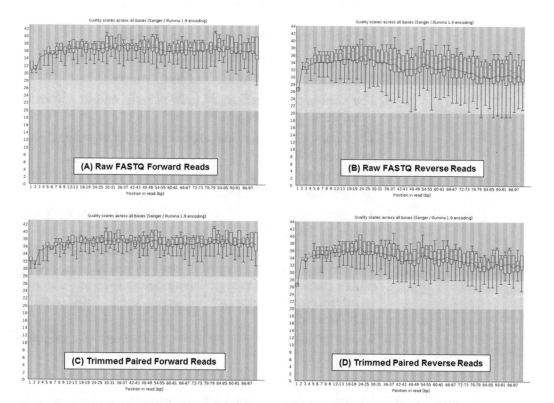

Fig. 1 FastQC per-base-quality for raw (**a, b**) and trimmed (**c, d**) paired reads. Each graph shows a box-and-whisker plot for the quality (−log10 error) for each base pair position along the reads. The quality (on average) drops along reads, is lower for the reverse read (e.g., comparing (**a**) to (**b**)), and is much improved after trimming (e.g., comparing (**a**) to (**c**)). Data for unpaired reads not shown

read; this is especially noticeable in the reverse reads (Fig. 1b). Any quality score below 20 is deemed to be poor-quality data. Although one error in 100 (score of 20) seems very low, in the context of $\sim 2.2 \times 10^6$ paired 100 bp reads yield $\sim 4.4 \times 10^8$ individual base calls, and therefore potentially yielding (in the order of) 10^6 erroneous calls. The other graphs in fastqc show more quality statistics related to the sample. The number of low-quality calls is reduced using a program called trimmomatic [3]:

```
$ TrimmomaticPE -phred33 \
    fastq/sample_1.fastq.gz fastq/sample_2.fastq.gz \
    trim/sample.p1.fastq.gz trim/sample.s1.fastq.gz \
    trim/sample.p2.fastq.gz trim/sample.s2.fastq.gz \
    ILLUMINACLIP:NexteraPE-PE.fa:3:20:10 SLIDINGWINDOW:4:30
    MINLEN:50
```

This command line trims off low-quality sequences from the paired-end input reads and outputs the resultant sequencing reads. In most cases the paired reads remain paired, but in some cases one of the paired reads fails the QC leaving a read without a mate, i.e., unpaired. These unpaired reads are output separately from the surviving paired reads.

The command line parameters for TrimmomaticPE, the paired-end version of trimmomatic, taken in order are:

1. -phred33 denotes fastq quality scoring method.
2. The raw input forward reads file (fastq/sample_1.fastq.gz).
3. The raw input reverse reads file (fastq/sample_2.fastq.gz).
4. The trimmed forward reads (still paired) output file name (trim/sample_p1.fastq.gz).
5. The trimmed forward reads (unpaired) output file name (trim/sample_s1.fastq.gz).
6. The trimmed reverse reads (still paired) output file name (trim/sample_p2.fastq.gz).
7. The trimmed reverse reads (unpaired) output file name (trim/sample_s2.fastq.gz).
8. QC filters: In this example, any recognized Illumina Nextera adapter sequences are removed; bases in a read after a 4 bp rolling quality score average falling below Q20 are removed (ILLUMINACLIP:NexteraPE-PE.fa:3:20:10   SLIDINGWINDOW:4:20).
9. Reads of less than 50 bp (after trimming) are removed (MINLEN:50).

The last line of trimmomatic output gives the number of reads passing QC, in this case 1.9×10^6 surviving out of 2.2×10^6 pairs (88%). In addition, 2.5×10^5 reads passed QC without their mate pair, becoming unpaired (or single end) reads. The four output fastq files can now be examined in fastqc as above. The per base pair quality score (used for the trimming, *see* Fig. 1c and d) shows higher average quality and lower variability at each position, the effect being most striking on the reverse reads (c.f. Fig. 1b and d).

3.2 Assemble

De novo assemblers are used to create large sequences (called contigs) from the trimmed reads. Assemblers, using various techniques, identify overlapping reads and by overlapping more and more reads create the contigs. The main parameter for this is called the k-mer (a measure of overlap) and must be chosen for each sample. The velvet de novo assembler [4] (*see* **Note 7**) has a two-step process: it first processes the input reads (called hashing) based on the k-mer and secondly it creates contigs from the hash. The (computationally intensive) job of VelvetOptimiser [11] is to run velvet for a range of k-mers and choose the best set of contigs created:

```
$ perl VelvetOptimiser.pl -s 45 -e 99 -f '-fastq.gz \
-shortPaired trim/sample.p1.fastq.gz trim/sample.p2.
   fastq.gz \
-short trim/sample.s1.fastq.gz trim/sample.s2.fastq.gz' \
-d velvet
```

The command line parameters are the following:

1. The start and end k-mers (-s 45 -e 99); k-mers must be odd. The original/pre-trimmed read length was 100 bp, so anything above 100 will create no contigs.

2. The command line parameters to be passed verbatim to velveth are enclosed in single quotes after -f:

   • -fastq.gz indicates the input format

   • -shortPaired indicates that the next two parameters are paired short read files (trim/sample.p1.fastq.gz and trim/sample.p2.fastq.gz).

   • –short indicates that the next parameters are single (unpaired)-end short read files (trim/sample.s1.fastq.gz and trim/sample.s2.fastq.gz).

3. All output files, including the contigs, are placed in the velvetthe end of the log file (called velvet directory (-d velvet).

For the example sample, the optimal k-mer is 63 where optimality is determined by a combination of statistics generated from the contigs, including N50, maximum, and total aggregate lengths. The N50 statistic reports the length of the contig that contains the "middle" base pair when all of the contigs are placed in length order from smallest to largest. These values are to be found at the end of the log file (called velvet/Log) and, for the example, are 485 contigs up to 250 kbp long, with combined length of 4.24 Mbp and an N50 of 108 kbp. Ideally there would be only one contig that covered the entire genome; in reality long contigs, high N50, and an aggregate contig length similar to that of *C. difficle* indicate a good assembly.

3.3   Order Contigs

To compare samples it is useful to order the contigs in a consistent manner. One method to do this is by matching contigs to a reference genome. The abacas [5] program does this using the nucmer [12] tool for the sequence alignment. The following command aligns our contigs created in Subheading 3.2 to the 630 *C. difficile* reference strain [1] downloaded in Subheading 2.3:

```
$ perl abacas.1.3.1.pl -r reference/630.fasta -q vel-
    vet/contigs.fa -p \
nucmer - c - d - N - l 1000 - o abacas/sample
```

This command line tells abacas:

1. The reference genome to compare to (-r reference/630.fasta).
2. The contigs to order (-q velvet/contigs.fa).
3. To use nucleotide matching (-p nucmer) instead of protein matching.
4. That the genome is circular (-c).
5. To call mummer with its default parameters (-d).
6. To produce an output file with no padding (N's) between contigs (-N).
7. To not include contigs less than 1000 bp long (-l 1000) as this makes the later visual comparisons easier.
8. To write all output files to the abacas directory and prefix each file name with "sample" (-o abacas/sample).

Abacas is a versatile tool and other options are available, to see them run perl abacas.1.3.1.pl -h.

The output can be assessed using standard Linux command line tools, for example wc velvet/sample.* will report the number of lines, words, and characters in each matching file and the fasta files should be of similar size to the genome, i.e., ~4×10^6 characters long.

When analyzing many samples it is advisable to order them all against the same reference genome as this will enable sample-to-sample comparisons. It can also be useful to order contigs against multiple reference genomes to maximize the number of contigs compared, as the differences in the references are likely to mean different contigs are used in the alignment.

3.4   Annotation of Contigs

The next step is to annotate the contigs with their likely genetic functional features, such as coding regions, genes, and RNA. The prokka [6] (short for prokaryotic annotation) program is ideal for this, combining BLAST [13] searches for common, conserved genes and hidden Markov models (via HMMer [14]) to identify more polymorphic genes. Running the following command will create a general feature format (GFF) annotation file composed of the identified genes and with the full sequence appended at the end:

```
$ prokka --outdir prokka --prefix sample \abacas/sample.
    NoNs.fasta
```

The ordered contig file with no padding (abacas/sample. NoNs.fasta created in step 3.3) is processed into files, all beginning with sample (from the --prefix option) in the prokka directory (--outdir option). Apart from the GFF file, this directory contains the same information in multiple formats, including GenBank format (prokka/sample.gbk) and a sequin format for uploading to the GenBank database [15]. Also included are .txt, .log, and .err files that contain statistics on the analysis, a full log, and any errors encountered, respectively. For this sample 3746 genes have been transferred compared to 3943 in the reference 630.embl file. Discrepancies can arise due to a number of possible reasons including sample genes containing deletions/insertions, incomplete genes at the start or end of contigs, and genes existing in silico that have not been confirmed.

3.5 Compare to Reference

The mutations in a sample are identified with respect to a reference genome. Genetic variations include single base pair differences (single-nucleotide polymorphisms or SNPs), insertions (extra DNA), and deletions (removal of DNA). More complex variations are not considered here but can be very important factors in determining C. *difficile* function, virulence, and resistance. They include repeat regions with different repeat counts and the multitude of possible genetic rearrangements (think: reversed section, jumping genes, etc.).

A standard command line BLAST generates the alignment information for the sample with respect to a given reference genome. First, a BLAST database for each reference is generated. This step only needs to be performed once per reference:

```
$ makeblastdb -in reference/630.fasta -dbtype nucl -out
    reference/630
```

With this command a nucleotide database (-dbtype nucl) is created from the reference genome (-in reference/630.fasta) and create the data in files called reference/630 (the -out option) with extensions .nhr, nin, and .nsq. Using these files, a nucleotide BLAST (-p blastn) is performed on the ordered, annotated sample (-i prokka/sample.gff):

```
$ blastall -p blastn -d reference/630 -i prokka/sample.
    fna -m 8 -F F \
-o sample.crunch
```

The output file (specified by -o as sample.crunch) is in a tabular-based format (-m 8) and without any low-complexity filtering (-F F). The crunch file provides information about areas of high identity between the reference and the sample; this file is used by Artemis Comparison Tool [8] (act) software to generate a graphical comparison. Each line shows an area of high identity, where the matching sections are in the two sequences and how alike they are with column three showing the percentage identity and column four the length of the region.

The hits identified in a blast can be filtered to remove poor matches, if required. The score of a match is determined from its length, how many mismatching bases exist, and how many gaps have been inserted to create the hit. The awk command line utility removes any hit with a score (in column 12) less than 1500, equating to keeping hits of ~800 bp or more:

```
$ awk '{if ($12 > 1500) {print}}' sample.crunch > sample.
  crunch.filter
```

The comparison can be visualized using act. From the annotated reference, the annotated sample, and their combined crunch file, act generates an interactive, searchable, visual interface to the data. The files can be loaded through the interactive menus or directly from the command line:

```
$ act reference/630.embl sample.crunch.filter prokka/
  sample.gff
```

In act the genomes are presented horizontally from left to right. The scrollbars on the right-hand side control the zoom level (up is more zoomed) and those along the bottom control the place on the genome viewed. The data can be zoomed in to single base pair resolution, with codons in all six reading frames (three forward and three reverse) included. Genes and other features are marked; *see* Fig. 2. Using the search facility (menu "GoTo," select "630.embl," select "Navigator"), specific features, genes, base pair positions, and ranges can be easily navigated to.

Areas in the reference that are missing from the assembled sample genome are easy to spot—these regions will be bounded on either side by different contigs. Likewise, deletions in comparison with the reference can be found where reference regions without any aligned sample contigs are bounded on either side by two halves of the same sample contig. Insertions are visually easy to spot as well, a sample contig will have both ends aligned together onto the reference genome, and the insertion will consist of the middle section of the contig. *See* Fig. 2, with a ~50 kbp insertion clearly visible at approximately 3,750,000 along the sample genome [10].

3.6 Identify Multi-Locus Strain Type (MLST) In Silico

Using mutation pattern in seven highly conserved genes, the MLST of a sample can be identified and placed in a wider *C. difficile* clade or lineage, with each clade exhibiting similar genetic and phenotypic profiles [16]. The alleles for these seven genes (*adk, atpA, dxr, glyA, recA, sodA,* and *tpi*) can be extracted from the contigs generated in Subheading 3.2 (or the ordered contigs from Subheading 3.3) to give an MLST for the sample. Missing or incomplete genes in the contigs can compromise the identification.

The mlst [9] command line tool automates searching for genes in contigs, identifying alleles, and assigning an MLST. It does this

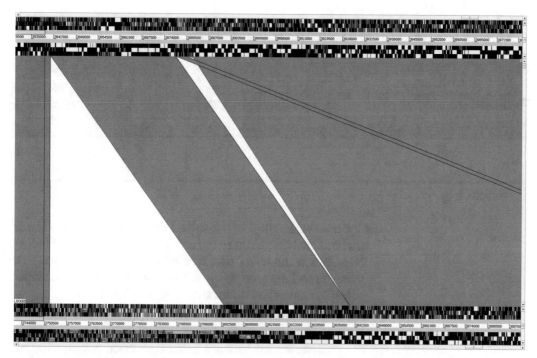

Fig. 2 A screenshot from the Artemis Comparison Tool (act) comparing the *C. difficile* 630 reference strain and the do novo-assembled, ordered, and annotated example sample. The section starting at ~3,750,000 shows a potential insertion in the data

for over 100 typeable species (see mlst --list). There are two MLST databases for *C. difficile*; the first is the pubMLST scheme (http://pubmlst.org/cdifficile/) and is used throughout these analyses. It can be run on multiple samples at once:

```
$  mlst --scheme cdifficile reference/630.fasta abacas/sample.
   NoNs.fasta
```

In this case, it runs on both the reference (reference/630.fasta) and the ordered sample (abacas/sample.NoNs.fasta) giving the genic allele, MSLT information in Table 1.

So both the reference and sample are from different MLSTs, indicating that the *C. difficile* 630 genome may not be a reasonable choice. *C. difficile* reference strain M68 (accession number FN668375) is also ST37 and therefore potentially a more sensible choice for ordering contigs in this method (and also for mapping analyses). At the time of writing, the seven genes together have 224 alleles and in combination their patterns form 274 MLSTs; this gives a fine granularity of sample typing for which in silico and in vivo tests give the same information.

Alternate method: Uploading the contigs fasta to an online MLST tool (such as http://cge.cbs.dtu.dk/ services/MLST/).

Table 1
In silico multi-locus strain types for the 630 reference and the example sample

File	MLST	adk	atpA	dxr	glyA	recA	sodA	tpi
Reference/630.fasta	54	1	4	7	1	1	3	3
Abacas/sample.fasta	37	3	7	3	8	6	9	11

4   Notes

1. One possible method is to install a Linux distribution on a virtual machine: enabling Linux to be run within a window on a Windows PC or Mac without any extra requirements (e.g., VirtualBox). On online Free Linux course is offered by the Linux foundation (https://training.linuxfoundation.org/free-linux-training).

2. *Important*: Whenever any program is run on the command line, the output must be read to check for correct operation. The programs used here are being developed continually, and this may lead to changes in required input file, command line parameters, or output files.

3. Most bioinformatic software have to be downloaded and installed by hand (i.e., not through a package manager). Some software can be run directly after extracting from a zip archive and some will need to be compiled. Instructions are available on the homepage of each piece of software. Compiling commonly requires extracting the data from an archive (.zip or .tar.gz) file using a variation on the following commands:

```
tar zxvf software-version.tar.gz
cd software-version
make
sudo make install
```

4. The convention of a fixed width typeface is used to indicate commands and options to be typed in verbatim.

5. There are a number of common file types that arise in bioinformatics. They are identifiable by their file extensions:

.gz	A compressed/zipped file can be seen in combination with other file extensions
.fastq	The raw data from the sequencer. Paired reads are split into two files: one for forward reads and the other for reverse reads. The order of the paired reads is the same in both files. Each read is composed of four lines: read name, called bases, comment, and encoded call quality. These files are normally compressed as well (.fastq.gz)
.fasta/.fa	A format for storing sequences. Each sequence starts with a name line beginning ">" followed by, on the next line, a string of A, C, G, T, or N characters, sometimes split over multiple lines

6. *Important*: The line continuation character is placed without spaces on either side of it for the purposes of printing a valid command on the page. When typing these commands into the command line, you do not need the continuation character or to move to a new line. For example in the first wget command the url can be typed whole as such:

```
http://www.ebi.ac.uk/Tools/dbfetch/dbfetch?db=embl&id=AM18035
5&style=raw
```

7. *Important*: When installing velvet it is important to modify the Makefile before compiling to increase the maximum k-mer. This value defaults to 31 but should be increased to an odd number greater than your longest read length, i.e., for up to 250 bp reads use 255. Velvet can be recompiled later if a larger value is needed.

References

1. Sebaihia M et al (2006) The multidrug-resistant human pathogen *Clostridium difficile* has a highly mobile, mosaic genome. Nat Genet 38(7):779–786

2. Andrews S (2015) FastQC. Available from: http://www.bioinformatics.babraham.ac.uk/projects/fastqc/

3. Bolger AM, Lohse M, Usadel B (2014) Trimmomatic: a flexible trimmer for Illumina sequence data. Bioinformatics 30(15):2114–2120

4. Zerbino DR, Birney E (2008) Velvet: algorithms for de novo short read assembly using de Bruijn graphs. Genome Res 18(5):821–829

5. Assefa S et al (2009) ABACAS: algorithm-based automatic contiguation of assembled sequences. Bioinformatics 25(15):1968–1969

6. Seemann T (2014) Prokka: rapid prokaryotic genome annotation. Bioinformatics 30(14):2068–2069

7. Camacho C et al (2009) BLAST+: architecture and applications. BMC Bioinformatics 10:421

8. Carver TJ et al (2005) ACT: the Artemis Comparison Tool. Bioinformatics 21(16):3422–3423

9. Seemann T (2015) MLST. Available from: https://github.com/tseemann/mlst

10. Cairns MD et al (2015) Genomic epidemiology of a protracted hospital outbreak caused by a toxin A-negative *Clostridium difficile* sublineage PCR ribotype 017 strain in London, England. J Clin Microbiol 53(10):3141–3147

11. Gladman S, Seemann, T (2012) VelvetOptimiser. Available from: http://bioinformatics.net.au/software.velvetoptimiser.shtml

12. Delcher AL, Salzberg SL, Phillippy AM (2003) Using MUMmer to identify similar regions in large sequence sets. Curr Protoc Bioinformatics. Chapter 10: Unit 10.3

13. Altschul SF et al (1990) Basic local alignment search tool. J Mol Biol 215(3):403–410

14. Eddy SR (1998) Profile hidden Markov models. Bioinformatics 14(9):755–763

15. Benson DA et al (2013) GenBank. Nucleic Acids Res 41(Database issue):D36–D42

16. Stabler RA et al (2012) Macro and micro diversity of *Clostridium difficile* isolates from diverse sources and geographical locations. PLoS One 7(3):e31559

Chapter 4

Clostridium difficile Genome Editing Using pyrE Alleles

Muhammad Ehsaan, Sarah A. Kuehne, and Nigel P. Minton

Abstract

Precise manipulation (in-frame deletions and substitutions) of the *Clostridium difficile* genome is possible through a two-stage process of single-crossover integration and subsequent isolation of double-crossover excision events using replication-defective plasmids that carry a counterselection marker. Use of a *codA* (cytosine deaminase) or *pyrE* (orotate phosphoribosyltransferase) as counter selection markers appears equally effective, but there is considerable merit in using a *pyrE* mutant as the host as, through the use of allele-coupled exchange (ACE) vectors, mutants created (by whatever means) can be rapidly complemented concomitant with restoration of the *pyrE* allele. This avoids the phenotypic effects frequently observed with high-copy-number plasmids and dispenses with the need to add antibiotic to ensure plasmid retention.

Key words *Clostridium difficile*, Pseudo-suicide, Allelic exchange, Allele-coupled exchange (ACE), Counterselection marker, *pyrE*, *codA*, Complementation, Overexpression

---

1 Introduction

Allelic exchange is an essential tool in the armory of the molecular biologist, allowing the precise manipulation of bacterial genomes through gene deletions, substitutions, and additions. The absence of high-frequency transfer in *Clostridium difficile* precludes the use of suicide vectors (plasmids that are unable to replicate in *C. difficile*) necessitating the use of so-called [1], "pseudo-suicide" vectors. Such plasmids carry a gene specifying resistance to an antibiotic (e.g., *catP*, encoding resistance to thiamphenicol) and are sufficiently replication defective for there to be a significant growth disadvantage in the presence of the appropriate antibiotic (e.g., thiamphenicol) compared to cells in which the plasmid, together with the antibiotic resistance gene (*catP*), has integrated. Such integrated clones grow faster, and produce larger colonies, on agar media supplemented with antibiotic (thiamphenicol), because all of the progeny carry a copy of the antibiotic resistance gene (*catP*). Cells carrying the antibiotic resistance gene (*catP*) on a non-integrated, defective, autonomous plasmid grow slower because in the presence of antibiotic they are limited by the rate at

Adam P. Roberts and Peter Mullany (eds.), *Clostridium difficile: Methods and Protocols*, Methods in Molecular Biology, vol. 1476, DOI 10.1007/978-1-4939-6361-4_4, © Springer Science+Business Media New York 2016

which the plasmid is segregated amongst daughter cells. Selection and re-streaking of the faster growing colonies allow the isolation of pure single-crossover integrants, as determined by appropriate PCR screening. The isolation of pure single-crossover populations is essential as the presence of substantive subpopulations of cells carrying autonomous plasmids can lead to high counts of spurious mutants in the presence of the counterselection agent.

The counterselection agent in the case of *codA* is 5-fluorocytosine (5-FC), which is converted to 5-fluorouracil (5-FU), a toxic derivative [1]. In the case of *pyrE*, counterselection is mediated by 5-fluoroorotic acid (FOA) which is also eventually converted into toxic product 5-fluorouracil (5-FU) in the form of 5-fluorouridylic acid (5-FUMP). 5-FU is a pyrimidine analogue that can be misincorporated into DNA and RNA in place of thymine or uracil, leading to interference in replication and transcription and thus to cell death [2]. Mutants of these genes require exogenous uracil for growth and are viable in medium containing 5-FOA [3], through the sequential actions of PyrE (orotate phosphor-ribosyltransferase) and PyrF (orotidine-5′-monophosphate decarboxylase). The *codA* marker may be used in a wild-type host, whereas the latter can only be deployed in a *pyrE* mutant background. Such a mutant is resistant to FOA, but becomes sensitive when a functional *pyrE* gene is introduced into the cell on a knockout (KO) vector. It is created using allele-coupled exchange (ACE), a highly effective and specialist form of allelic exchange [4] which brings about inactivation of *pyrE* by its replacement with a mutant allele lacking approximately 300 bp from the 3′ end of the structural gene. Crucially, the design of the created *pyrE* mutant strain is such that its mutant *pyrE* allele can be rapidly (2 days) restored to wild-type using an appropriate ACE correction vector allowing the specific in-frame deletion mutant to be characterized in a clean, wild-type background. Moreover, this facility provides in parallel the opportunity to complement the mutant at an appropriate gene dosage, through insertion of a wild-type copy of the gene, into the genome under the control of either its native promoter or the strong P_{fdx} promoter (derived from the ferredoxin gene of *Clostridium sporogenes*), concomitant with restoration of the *pyrE* allele back to wild-type [3].

Either counterselection marker appears equally effective [2], but the benefits of the presence of the *pyrE* locus are such that there is a rational argument for using *pyrE* mutant hosts, and their cognate ACE correction vectors, with any particular mutagen, including the ClosTron and any of the available clostridial, negative selection markers [1, 2, 5–9]. Through the use of ACE vectors, mutants created in such strains (by whatever means) can be rapidly complemented. This avoids the phenotypic effects frequently observed with high-copy-number plasmids and dispenses with the need to add antibiotic to ensure the retention of the complementing plasmid. Moreover, the *pyrE* allele represents an ideal position where other application-specific modules may be inserted into clostridial genomes, such as a sigma factor to allow deployment of a *mariner* transposon [10], hydrolases for degrading complex carbohydrates [11], or therapeutic genes in cancer delivery vehicles [12].

2   Materials

2.1   Culture Media

1. L Broth Medium (LB): Add the following to 800 ml of dH_2O: 10 g tryptone extract, 5 g yeast extract, and 5 g NaCl. Dissolve, and adjust the final volume to 1 l. Add 1.5 % w/v bacteriological agar for solid medium. Sterilize by autoclaving at 121 °C for 15 min. LB is routinely used for *Escherichia coli* cloning and plasmid maintenance [13].

2. Brain–heart infusion supplement medium (BHIS): This medium is the commercially available BHI medium (Oxoid) 37 g/l supplemented with 1 g/l of l-cysteine and 5 g/l of yeast extract. Sterilize by autoclaving at 121 °C for 15 min. This medium is routinely used for culturing *C. difficile* [14].

3. *Clostridium difficile* minimal medium (CDMM): This is a defined minimal medium used for the selection of cells in which the second crossover event has taken place, supplemented with FOA in the case of allelic exchange using *pyrE* as a negative selection marker, or with 5-FC when *codA* is used as the counterselection marker. It is prepared by making the following stock solutions in water:
   Amino acid solution (5×): Dissolve in 200 ml of dH_2O: 10.0 g Cas-amino acids, 0.5 g tryptophan, and 0.5 g cysteine. *Salt solution (10×)*: Dissolve in 100 ml of dH_2O: 0.9 g KH_2PO_4, 5.0 g Na_2HPO_4, 0.9 g NaCl, and 5.0 g $NaHCO_3$. *Trace salt solution (50×)*: Dissolve in 100 ml of dH_2O: 130 mg $CaCl_2 \cdot 2H_2O$, 100 mg $MgCl_2 \cdot 6H_2O$, 50 mg $MnCl_2 \cdot 4H_2O$, 200 mg $(NH_4)_2SO_4$, and 5 mg $CoCl_2 \cdot 6H_2O$. *FeSO4·7H2O solution (100×)*: Dissolve 40 mg of $FeSO_4 \cdot 7H_2O$ in 100 ml anaerobic dH_2O. *Vitamin solution (100×)*: Dissolve 10 mg of each of the following vitamins in 100 ml of dH_2O: Calcium-d-pantothenate, pyridoxine, and d-biotin. *Glucose (20%)*: d-Glucose 20 g per 100 ml and sterilize by filtration/autoclaving.
   To make 1 l of CDMM, mix 200 ml of 5× amino acid solution with 100 ml of 10× salt solution, 50 ml of 20% glucose, 20 ml of 50× trace salt solution, 10 ml of 100× iron solution, and 10 ml of 100× vitamins with 610 ml sterile dH_2O [15]. For agar plates, use 1.5% bacteriological agar. Liquid medium and agar plates are required to be reduced at least 12 h and 4 h, respectively, before use (*see* **Note 1**).

2.2   Antibiotic and Other Supplements

The listed antibiotics are used when required at the following concentrations: 25 µg/ml chloramphenicol (Cm) in agar and 12.5 µg/ml in liquid (from a stock solution of 25 mg/ml in ethanol),

15 µg/ml thiamphenicol (Tm) (from a stock solution of 15 mg/ml in a 1:1 mix of ethanol and dH$_2$O), 250 µg/ml d-cycloserine, and 8 µg/ml cefoxitin (CC). The latter are made from a combined stock solution of 25 mg/ml cycloserine and 0.8 mg/ml cefoxitin in dH$_2$O or cycloserine separately, as required. Cm is always used to select for *catP* in *E. coli*, whereas the same gene is selected for in clostridia using Tm. CDMM is supplemented with 2 mg/ml fluoroorotic acid (FOA) (stock 100 mg/ml in dimethyl sulfoxide, DMSO), and 5 µg/ml uracil (stock 1 mg/ml dH$_2$O) when using *pyrE* as the negative selection marker while for *codA*, 50 µg/ml 5-fluorocytosine (5-FC) is used (stock 10 mg/ml in dH$_2$O). Cm is stored at −20 °C; all other antibiotics at 4 °C while stocks for FOA and 5-FC are prepared fresh before use.

2.3 Molecular Biology Reagents, Strains, and Plasmids

1. *E. coli* strain TOP10 (Invitrogen) is used for cloning and plasmid maintenance [genotype: F-*mcrA*, Δ(*mrr-hsdRMS-mcrBC*), *Φ80lacZΔM15*, Δ*lacX74*, *recA1*, *araD139*, Δ(*ara-leu*)7697, *galU galK rpsL* (Str^R), *endA1* λ-, *nupG*], and strain CA434 [genotype: *thi-1*, *hsdS20* (r-B, m-B), *supE44*, *recAB*, *ara-14*, *leuB5*, *proA2*, *lacY1*, *galK*, *rpsL20*, *xyl-5*, *mtl-1*—R702 (Tc^R) Tra$^+$, Mob$^+$] as the donor for conjugative plasmid transfer.

2. Restriction endonucleases and DNA ligase can be purchased from NEB or Promega and used under the conditions recommended by the manufacturer. All DNA samples are electrophoresed on standard agarose gels at 0.8% (w/v) and visualized under UV using a chosen imaging system.

3. Plasmids used for KO are the *pyrE*-based vectors pMTL-YN3 and pMTL-YN4 and the *codA*-based vector pMTL-SC7215 and pMTL-SC7315. Plasmids pMTL-YN3 and pMTL-SC7315 are used for making in-frame deletions and substitutions in *C. difficile* 630Δ*erm* whereas pMTL-YN4 and pMTL-SC7215 are employed in strain *C. difficile* R20291. The former pair of plasmids carries the pCB102 replicon, whereas the latter two plasmids are based on the replication region of plasmid pBP1 [16] (*see* **Note 2**).

Fig .1 (continued) of the *oriT* region of plasmid RP4; and Rep+ve, an unstable variant of the pCB102 replicon (pMTL-YN1; for use in *C. difficile* Δ*erm*Δ*pyrE*) or pBP1 (pMTL-YN2; for use in *C. difficile* R20291Δ*pyrE*). Plasmids pMTL-YN1C and pMTLYN2C have an additional segment of DNA inserted between the left-hand homology arm (LHA) and the right-hand homology arm (RHA) which carries a transcriptional terminator (T1) of the ferredoxin gene of *Clostridium pasteurianum*; a copy of the *lacZ'* gene encoding the alpha fragment of the *E. coli* β-galactosidase, and a multiple cloning site (MCS) region derived from plasmid pMTL20 [17]. They are used to insert cargo DNA (cloned into the MCS) into the genome concomitant with restoration of the *pyrE* allele to wild-type, most commonly a functional copy of a gene inactivated elsewhere in the genome for complementation studies. Plasmids pMTL-YN1X and pMTL-YN2X are similar to pMTL-YN1C and pMTL-YN2C, respectively, except that they carry the promoter region (P*fdx*) of the *C. sporogenes* ferredoxin gene [3] positioned immediately before the *lacZ*-encoding region. This allows the effect of overexpressing the introduced cargo gene to be assessed

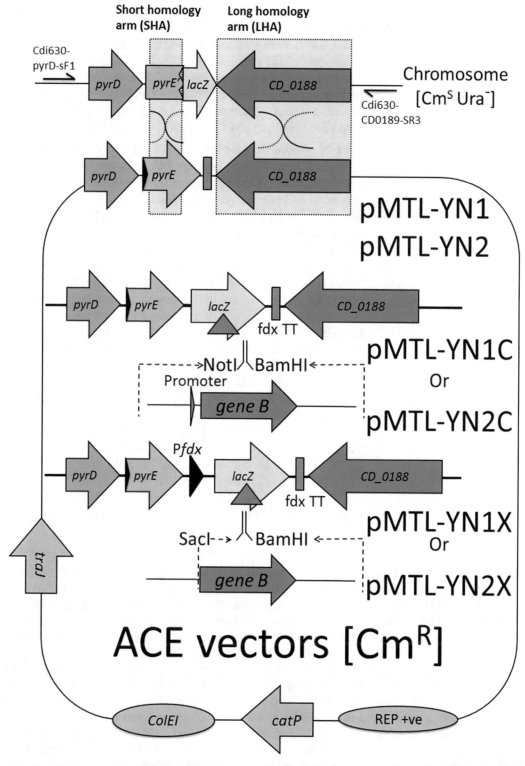

Fig. 1 The *pyrE* ACE correction, complementation and overexpression vectors. All vectors carry identical components between their FseI and SbfI restriction sites: *catP*, the *catP* gene of *Clostridium perfringens* conferring thiamphenicol resistance; ColE1, the replication region of the *E. coli* plasmid ColE1; *traJ*, the transfer function

4. A suite of *pyrE* ACE vectors are available (Fig. 1) to either correct the mutant *pyrE* allele of deletion mutants made in strain 630Δ*erm*Δ*pyrE* and *C. difficile* R20291Δ*pyrE* back to wild-type (pMTL-YN1 and pMTL-YN2, respectively); simultaneously complement an inactivated gene concomitant with restoration of prototrophy (pMTL-YN1C and pMTL-YN2C); or bring about overexpression of the complementing gene (pMTL-YN1X and pMTL-YN2X) (*see* **Note 3**).

5. Pairs of oligonucleotide primers are used to distinguish wild-type cells from single- and double-crossover mutants using standard PCR screening. One primer pair which flanks the predicted KO region, given the generic names SEQ-FWD and SEQ-REV in Fig. 2, is designed to result in a large PCR DNA fragment in the case of a wild-type cell, and a DNA fragment of a much smaller, predicted size if the clone is a double-cross-over mutant. A further primer pair comprises of one or other of these flanking primers in combination with a primer complementary to the vector backbone, and not present in the target chromosome. Generally speaking two primers are available complementary to either strand of the vector, e.g., in the case of the *codA* vectors pMTL-SC7215 and pMTL-SC7315 [1] primers SC7-F (5′-GACGGATTTCACATTTGCCGTTTT GTAAACGAATTGCAGG-3′) and SC7-R (5′-AGATCCTT TGATCTTTTCTACGGGGTCTGACGCTCAG TGG-3′). If the KO cassette is inserted between AscI and SbfI sites, then primer pMTL-ME2-Seq-F (5′-CTCCATCAAGA VAGAGCGAC-3′) in combination with primer SEQ-REV could be used in the case of pMTL-YN3 and pMTL-YN4 while primer pMTL-ME2-Seq-R (5′-CTTTCTATTCAGCAC TGTTATGCC-3′) could only be used in combination with the primer SEQ-FWD in the case of pMTL-YN3 (*see* **Note 4**).

Fig .2 (continued) than if integration had been mediated by the RHA. Single-crossover integrants are then streaked onto BHIS supplemented with 20 μg/ml uracil, but lacking Tm followed by plating as a dilution series onto medium CDMM supplemented with 5-fluoroorotic acid (FOA) or 5-fluorocytosine (5-FC) [C]. FOA^R- and FC^R-resistant colonies are then patch plated for plasmid loss onto BHIS with and without 20 μg/ml uracil and 15 μg/ml Tm. If plasmid excision takes place via homologous recombination between the two copies of LHA, then the wild-type is regenerated together with an autonomous copy of the original KO plasmid carrying the mutant allele. If plasmid excision takes place via homologous recombination between the two copies of RHA (as illustrated in [C]), then the desired mutant is generated along with an autonomous copy of the KO plasmid carrying a wild-type allele. FOA^R Tm^S or FC^R Tm^S colonies are screened by PCR for double-crossover in-frame deletions using the flanking primer pair SEQ-FWD and SEQ-REV which will generate a smaller band in the case of a deletion mutant compared to wild-type [D]. Plasmid components are *catP*, the *catP* gene of *Clostridium perfringens* conferring thiamphenicol resistance; *Csp-pyrE*, the *pyrE* gene of *Clostridium sporogenes*; ColE1 RNAII, the replication region of the *E. coli* plasmid ColE1; *traJ*, transfer function of the *oriT* region of plasmid RP4, the Rep+ve is either an unstable variant of the pCB102 replicon (pMTL-YN3; for use in *C. difficile* Δ*erm*Δ*pyrE*) or pBP1 (pMTL-YN4; for use in *C. difficile* R20291 Δ*pyrE*)

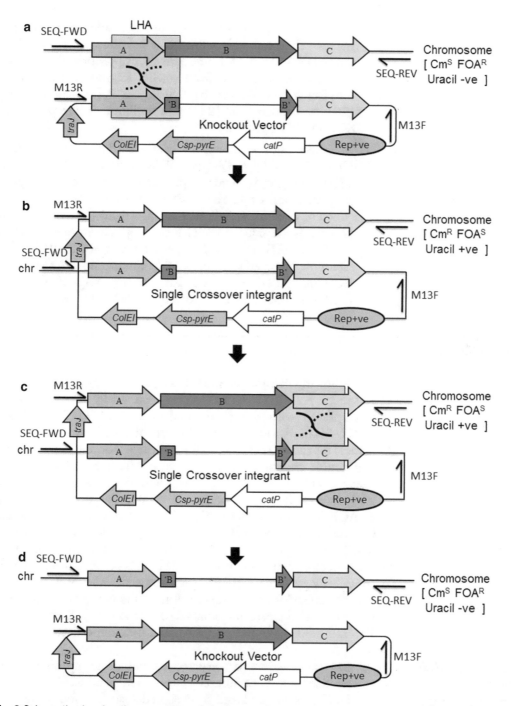

Fig. 2 Schematic showing the generation of single- and double-crossover integrants and the location of PCR screening primers. The process of mutant generation in gene B is represented in four phases. [A] The KO plasmid undergoes homologous recombination via the LHA and the complementary sequence in the genome to generate a single-crossover integrant as illustrated in [B]. Selection is based on faster growing, large colonies on medium supplemented with Tm. Its identity as a single-crossover integrant is confirmed using the primer pairs SEQ-FWD and M13F or SEQ-REV and M13R. The relative size of the DNA fragment obtained identifies at which homology arm integration took place. In the example integration has taken place at the LHA. As a consequence, SEQ-FWD and M13F (reverse primer from KO plasmid) will generate a smaller PCR fragment

6. The KO cassettes can be made and assembled by a variety of means. They can be commercially synthesized, as either the entire DNA fragment or alternatively, if appropriately designed, they can be assembled from smaller fragments using procedures such as G-Blocks [18], USER cloning [19], ligase cycling [20], or Golden Gate [21]. The traditional route is through SOE PCR (*see* **Note 5**).

7. The following Qiagen kits are used according to the manufacturer's instructions: Qiaquick PCR purification kit (Cat no. 28104), Qiaprep plasmid miniprep kit (Cat no. 27106), Qiaquick gel purification kit (Cat no. 28704), DNeasy blood and tissue kit (Cat no. 69506), and Proteinase K, 10 ml (Cat no. 19133). Other kits are equally useful for example from Sigma-Aldrich GenElute™ HP Plasmid Miniprep Kit Cat no. NA0160-1KT, GenElute™ Bacterial Genomic DNA Kits Cat no. NA2120-1KT, GenElute™ PCR Clean-UP Kit Cat no. NA1020-1KT, and GenElute™ Gel Extraction Kit Cat no. NA1111-1KT.

---

3   Methods

The following method section is based on the use of the *pyrE*-based KO vector pMTL-YN3 (pMTL-YN4). Essentially the same strategy is employed with the *codA*-based vectors pMTL-SC7215 and pMTL-SC7315, but involves the use of a different cloning site (PmeI) for the KO cassette, different primers for screening of single and double crossovers, and of course a different counter selection agent, 5-FC, in place of FOA. The method also describes how the *pyrE* allele of the mutant host is converted back to wild-type using an ACE correction vector (pMTL-YN1 and pMTL-YN2 for strains 630Δ*erm*Δ*pyrE* and R20291Δ*pyrE,* respectively). It additionally details how the knocked out gene can be complemented using the ACE complementation vectors pMTL-YN1C and pMTL-YN2C (630Δ*erm*Δ*pyrE* and R20291Δ*pyrE,* respectively) as well as how to test the effect of the overexpression of the complementing gene using the ACE overexpression vectors pMTL-YN1X and pMTL-YN2X in 630Δ*erm*Δ*pyrE* and R20291Δ*pyrE,* respectively.

3.1   Design of KO Cassette and Incorporation into the KO Vector

1. KO cassettes are constructed/assembled comprising equal-sized left and right homology arms (LHA and RHA) of at least 500 bp each (*see* **Note 6**) designed such that following their fusion only the first two to three codons of the target gene are present, joined in-frame to its last two to three codons.

2. Design (*see* **Note 7**) and order the necessary oligonucleotides (15–30 bases in length and with approximately 50 % G + C residues) from a suitable supplier (e.g., Eurofins Genomics or Sigma-Aldrich) and make 10 pmol dilutions of each. See the

example in Fig. 3 for a graphic representation of the primers used: SbfI-OUTER-FWD and SOE-INNER-REV for LHA and SOE-INNER-FWD and AscI-OUTER-REV for the RHA.

3. Assemble a PCR reaction of 25 μl comprising 12.5 μl of PCR 2× Buffer E PreMix (Failsaife™, Cambio Ltd); 1 μl each of the 10 pmol forward and reverse primers; 2 μl genomic DNA template (100–200 ng); 8 μl dH$_2$O; and 0.25–0.5 μl of a proofreading polymerase. The PCR reaction mixes are prepared and stored on ice in triplicate.

4. Use the following PCR cycle conditions: Denature at 95 °C for 30 s followed by 30 cycles of 95 °C for 30 s, 55 °C for 1 min, and 72 °C for 1 min/kb with a final extension at 72 °C for 5–10 min.

5. In the second step of SOE PCR [22], both the products from the first PCRs are used as template with flanking primers (SbfI-OUTER-FWD and AscI-OUTER-REV) to generate the KO cassettes.

6. Restriction sites are included in the forward primer (SbfI-OUTER-FWD) of the LHA and reverse primer (AscI-

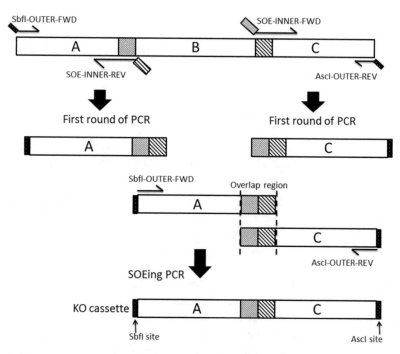

Fig. 3 Schematic representation of the construction of a KO cassette by SOEing PCR. Two regions (A and C) flanking the region to be deleted (B) are joined by SOEing PCR. The fusion is mediated by an overlap region of the two strands of PCR products that were created with the use of primers (Sbfl-OUTER-FWD and SOE-INNER-REV, and SOE-INNER-FWD and AscI-OUTER-REV). The 3′-region of A is complementary to the 5vv-region of C. A recombinant product is formed when this overlap is extended in a second amplification reaction using the forward and reverse outer primers (Sbfl-OUTER-FWD and AscI-OUTER-REV)

OUTER-REV) of the RHA so that after PCR amplification or synthesis, the KO cassettes can be digested and cloned into the vectors pMTL-YN3 or pMTL-YN4 between the SbfI and AscI restriction sites (*see* **Note 8**).

7. The PCR product is electrophoresed on an 0.8% agarose gel to verify the correct size (e.g., 1500 bp if the two homology arms are 750 bp in size) followed by purification using Qiaquick gel purification (Qiagen). Typically this results in between 50 and 90 ng DNA per µl in a final volume of 30–40 µl in Qiagen elution buffer (10 mM Tris–HCl, pH 8.0) or dH$_2$O. The KO vector and KO cassettes are then digested with restriction enzymes ready for ligation (*see* **Note 9**). Reactions are performed in a final volume of 20 µl, using vector:insert ratios of 1:1 or 1:3, 1× T4 DNA ligase buffer, and 10 U of T4 DNA ligase followed by incubation at 4 °C overnight or at room temperature for 3 h if using the Rapid DNA Ligation System from Promega (*see* **Note 10**).

8. Following reaction completion the ligation mixtures are transformed into *E. coli* TOP10 either by heat shock at 42 °C for 45 s or electroporation using 2 mm electroporation cuvettes. After recovery the cells are plated onto medium supplemented with 25 µg/ml Cm to select for transformants. Blue-white selection using Xgal can be performed (if cloning in the MCS) as the empty KO vector carries a cargo region encoding the LacZα fragment which will be replaced by the KO cassette.

9. After 24–48 h, screen and verify the transformants for the correct-sized insert by colony PCR using specific primers.

10. Inoculate six separate colonies in 5 ml LB broth supplemented with 12.5 µg/ml Cm and incubate overnight at 37 °C. In parallel, restreak each onto fresh LB agar medium supplemented with 25 µg/ml Cm and incubate for 24–48 h, for safekeeping.

11. Extract the plasmid DNA from the purified transformant colonies using a standard commercial kit and verify the clones by restriction digestion. Finally verify that the clones that give the correct restriction pattern for the inserted KO cassette are authentic by performing Sanger nucleotide sequencing on the plasmid.

3.2 Conjugation and Isolation of Single-Crossover Clones

1. Transfer of plasmid DNA into *C. difficile* is accomplished using conjugation from an *E. coli* donor essentially as described by Purdy et al. [23]. The system is reliant on the presence of an *oriT* fragment on the KO vectors and their mobilization by the IncPβ conjugative plasmid R702 carried by the *E. coli* donor CA434 [23]. Accordingly, the *E. coli* donor CA434 strain is transformed with the KO plasmid and transformants are selected on medium supplemented with Cm (25 µg/ml). The resultant transformants are grown overnight in 5 ml of LB medium supplemented with an appropriate antibiotic (here 12.5 µg/ml Cm) to ensure that the plasmid is retained.

2. In parallel, the *C. difficile* Δ*pyrE* recipient strain is grown overnight at 37 °C in 1 ml of rich medium (BHIS) supplemented with 20 µg/ml uracil under anaerobic conditions.

3. Pellet 1 ml of CA434 overnight culture harboring the KO plasmid at 1500×*g* in a benchtop microfuge for 1 min, wash the pellet in 0.5 ml PBS, and spin as before. Take the pellet into the anaerobic cabinet.

4. In the anaerobic cabinet, resuspend the CA434 pellet in 200 µl of an overnight culture of the *C. difficile* Δ*pyrE* recipient. Aliquot the mating mixture onto one nonselective BHIS plate as eight individual drops of 25 µl. Do not invert the plate. Incubate at 37 °C for between 8 and 24 h depending on the *C. difficile* strain.

5. Using a disposable loop scrape the bacterial growth off the plate and resuspend in 1 ml of PBS. Plate the cells (200 µl per plate) on selective medium, 15 µg/ml of Tm, BHIS to select for inheritance of the KO vector carrying *catP* and including a counterselection agent directed against the *E. coli* CA434 donor, usually 250 µg/ml and 8 µg/ml cycloserine and cefoxitin (CC), respectively. Plates are anaerobically incubated for 1–3 days at 37 °C.

6. Examine the plates and restreak transconjugants on the same medium (BHIS, CC, Tm15). Incubate as described above. Transconjugants should regrow within 24 h.

7. Identify transconjugant colonies that are visibly larger in size (*see* **Note 11**). These are most likely single-crossover integrants which have a growth advantage over cells carrying the segregationally unstable, autonomous, pseudo-suicide plasmids [1] due to integration of the plasmid-encoded antibiotic resistance marker (*catP*) into the genome. Streak a random selection of such larger colonies onto BHIS plates supplemented with 15 µg/ml Tm and incubate anaerobically for 24 h at 37 °C. Restreak each clone again on the same selective plates to purify them and set up 1 ml BHIS overnight culture supplemented with Tm (12.5 µg/ml) (*see* **Note 12**).

8. The following day, streak the overnight cultures onto BHIS plates supplemented with 15 µg/ml Tm, 250 µg/ml, and 8 µg/ml cycloserine and cefoxitin (CC), respectively, for safe keeping and then extract genomic DNA using a standard genomic extraction kit, e.g., DNeasy blood and tissue kit (Cat no. 69506), following the manufacturer's instructions.

9. It is crucial to isolate pure single-crossover integrants at this stage as contamination with transconjugants (cells which contain independently replicating KO plasmid) will cause unacceptable background when plating on medium supplemented with the counterselective agent, FOA or 5-FC. To verify the

purity of single-crossover integrants, undertake PCR using two primer pairs; the first pair includes the forward primer from the KO plasmid outside the LHA or RHA and the reverse primer from the chromosome outside the RHA and the second pair consists of flanking primers from the chromosome outside the LHA and RHA. If any clone is a pure single-crossover integrant, it will be verified by the amplification of a specifically sized band when the first pair of primers is used but no wild-type band will be present in the second pair of primers.

3.3 Isolation of Double-Crossover Clones

1. Once a pure single-crossover integrant has been isolated, it is restreaked onto BHIS supplemented with 20 µg/ml uracil, but lacking Tm, and incubated for 4 days to allow the cells to undergo a rare second recombination event resulting in excision of the integrated plasmid. This can be mediated by either homology arm (LHA or RHA) generating either a mutant or wild-type cell.

2. Collect all of the growth using a sterile loop, resuspend in 500 µl of PBS, make serial dilutions in PBS (to 10^{-6}), and plate 100 µl of each dilution onto CDMM agar plates supplemented with 2 mg/ml FOA and 20 µg/ml uracil.

3. After 48 h of anaerobic incubation at 37 °C, patch plate FOA^R clones onto BHIS agar plates supplemented with 15 µg/ml Tm and 20 µg/ml uracil and onto BHIS agar plates supplemented with only 20 µg/ml uracil. Those cells which grow on the latter media, but not the former, will have lost the excised KO plasmid.

4. Set up overnight cultures in 1 ml of BHIS supplemented with 20 µg/ml uracil of the identified FOA^R and Tm^S clones.

5. After overnight growth, restreak each clone onto BHIS agar plates supplemented with 20 µg/ml uracil for safekeeping and extract genomic DNA from liquid culture to analyze by PCR using the primer pairs flanking the intended deletion site, e.g., SEQ-FWD and SEQ-REV (Fig. 2). Mutants will yield a small PCR fragment, whereas wild-type revertants will generate a large DNA fragment. Confirm the authenticity of any small mutant fragments by Sanger sequencing (*see* **Note 13**).

3.4 Correction Back to pyrE+

1. After the verification of the in-frame deletion mutant in the host *C. difficile* Δ*pyrE* strain, the mutant *pyrE* allele is corrected back to wild-type to allow the analysis of the phenotype of the newly made in-frame deletion in an otherwise wild-type background. Dependant on the strain, this is accomplished using the ACE correction vectors pMTL-YN1 (strain *630ΔermΔpyrE*) *or* pMTL-YN2 (strain R20291Δ*pyrE*).

2. Transform the donor strain CA434 with vectors pMTL-YN1 or pMTL-YN2, and conjugate into the KO mutant as described above.

3. Select the bigger transconjugants from BHIS plates supplemented with 15 μg/ml Tm, 250 μg/ml, and 8 μg/ml cycloserine and cefoxitin (CC), respectively, and 20 μg/ml uracil after anaerobic incubation for 24–48 h at 37 °C and purify by streaking twice to single colonies on the same agar medium.

4. Streak a loop full from each clone of the pure single-crossover integrants onto CDMM lacking uracil supplementation and incubate anaerobically for 24–48 h at 37 °C.

5. Set up overnight cultures of selected clones, extract genomic DNA, and verify by PCR using flanking primers Cdi630pyrD-sF1 (5′-AGAGAAGGAATAAAAAGTTTAGACGAAATAA GAGG-3′) and Cdi630-CD0189-SR3 (5′-CCAAGCTCTATG ACAGACAGCTCATTGTTTAGAAC-3′) which are complementary to regions upstream of the *pyrE* locus and downstream of CD0189 (Fig. 1). Verify the PCR product by Sanger sequencing. Also restreak the clones for safekeeping.

6. Finally compare this strain to wild-type for any phenotypic variation.

3.5 Complementation and Overexpression in the Chromosome

1. Regardless of which counterselection marker is used (*codA* or *pyrE*) the use of a *pyrE* strain as the host for mutagenesis provides the parallel opportunity to complement the mutant at an appropriate gene dosage, through insertion of a wild-type copy of the gene, under the control of either its native promoter or the strong P*fdx* promoter (derived from the ferredoxin, *fdx*, gene of *C. sporogenes*), concomitant with restoration of the *pyrE* allele back to wild-type [2–4] (*see* **Note 3**).

2. Amplify your gene(s) including its native promoter either by PCR or DNA synthesis flanked by appropriate restriction sites (e.g., NotI and BamHI) and clone between those sites in vectors pMTL-YN1C and pMTLYN2C, for strains *C. difficile* 630Δ*erm*Δ*pyrE* and *C. difficile* R20291Δ*pyrE*, respectively. Similarly for overexpression purpose, clone your gene without its native promoter into appropriate sites downstream of the P*fdx* promoter of pMTL-YN1X and pMTL-YN2X. The gene should ideally be amplified with its native ribosome-binding site and, through the incorporation of appropriate nucleotide sequences into the primers, cloned between the SacI and BamHI sites of either vector (*see* **Note 14**). Verify the vectors by restriction digestion and Sanger sequencing followed by transformation into the donor strain CA434.

3. Conjugate CA434 with respective *C. difficile* strains and follow the steps as described for repairing of the *pyrE* mutant back to wild-type and by this way the complemented or overexpressed gene is integrated into gene downstream of the now repaired *pyrE* gene.

4   Notes

1. CDMM can be prepared on the bench. It is important to keep the iron solution frozen at –20 °C and only defrost when needed. The CDMM plates should be prepared freshly and given enough time to reduce in the anaerobic cabinet (12–24 h) before being used.

2. The pCB102 replicon is more unstable in *C. difficile* 630Δ*erm* than that of pBP1, whereas the opposite is true for *C. difficile* R20291. While pMTL-SC7315 carries the native pCB102 replicon, plasmid pMTL-YN3 carries a variant pCB102 replicon in which a frame-shift has been introduced into *repH* which results in an even more unstable plasmid [1, 3].

3. The extra effort involved in the deployment of ACE vectors compared to the use of autonomous complementation vectors is minimal. They require the same amount of effort in terms of construction and transfer into the desired bacterial host. Mutants transformed with autonomous complementation plasmids need to be purified by restreaking, whereas an ACE complementation transformant merely needs to be restreaked onto a minimal plate lacking uracil, and those colonies that grow purified by restreaking. The extra effort, therefore, equates to the time it takes for uracil prototrophic colonies to develop, ca. 2–3 days in the case of *C. difficile*. The efficiency of ACE is such that success is assured and moreover false positives cannot arise as reversion of the *pyrE* deletion is impossible. Although the effort required for ACE-mediated complementation is minimal, the benefits are considerable. It avoids the phenotypic effects frequently observed with high-copy-number plasmids and dispenses with the need to add antibiotic to ensure the retention of the complementing plasmid. Such antibiotic addition can affect phenotype and necessitate the inclusion in any phenotypic assessments of the mutant a vector-only control. The benefits of the presence of the *pyrE* locus are such that there is a rational argument for using *pyrE* mutant hosts, and their cognate ACE correction vectors with any particular mutagen, including *codA* [1] and the ClosTron [24].

4. If the KO cassette is cloned between unique restriction sites within the MCS of pMTL-YN1C/X or pMTL-YN2C/X, then a further option is to make use of the widely employed M13R (5′-CAGGAAACAGCTATGACC-3′) and M13F (5′-GTAAAACGACGGCCAG-3′) primers. These cannot be used if the KO cassette is inserted between AscI and SbfI, as the complementary regions to these primers will be deleted as a consequence of insertion of the KO cassette (see plasmid maps in Fig. 2). In this schematic, the primer pair SEQ-FWD and M13F will generate a PCR DNA fragment if the clone is a

single-crossover integrant. Moreover the size of the DNA fragment obtained indicates which of the two homology arms mediated plasmid integration. Thus, in the above example, if recombination has occurred between the chromosome and the LHA of the vector, then the PCR fragment generated is smaller than that which results from an integrant via the RHA. The opposite will be true if SEQ-REV and M13R are employed.

5. Traditionally KO cassettes may be individually generated (PCR) as separate left and right homology arms (LHA and RHA) that are sequentially cloned using created (part of the primer) restriction sites into corresponding vector restriction sites. Alternatively, the two DNA fragments comprising the LHA and RHA may be joined prior to cloning using splicing overlap extension PCR (SOE) [22] using a proofreading DNA polymerase, such as the enzyme Failsafe and 2× buffer E from Cambio Ltd or Phusion® High-Fidelity DNA Polymerase from New England Biolabs (NEB). For plasmids pMTL-SC7215 and pMTL-SC7315 the KO cassettes are cloned at the unique PmeI site. In the case of pMTL-YN3 and pMTL-YN4, they can either be cloned between the unique AscI and SbfI sites or between one or more sites that are unique in the MCS. The latter include the six-base recognition sequences, BamHI, NcoI, NotI, NdeI, NheI, SmaI, XmaI, XbaI, XhoI, and StuI. As the restriction enzymes AscI and SbfI have eight-base recognition sequences, they are less likely to cleave the LHA and RHA regions, and so their use is preferred.

6. While homology arms of 500 bp are effective, efficiency of the process increases with size, with sizes of either 750 or 1000 bp now routinely being used in this laboratory.

7. The primers used incorporate at their proximal (LHA) and distal (RHA) ends the nucleotides necessary to create restriction enzyme recognition sites that enable the final KO cassette to be cloned into the appropriate KO vector, e.g., sites compatible with PmeI for plasmids pMTL-SC7215 and pMTL-SC7315 and the restriction enzyme sites AscI and SbfI (or any of the various unique restriction enzymes in the MCS) for the plasmids pMTL-YN3 and pMTL-YN4. The distal primers of the LHA and the proximal primers of the RHA are designed to possess 20–25 overlapping nucleotides (dependent on GC content and melting temperature) to allow the subsequent fusion of the two amplified fragments by SOE PCR.

8. The *codA*-based vectors, pMTL7215/pMYL7315, can be used for gene KO in any *C. difficile* recipient, including wild-type backgrounds, whereas the *pyrE*-based KO vectors (pMTL-YN3 and pMTL-YN4) must be used in a *pyrE* background. Such mutants of strains 630Δ*erm* (CRG1496) and R20291 (CRG2359) have been previously made [3]. In the

case of other *C. difficile* hosts, *pyrE* mutants are easily created using ACE vectors equivalent to pMTL-YN18 [3] in which the LHA and SHA are, if necessary, exchanged with regions that are 100 % homologous to the *pyrE* locus in the target host.

9. To prevent self-ligation of the vector (important in the case of PmeI-cleaved pMTL-SC7215 and pMTL-SC7315), it is advisable to dephosphorylate the vector. Our laboratory uses Antarctic Phosphatase (AP) from NEB Biolabs, but other sources can be used. In essence, the linearized vector (100–200 ng in approximately 10 μl) is made up to a final volume of 20 μl using 10× AP buffer (NEB Biolabs) and following the addition of 5 U of AP enzyme, incubated at 37 °C for 30–60 min.

10. While the protocol is written, using Qiagen kits (Qiaquick PCR purification kit Cat no. 28104, Qiaprep plasmid miniprep kit Cat no. 27106, Qiaquick gel purification kit Cat no. 28704, DNeasy blood and tissue kit Cat no. 69506, and Proteinase K, 10 ml Cat no. 19133, any other kits for example Sigma-Aldrich GenElute™ HP Plasmid Miniprep Kit Cat no. NA0160-1KT, GenElute™ Bacterial Genomic DNA Kits Cat no. NA2120-1KT, GenElute™ PCR Clean-UP Kit Cat no. NA1020-1KT and GenElute™ Gel Extraction Kit Cat no. NA1111-1KT could equally be used.

11. If you do not see larger, faster growing colonies when restreaking to purify a single-crossover clone, do not restreak more than three times. In this case we recommend to start again at the initial conjugation step.

12. Not all strains display equally larger, faster growing colonies. In strain 630 the difference between transconjugants and single-crossover clones is very obvious, whereas in R20291 the size difference is less visible. It is therefore advisable to use as a comparative control cells carrying just the empty KO vector to compare size differences.

13. Theoretically, your double-crossover clones should comprise a 50:50 mix of wild-type revertant clones (i.e., clones which still have the wild-type allele) and recombinant clones (i.e., clones in which the wild-type allele has been exchanged for your recombinant allele).

14. Plasmids pMTL-YN1X and pMTL-YN2X both contain a NdeI following the *fdx* RBS and encompassing the start codon of the *lacZ'* gene. While in other vectors such a site is frequently used to conveniently clone genes lacking both a promoter and RBS, it is not easily possible in this case as the LHA of these vectors also contains an NdeI restriction site.

Acknowledgments

The authors acknowledge the financial support of the UK Medical Research Council (G0601176) and the UK Biotechnology and Biological Sciences Research Council (BB/L013940/1 and BB/G016224/1).

References

1. Cartman ST, Kelly ML, Heeg D, Heap JT, Minton NP (2012) Precise manipulation of the *Clostridium difficile* chromosome reveals a lack of association between the *tcdC* genotype and toxin production. Appl Environ Microbiol 78(13):4683–4690. doi:10.1128/AEM.00249-12

2. Ehsaan M, Kuit W, Zhang Y, Cartman ST, Heap JT, Winzer K, Minton NP (2016) Mutant generation by allelic exchange and genome resequencing of the biobutanol organism *Clostridium acetobutylicum* ATCC 824. Biotechnol Biofuels 9:4. doi:10.1186/s13068-015-0410-0

3. Ng YK, Ehsaan M, Philip S, Collery MM, Janoir C, Collignon A, Cartman ST, Minton NP (2013) Expanding the repertoire of gene tools for precise manipulation of the *Clostridium difficile* genome: allelic exchange using *pyrE* alleles. PLoS One 8(2):e56051. doi:10.1371/journal.pone.0056051

4. Heap JT, Ehsaan M, Cooksley CM, Ng YK, Cartman ST, Winzer K, Minton NP (2012) Integration of DNA into bacterial chromosomes from plasmids without a counter-selection marker. Nucleic Acids Res 40(8):e59. doi:10.1093/nar/gkr1321

5. Tripathi SA, Olson DG, Argyros DA, Miller BB, Barrett TF, Murphy DM, McCool JD, Warner AK, Rajgarhia VB, Lynd LR, Hogsett DA, Caiazza NC (2010) Development of *pyrF*-based genetic system for targeted gene deletion in *Clostridium thermocellum* and creation of a *pta* mutant. Appl Environ Microbiol 76(19):6591–6599. doi:10.1128/AEM.01484-10

6. Nariya H, Miyata S, Suzuki M, Tamai E, Okabe A (2011) Development and application of a method for counterselectable in-frame deletion in *Clostridium perfringens*. Appl Environ Microbiol 77(4):1375–1382. doi:10.1128/AEM.01572-10

7. Dusseaux S, Croux C, Soucaille P, Meynial-Salles I (2013) Metabolic engineering of *Clostridium acetobutylicum* ATCC 824 for the high-yield production of a biofuel composed of an isopropanol/butanol/ethanol mixture. Metab Eng 18:1–8. doi:10.1016/j.ymben.2013.03.003

8. Argyros DA, Tripathi SA, Barrett TF, Rogers SR, Feinberg LF, Olson DG, Foden JM, Miller BB, Lynd LR, Hogsett DA, Caiazza NC (2011) High ethanol titers from cellulose by using metabolically engineered thermophilic, anaerobic microbes. Appl Environ Microbiol 77(23):8288–8294. doi:10.1128/AEM.00646-11

9. Al-Hinai MA, Fast AG, Papoutsakis ET (2012) Novel system for efficient isolation of *Clostridium* double-crossover allelic exchange mutants enabling markerless chromosomal gene deletions and DNA integration. Appl Environ Microbiol 78(22):8112–8121. doi:10.1128/AEM.02214-12

10. Zhang Y, Grosse-Honebrink A, Minton NP (2015) A universal mariner transposon system for forward genetic studies in the genus *Clostridium*. PLoS One 10(4):e0122411. doi:10.1371/journal.pone.0122411

11. Kovacs K, Willson BJ, Schwarz K, Heap JT, Jackson A, Bolam DN, Winzer K, Minton NP (2013) Secretion and assembly of functional mini-cellulosomes from synthetic chromosomal operons in *Clostridium acetobutylicum* ATCC 824. Biotechnol Biofuels 6(1):117. doi:10.1186/1754-6834-6-117

12. Heap JT, Theys J, Ehsaan M, Kubiak AM, Dubois L, Paesmans K, Mellaert LV, Knox R, Kuehne SA, Lambin P, Minton NP (2014) Spores of Clostridium engineered for clinical efficacy and safety cause regression and cure of tumors in vivo. Oncotarget 5(7):1761–1769. doi:10.18632/oncotarget.1761

13. Shubeita HE, Sambrook JF, McCormick AM (1987) Molecular cloning and analysis of functional cDNA and genomic clones encoding bovine cellular retinoic acid-binding protein. Proc Natl Acad Sci U S A 84(16):5645–5649

14. Smith CJ, Markowitz SM, Macrina FL (1981) Transferable tetracycline resistance in *Clostridium difficile*. Antimicrob Agents Chemother 19(6):997–1003

15. Cartman ST, Minton NP (2010) A mariner-based transposon system for in vivo random mutagenesis of *Clostridium difficile*. Appl Environ Microbiol 76(4):1103–1109. doi:10.1128/AEM.02525-09

16. Heap JT, Pennington OJ, Cartman ST, Minton NP (2009) A modular system for Clostridium shuttle plasmids. J Microbiol Methods 78(1):79–85. doi:10.1016/j.mimet.2009.05.004

17. Chambers SP, Prior SE, Barstow DA, Minton NP (1988) The pMTL *nic*⁻ cloning vectors. I. Improved pUC polylinker regions to facilitate the use of sonicated DNA for nucleotide sequencing. Gene 68(1):139–149. doi:10.1016/0378-1119(88)90606-3

18. Gibson DG, Young L, Chuang RY, Venter JC, Hutchison CA III, Smith HO (2009) Enzymatic assembly of DNA molecules up to several hundred kilobases. Nat Methods 6(5):343–345. doi:10.1038/nmeth.1318

19. Lund AM, Kildegaard HF, Petersen MB, Rank J, Hansen BG, Andersen MR, Mortensen UH (2014) A versatile system for USER cloning-based assembly of expression vectors for mammalian cell engineering. PLoS One 9(5): e96693. doi:10.1371/journal.pone.0096693

20. de Kok S, Stanton LH, Slaby T, Durot M, Holmes VF, Patel KG, Platt D, Shapland EB, Serber Z, Dean J, Newman JD, Chandran SS (2014) Rapid and reliable DNA assembly via ligase cycling reaction. ACS Synth Biol 3(2):97–106. doi:10.1021/sb4001992

21. Engler C, Marillonnet S (2011) Generation of families of construct variants using golden gate shuffling. Methods Mol Biol 729:167–181. doi:10.1007/978-1-61779-065-2_11

22. Warrens AN, Jones MD, Lechler RI (1997) Splicing by overlap extension by PCR using asymmetric amplification: an improved technique for the generation of hybrid proteins of immunological interest. Gene 186(1):29–35. doi:10.1016/S0378-1119(96)00674-9

23. Purdy D, O'Keeffe TAT, Elmore M, Herbert M, McLeod A, Bokori-Brown M, Ostrowski A, Minton NP (2002) Conjugative transfer of clostridial shuttle vectors from *Escherichia coli* to *Clostridium difficile* through circumvention of the restriction barrier. Mol Microbiol 46(2):439–452. doi:10.1046/j.1365-2958.2002.03134.x

24. Minton NP, Ehsaan M, Humphreys CM, Little GT, Baker J, Henstra AM, Liew F, Kelly ML, Sheng L, Schwarz K, Zhang Y (2016) A roadmap for gene system development in Clostridium. Anaerobe. 2016 May 24. pii: S1075-9964(16)30064-6. doi:10.1016/j.anaerobe.2016.05.011

Chapter 5

Use of mCherryOpt Fluorescent Protein in *Clostridium difficile*

Eric M. Ransom, David S. Weiss, and Craig D. Ellermeier

Abstract

Here we describe protocols for using the red fluorescent protein mCherryOpt in *Clostridium difficile*. The protocols can be readily adapted to similar fluorescent proteins (FPs), such as green fluorescent protein (GFP) and cyan fluorescent protein (CFP). There are three critical considerations for using FPs in *C. difficile*. (1) Choosing the right color: Blue and (especially) red are preferred because *C. difficile* exhibits considerable yellow-green autofluorescence. (2) Codon optimization: Most FP genes in general circulation have a GC content of ~60%, so they are not well expressed in low-GC bacteria. (3) Fixing anaerobically grown cells prior to exposure to O_2: The FPs under consideration here are non-fluorescent when produced anaerobically because O_2 is required to introduce double bonds into the chromophore. Fixation prevents *C. difficile* cells from becoming degraded during the several hours required for chromophore maturation after cells are exposed to air. Fixation can probably be omitted for studies in which maintaining cellular architecture is not important, such as using mCherryOpt to monitor gene expression.

Key words Anaerobic fluorescence, Peptoclostridium, Paraformaldehyde, Formaldehyde, GFP, RFP, Translational fusion, Reporter, Fixation, Clostridia

1 Introduction

Fluorescent reporter proteins are powerful tools for studying protein localization, cellular structure, protein dynamics, and gene expression [1–3]. Several features of fluorescent proteins (FPs) have contributed to their popularity. Unlike enzymatic reporters of gene expression, there is no requirement to permeabilize cells or add an exogenous substrate. This makes FPs especially attractive for high-throughput screens. FPs come in a variety of colors, making it possible to determine the subcellular localization of two or more proteins in the same cell. Moreover, they are often bright enough to be visualized during fluorescence microscopy even when fused to proteins of low abundance. Because FPs can be visualized in live cells, they allow investigation of protein dynamics in

Adam P. Roberts and Peter Mullany (eds.), *Clostridium difficile: Methods and Protocols*, Methods in Molecular Biology, vol. 1476, DOI 10.1007/978-1-4939-6361-4_5, © Springer Science+Business Media New York 2016

real time, at least in organisms that require (or tolerate) exposure to air. A further attractive feature is that FPs can double as tags for protein purification and immunofluorescence.

Besides these advantages, there are some notable limitations to FP technology. FPs are relatively insensitive as reporters of gene expression because, unlike enzymatic reporters, they do not allow for signal amplification. In addition, chromophore maturation can require several hours and FPs often have long half-lives, making them poorly suited to study the kinetics of gene induction or repression. Another potential problem with FP tags is that they sometimes interfere with the function of the protein they are fused to [4]. This can lead to localization artifacts. Finally, because widely used FPs require O_2 for chromophore maturation [5], they are not suitable for live-cell studies of strict anaerobes such as *Clostridium difficile*. This limitation may be overcome by using flavin-based FPs that do not require O_2 [6, 7].

Here we describe procedures for using a red fluorescent protein called mCherryOpt for studies of protein localization and gene expression in *C. difficile* [8]. This application is possible because FPs produced anaerobically can acquire fluorescence after cells are exposed to air [5, 9]. We have extended this observation by showing that chromophore maturation occurs even in fixed cells, making it possible to preserve native patterns of protein localization after the cells are removed from the anaerobic chamber [8, 10]. Both CFPopt [11] and mCherryOpt [8] work well in *C. difficile*, but mCherryOpt is preferable for most applications because it is brighter and matures more quickly, and there is less interference from the organism's intrinsic autofluorescence.

2 Materials

2.1 Plasmid Constructions in *Escherichia coli*

1. pDSW1728 and/or pRAN473 plasmid DNA: These plasmids are derivatives of pRPF185 [12]. Plasmid DNA is available from the authors and DNA sequences have been deposited in Genbank (pDSW1728, $P_{tet}mCherryOpt$, accession number KT371995; pRAN473, $P_{tet}:mCherryOpt$-MCS, accession number KT371996).

2. Gene-specific oligonucleotide primers.

3. Restriction enzymes and buffers.

4. T4 DNA ligase and buffer.

5. Supplies for agarose gel electrophoresis.

6. Competent *E. coli* cloning host: We use OmniMAX 2 T1^R (Life Technologies), but just about any standard cloning strain will suffice.

7. LB medium: 10 g/l tryptone, 5 g/l yeast extract, and 10 g/l NaCl. Add 15 g/l agar for plates.

8. LB Cm10 plates: LB plates containing 10 μg/ml chloramphenicol for selection and maintenance of *E. coli* transformants carrying pDSW1728, pRAN473, and their derivatives.

2.2 Transfer of pDSW1728 or pRAN473 Derivatives to C. difficile by Conjugation

1. Chemically competent *E. coli* conjugation donor strain: We use HB101/pRK24 [13].

2. *C. difficile* conjugation recipient: We have succeeded in producing mCherryOpt in all *C. difficile* strains tested so far: JIR8094, R20291, CD630, CD196, NAP07, and NAP08.

3. LB media: See above.

4. LB Amp100 plates: LB plates containing 100 μg/ml ampicillin for selection and maintenance of HB101/pRK24.

5. LB Amp100 Cm10 plates: LB plates containing 100 μg/ml ampicillin and 10 μg/ml chloramphenicol for selection and maintenance of HB101/pRK24 transformants carrying derivatives of pDSW1728 or pRAN473.

6. TY media: 30 g/l Tryptone, 20 g/l yeast extract, and 0.1% cysteine. Add 20 g/l agar for plates.

7. TY Thi10 Kan50 Cef16: TY containing 10 μg/ml thiamphenicol, 50 μg/ml kanamycin, and 16 μg/ml cefoxitin are used to select for *C. difficile* exconjugants and counter-select against the *E. coli* donor.

2.3 Growth of C. difficile Exconjugants for Studies of Gene Expression and Protein Localization Using mCherryOpt Plasmid Constructs

1. TY Thi10: TY containing 10 μg/ml thiamphenicol to select for pDSW1728, pRAN473, or their derivatives. Note that other growth media may be more appropriate depending on the nature of the experiment.

2. Anhydrotetracycline (ATc; Sigma) is used for induction of genes under control of the P_{tet} promoter [12]. Prepare a 1 mg/ml ATc stock solution by dissolving the powder in 50% ethanol and storing at −20 °C in the dark. Sterilization is not necessary on account of the high ethanol concentration.

2.4 Fixation Reagents

1. 16% (wt/vol) paraformaldehyde aqueous solution (methanol-free; catalog #AA433689M, Alfa Aesar, Ward Hill, MA): Paraformaldehyde is hazardous. Wear protective gear and work with concentrated stocks in a fume hood (*see* **Notes 1** and **2**).

2. 1 M $NaPO_4$ buffer (pH 7.4).

3. Phosphate-buffered saline (PBS): 137 mM NaCl, 2.7 mM KCl, 10 mM Na_2HPO_4, and 1.8 mM KH_2PO_4. Adjust pH to 7.4.

4. Anaerobic 1.5 ml microcentrifuge tubes: one per sample.

2.5 Detection and Quantification of mCherryOpt in C. difficile

2.5.1 Fluorescence Microscopy

1. Glass microscope slides (catalog #3800240, precleaned, $1'' \times 3'' \times 0.04''$, frosted ground, Leica, Richmond, IL).

2. Cover slips (catalog #3845500, precleaned, $22'' \times 22''$ #1, Leica, Richmond, IL).

3. 1% (wt/vol) agarose (Gibco) in water for immobilization pads.

4. Fluorescence microscope with sensitive digital camera camera and appropriate filters: We use an Olympus BX60 microscope equipped with a 100 UPlanApo objective (numerical aperture, 1.35). Images are captured using a black-and-white Spot 2-cooled charge-coupled device camera (Diagnostic Instruments, Sterling Heights, MI) with a KAF1400E chip (class 2), a Uniblitz shutter, and a personal computer with Image-Pro software (Media Cybernetics, Silver Spring, MD). Our filter sets for fluorescence imaging are from Chroma Technology Corp. (Brattleboro, VT). For mCherryOpt the filter set (catalog no. 41004) comprises a 538 to 582 nm excitation filter, a 595 nm dichroic mirror (long pass), and a 582 to 682 nm emission filter. For CFPopt the filter set (catalog no. 31044v2) comprises a 426 to 446 nm excitation filter, a 455 nm dichroic mirror (long pass), and a 460 to 500 nm emission filter (band pass).

2.5.2 Fluorometer (Fluorescent Plate Reader)

1. A microplate reader capable of monitoring optical density (OD) and red fluorescence. We use a Tecan Infinite M200 Pro plate reader. For mCherryOpt the following software settings work well: OD_{600} with the number of flashes = 25; fluorescence excitation = 554, emission = 610, mode = top, Z-position = 20,000 μm, number of flashes = 25, gain = 100 manual, and integration time = 20 μs.

2. Microplates compatible with the reader: We use 96-well tissue culture plates from Advangene (CC Plate-PS-96S-F-C-S).

2.5.3 Flow Cytometry

1. Flow cytometer: We use a Becton Dickinson LSR II with the following settings: 561 nm excitation, photomultiplier tube C, and band-pass filters 610/20.

2. Cell strainers with 70 μm cutoff such as Falcon cat. #352350.

3. Sterile 50 ml conical centrifuge tubes such as Falcon cat. # 352098.

4. Sterile 5 ml round-bottom polystyrene tubes such as Falcon cat. #352054.

---

3 Methods

Use of mCherryOpt reporters can be divided into five stages: construction of a reporter plasmid in *E. coli*, transfer of the plasmid to *C.*

difficile by conjugation, growth of the exconjugant, fixation of the cells followed by exposure to air to allow chromophore maturation, and, finally, analysis of mCherryOpt fluorescence by microscopy, fluorometry (fluorescent plate reader), and/or flow cytometry. The procedures outlined below are intended to guide investigators through each of these steps. We also included a section on critical parameters of the assays and troubleshooting. Although the protocols are written with reference to mCherryOpt, they are readily adapted to CFPopt. In writing up these procedures, we assumed a basic familiarity with molecular biology and methods for cultivating *C. difficile*. Investigators who need more background are referred to Current Protocols in Molecular Biology [14] and other chapters in this manual.

3.1 Guidelines for Constructing mCherryOpt Promoter Fusions

To monitor gene expression, investigators will want to construct a derivative of pDSW1728. This plasmid has tetracycline-inducible promoter upstream of mCherryOpt (P_{tet}::*mCherryOpt*) flanked by restriction sites for NheI and SacI, which can be used to replace P_{tet} promoter with a promoter of choice. Key features of pDSW1728 are shown in Fig. 1.

1. Purified pDSW1728 DNA should be digested with NheI and SacI.

2. Design oligonucleotide primers to amplify the promoter region of interest by PCR with *C. difficile* genomic DNA as the template. The 5′ and 3′ primers should include NheI and SacI sites, respectively, to facilitate downstream cloning steps. Alternatively, if ligation-free cloning methods such as Gibson Assembly [15] will be used, the primers must include appropriate regions of homology to the target vector. Because pDSW1728 supplies an optimized Shine-Dalgarno for *mCherryOpt*, there is no need to include one in the 3′ primer.

3. Clone the promoter fragment into pDSW1728 using traditional ligase-dependent cloning or ligase-independent methods such as Gibson Assembly [15].

4. Once putative clones are identified, verify the DNA sequence of the insert using the following sequencing primers: RP298 (5′-CAAATTCATGTCCATTAACAGATCCTTCC-3′) and RP206 (5′-CAAATTCATGTCCATTAACAGATCCT TCC-3′). The sites to which these primers bind are depicted in Fig. 1.

3.2 Guidelines for Constructing mCherryOpt Gene Fusions

To monitor protein localization, investigators will want to construct a derivative of pRAN473. This plasmid allows for fusing mCherryOpt to the N-terminus of a protein of interest. It has a P_{tet} promoter and a multiple cloning site at the 3′ terminus of *mCherryOpt* (P_{tet}::*mCherryOpt*-MCS). A schematic diagram of pRAN473 is provided in Fig. 2.

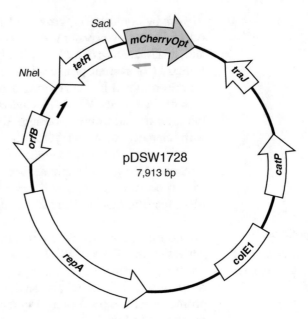

Fig. 1 Schematic diagram of pDSW1728. The P_{tet} promoter can be replaced with a promoter of interest using the NheI and SacI restriction sites. The approximate locations of two sequencing primers are indicated with *half arrows*. For additional details *see* ref. 8

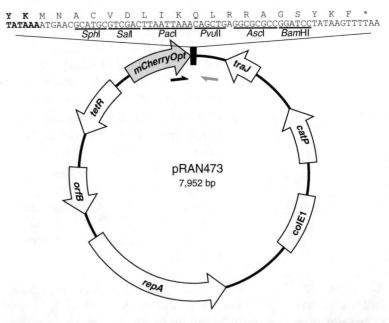

Fig. 2 Schematic diagram of pRAN473. The sequence above the plasmid shows the last two codons of mCherryOpt (in *bold*) followed by the multiple cloning site for constructing gene fusions. The approximate locations of two sequencing primers are indicated with *half arrows*. For other details *see* ref. 8

1. Purified pRAN473 DNA should be digested with the enzymes of choice.

2. Design oligonucleotide primers to amplify the gene of interest. Figure 2 shows the reading frame across the multiple cloning site of pRAN473 to facilitate constructing fusions that are in frame with *mCherryOpt*. We often incorporate three asparagine (Asn) codons into the 5′ primer to create an extended linker between mCherryOpt and the target protein. For example, to use the SalI site in pRAN473 to fuse mCherryOpt to the N-terminus of a target protein, the 5′ PCR primer for amplifying the target gene would have the general structure: 5′-XXX<u>GTCGAC</u>*AACAACAAC*ATG(N18)-3′. Here XXX denotes bases added to facilitate restriction digestion, the SalI site is underlined, the sequence encoding the three Asn residues is italicized, ATG is the start codon for the target gene, and the series of Ns reflects bases that anneal to the target gene (and can be extended if necessary for better annealing). The 3′ primer typically captures the last ~7 codons of the target gene (including the stop codon) followed by a restriction site for cloning (e.g., BamHI) and three bases to facilitate restriction digestion, for example: 5′-XXX<u>GGATCC</u>TTA(N18)-3′.

3. Clone the target gene into pRAN473 using traditional ligase-dependent cloning or ligase-independent methods such as Gibson Assembly [15]. We use OmniMAX 2 T1^R as the *E. coli* cloning host strain. Other standard cloning strains will work too. The advantage of OmniMAX 2 T1^R is that it is Tet^R, which facilitates screening for ATc-dependent red fluorescence to verify expression of new constructs before moving them into *C. difficile*.

4. Screen for plasmids that contain the desired insert by restriction digest, and then verify that the insert is in the correct reading frame and free of undesired mutations by DNA sequencing. We use the following sequencing primers: RP298 (5′-CAAATTCATGTCCATTAACAGATCCTTCC-3′) and RP206 (5′-CAAATTCATGTCCATTAACAGATCCTTCC-3′). These primers bind to sites flanking the insertion as depicted in Fig. 2.

3.3 Conjugation

Prior to initiating the conjugation procedure described below, it will be necessary to transform your mCherryOpt construct(s) from Subheading 3.1 or 3.2 into *E. coli* HB101/pRK24 or some other *E. coli* conjugation donor strain. We select and maintain transformants on LB plates containing 100 μg/ml ampicillin (for pRK24) and 10 μg/ml chloramphenicol (for mCherryOpt constructs). For greater detail on moving plasmids from *E. coli* to *C. difficile* by conjugation, *see* Subheading 3.2, **step 4**, of Heap et al. [16].

1. Centrifuge 1 ml of an overnight culture of the *E. coli* donor at $3000 \times g$ for 1 min to collect the cells.

2. Remove the supernatant and suspend the cell pellet in 1 ml of reduced TY (containing cysteine) from the anaerobic chamber.

3. Spin down the cells again at $3000 \times g$ for 1 min and remove the supernatant.

4. Transfer the microfuge tube containing the *E. coli* cell pellet into an anaerobic chamber maintained at 37 °C.

5. Gently suspend the *E. coli* cell pellet in 100 µl of an overnight culture of *C. difficile*. Spot the mixture on a TY plate with no antibiotics.

6. Incubate the plate overnight (or for at least 6 h), and then collect cells from the plate in 1 ml of TY broth.

7. Spread 500 µl on a TY Thi10 Kan50 Cef16 plate. Incubate overnight.

8. Streak individual colonies onto TY Thi10 Kan50 Cef16 and incubate overnight.

3.4 Growth of C. difficile/pDSW1728 Derivatives to Monitor Gene Expression

1. Working in an anaerobic chamber, use a colony of the desired exconjugant to inoculate 3 ml of TY Thi10. Grow overnight at 37 °C. As a control also inoculate a culture of *C. difficile*/ pDSW1728.

2. In the morning, subculture cells 1:100 by adding 30 µl of the overnight culture to 3 ml of TY Thi10. The control strain should be subcultured *in duplicate*.

3. When the OD_{600} reaches 0.6 (~4 h) add ATc to a final concentration of 500 ng/ml to one of the cultures of *C. difficile*/pDSW1728. This is your positive control. The duplicate culture should not receive any inducer and serves as your negative control.

4. After 1 h, fix an aliquot of each culture for later analysis of mCherryOpt fluorescence (*see* Subheading 3.5).

5. After allowing for chromophore maturation (*see* **Note 3**), evaluate the level of mCherryOpt fluorescence by microscopy, fluorometry, and/or flow cytometry. These methods are discussed below (Subheadings 3.6–3.9).

6. Variations: This protocol is intended for illustration purposes only. Other growth media can be substituted for TY. To evaluate expression at different growth phases, samples can be fixed at different ODs. To evaluate the importance of a putative regulatory element, the reporter plasmid can be introduced into a *C. difficile* mutant and its corresponding parental wild type. To query a stress response, samples should be fixed before and after the stress (e.g., addition of NaCl).

3.5 Growth of C. difficile/pRAN473 Derivatives to Monitor Protein Localization

1. Working in an anaerobic chamber, use a colony of the desired exconjugant to inoculate 3 ml of TY Thi10. Grow overnight at 37 °C. As a control also inoculate a culture of *C. difficile*/pRAN473.

2. In the morning, subculture cells 1:100 by adding 30 μl of the overnight culture to 3 ml of TY Thi10. Because the appropriate level of expression of the *mCherryOpt* fusion has to be determined empirically, this strain should be used to set up five parallel cultures, which will ultimately be induced with five different concentrations of ATc. The control strain should be subcultured *in duplicate*.

3. When the OD_{600} reaches 0.6 (~4 h) induce the experimental cultures by adding ATc at 0, 50, 100, 200, and 400 ng/ml (final concentrations). Induce the control with 0 and 400 ng/ml ATc. Be aware that ATc can retard growth even at 100 ng/ml (*see* **Note 4**).

4. After 1 h fix, aliquot each culture for later analysis of mCherryOpt fluorescence (*see* Subheading 3.5).

5. Variations: This protocol is intended for illustration purposes and is designed to help the investigator hone in on an appropriate induction regimen. In many cases it will not be biologically meaningful to monitor protein localization in cells growing exponentially in TY.

3.6 Fixation

1. While cells are growing, prepare a 5× fixation master mix (made fresh daily) consisting of 20 μl of 1 M $NaPO_4$ and 100 μl of 16% paraformaldehyde per sample. Paraformaldehyde is hazardous. Wear protective gear and work with concentrated stocks in a fume hood (*see* **Note 1**). Earlier versions of our fixative mixture included glutaraldehyde [8, 10], but we have since found that this can be omitted.

2. Transfer the 5× fixation master mix into the anaerobic chamber.

3. When it is time to fix cells, transfer 500 μl of culture to an anaerobic 1.5 ml microcentrifuge tube.

4. To this, add 120 μl of 5× fixation master mix.

5. Mix briefly by pipetting, vortexing, or simply inverting the tube by hand about eight times.

6. Once samples are in fixative, remove from anaerobic chamber. Incubate in the dark for 30 min at room temperature followed by 30 min on ice. Fixation times up to at least 2 h are acceptable.

7. Centrifuge for 1 min >$15,000 \times g$ to pellet cells.

8. In a fume hood, use a pipette to remove media containing fixative and discard in an appropriate waste container. Subsequent steps can be done at the bench.

9. Wash the cells by suspending the pellet in 1 ml PBS with the aid of a vortex mixer. Then centrifuge to collect the cell pellet, discarding the PBS supernatant. Repeat these steps for a total of three washes.

10. Suspend the final cell pellet in 30 μl of PBS.

11. Store in the dark at room temperature or 4 °C to allow for chromophore maturation. mCherryOpt fluorescence can generally be detected within 30 min and reaches a maximum in about 3 h [8], but we generally find it convenient to wait overnight (*see* **Note 3**).

3.7 Analysis by Fluorescence Microscopy

The high resolution of fluorescence microscopy is useful for determining the subcellular location of a protein. In addition, fluorescence microscopy can reveal whether a pattern of expression or localization is uniform across a population.

1. Cells should be immobilized for microscopy. We accomplish this using agarose pads. First, place a strip of masking tape at each end of a microscope slide, leaving a gap of ~2 cm (Fig. 3). Next, melt an aliquot of 1 % agarose (in water) and spot 30 μl onto the slide between the strips of tape. Quickly place a second microscope slide on top to form a sandwich. The pool of agarose will spread to fill the region bounded by the strips of tape. Wait for at least 20 min for the agarose to solidify, and then gently separate the microscope slides without damaging the agarose pad. It does not matter which of the two glass slides the pad sticks to, but sometimes different regions of the pad stick to different slides, which can cause the pad to tear. For this reason, we generally prepare several extra pads. Agarose pads are only useful for a few hours because they tend to dry out. We discard unused pads at the end of the day, and we do not separate the cover slips to expose a pad until immediately before use.

2. Spot 1 μl of fixed cells onto the agarose pad and apply a cover slip.

3. Proceed to the microscope for imaging. We assume that the investigator has access to a high-quality microscope system equipped for fluorescence. If this describes you, skip the rest of this paragraph.

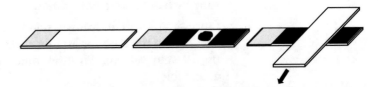

Fig. 3 Schematic diagram for preparing an agarose pad for microscopy. To a clean glass slide affix two pieces of tape. Between these spot 30 μl of molten 1 % agarose and immediately cover with a second microscope slide. Wait for at least 20 min for the agarose to solidify. Pull the top slide towards you when ready to use. The agarose pad usually sticks to the top slide

But if you do your microscopy with the help of a colleague or core facility that is set up for eukaryotes, the following discussion of critical parameters might prove helpful. (1) Bacteria are small, so you will need a 100× oil-immersion objective. The objective should have a high numerical aperture (e.g., 1.35) and PlanApo correction. (2) The filter set should be well matched to the characteristics of mCherry. Note that mCherryOpt is identical to mCherry in this context; "opt" refers to codon usage. (3) A sensitive, high-resolution digital camera is needed because many bacterial proteins are produced at low levels. You cannot compensate for weak fluorescence by binning because you will lose too much resolution. Nor can you compensate by overproducing the fusion protein because that is apt to cause mislocalization. You should not use photographic exposure times longer than several seconds because mCherryOpt will bleach.

4. Place your slide on the microscope stage, add a drop of immersion oil to the top of the cover slip, and focus on your cells under phase contrast. We recommend starting with phase because mCherryOpt bleaches too quickly to find cells under fluorescence.

5. Take a picture under phase. The exposure time is likely to be <1 s, but microscopes vary.

6. Switch to the mCherry filter set and capture a fluorescence image. The exposure time is likely to be in the range of 0.5–6 s. You should now have matched phase contrast and fluorescence images of the same field of cells.

7. Figure 4 shows examples of mid-cell localization of a cell division protein (P$_{tet}$::*mldA-mCherryOpt*) and forespore-specific gene expression (P$_{spoIIR}$::*mCherryOpt*).

3.8 Analysis Using a Fluorometer (Fluorescent Plate Reader)

A fluorometer provides a quick and highly quantitative way to measure the total fluorescence of a large population of cells.

1. To the fixed cells from Subheading 3.4 (30 μl, in PBS) add 170 μl of PBS and then transfer the entire 200 μl to a single well of a 96-well plate. One of the fixed samples should be an uninduced or empty vector control strain. A well containing 200 μl of PBS is used to blank the instrument.

2. Note that because it is not necessary to preserve cellular architecture to read total mCherryOpt fluorescence, it may be possible to omit the fixation step. But in this case the media should be replaced with PBS to reduce background fluorescence. It is probably advisable to conduct a pilot experiment with your particular strain(s) to compare fixed to unfixed samples.

3. Cover the plate and proceed with the readings as per the instructions for your instrument. Record both fluorescence and optical density, which you will need to normalize between samples.

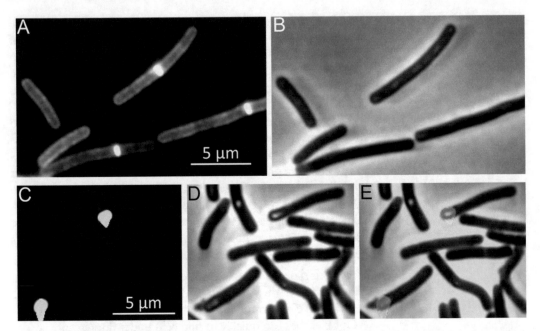

Fig. 4 Representative micrographs showing septal localization of a cell division protein and forespore-specific gene expression. (**a, b**) *C. difficile*/pRAN535 (P*tet*:: *mCherryOpt-mldA*) grown in TY Thi10 was induced for 1 h with 80 ng/ml ATc. Cells were fixed and processed as described herein, and then photographed under fluorescence (**a**) and phase contrast (**b**). (**c–e**) *C. difficile*/pRAN739 (P*spoIIR*::*mCherryOpt*) was grown on a TY Thi10 plate for 48 h. Cells were recovered from the plate by suspending in 2 ml of PBS. Subsequent fixation and processing steps were as described herein. (**c**) Fluorescence micrograph. (**d**) Phase contrast. (**e**) Overlay

4. To verify the linearity of the instrument, we recommend reading a dilution series of an induced (i.e., fluorescent) sample.

5. Figure 5a shows an example of the dose dependency of the tetracycline-inducible promoter (P*tet*::*mCherryOpt*) as measured using a plate reader.

3.9 Analysis by Flow Cytometry

Flow cytometry provides excellent quantitation and information on the uniformity of fluorescence across a large sample of cells, often numbering in the millions. In combination with a cell sorter, this method can be used to isolate different subsets of cells such as fluorescent vs. non-fluorescent for further analyses.

1. Recall that the fixed cells from Subheading 3.4 were ultimately suspended in 30 μl of PBS. Add 5 μl of fixed cells to 0.5 ml of PBS in a microfuge tube.

2. Transfer the sample to a cell strainer (70 μm cut-off) and let flow through under gravity into a 50 ml conical centrifuge tube.

3. Transfer the filtered sample into a 5 ml polystyrene round-bottom tube. The sample is then ready for flow cytometry.

4. Figure 5b shows an example of the dose dependency of the tetracycline-inducible promoter (P*tet*::*mCherryOpt*) as measured by flow cytometry.

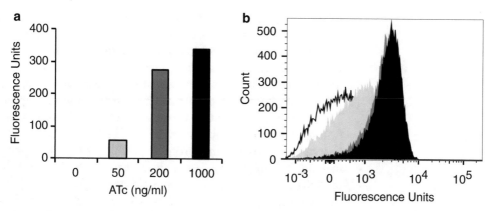

Fig. 5 Dose-dependent expression of P$_{tet}$::*mCherryOpt* induced with ATc. *C. difficile*/pDSW1728 grown in TY Thi10 was induced for 1 h with various concentrations of ATc as shown. Cells were fixed and processed as described herein, and then analyzed using a fluorescent plate reader (**a**) or flow cytometry (**b**)

3.10 Critical Parameters and Troubleshooting

1. *No transformants (or only incorrect transformants) when constructing plasmids in E. coli.* Some derivatives of pDSW1728 and pRAN473 may be toxic in *E. coli*, where the plasmids have a high copy number of about 200 per genome. Growing *E. coli* transformants at lower temperatures can help, as can using *E. coli* strains engineered to lower the copy number of ColE1-related plasmids (e.g., ABLE K from Agilent Technologies).

2. *Cells are not fluorescent.* Anti-mCherry antibodies are available from a number of commercial suppliers and can be used to determine whether mCherryOpt (or an mCherryOpt fusion protein) is being produced. If not, recover the plasmid and double-check it for mutations. Also, if the construct uses the P$_{tet}$ promoter, determine whether *E. coli* transformants induced with ATc are fluorescent—this can be done with cells grown aerobically and thus bypasses potential problems arising during fixation. If mCherryOpt is produced as determined by Western blotting but does not fluoresce, verify that the microscope/plate reader/flow cytometer is functioning properly.

3. *FPs as reporters of gene expression.* FPs are not well suited for studying the kinetics of gene expression because they acquire fluorescence slowly and have long half-lives. Thus, there is a significant lag between induction of a gene and the appearance of fluorescence and an even longer lag between repression of a gene and disappearance of fluorescence. Nevertheless, FPs are very useful for studying the conditions under which a promoter is activated, the regulatory factors controlling expression from that promoter, and identifying small molecules that modulate gene expression.

4. *FP tags in protein localization experiments*. Tagging a protein can alter its behavior. For this reason, it is generally advisable to use complementation to determine whether your fusion retains (near) wild-type activity. It is also advisable to verify that the fusion protein is largely intact. Anti-mCherry antibodies suitable for Western blotting are available from multiple suppliers. There are several options for addressing problems related to fusion protein function and stability. (1) Move the tag to the C-terminus of the target protein. (2) Alter the linker, perhaps making it longer. (3) Try a different tag, such as CFPopt, tdTOMATO, a SNAP tag, or an epitope tag [10, 17–19]. Note that a tagged protein might mislocalize if it is overproduced. Antibody against the target protein can be used in Westerns to determine whether the fusion protein is produced at physiological levels. Antibody against the target protein might also be used in immunofluorescence microscopy to localize that protein, obviating the need for tags altogether. A drawback of immunofluorescence in bacteria is that it is technically challenging and antibody of sufficient quality is often not available.

4 Notes

1. Paraformaldehyde is hazardous and should be handled with caution. Gloves, lab coat, safety goggles, and use of a fume hood when aliquoting stock solutions are strongly recommended.

2. Paraformaldehyde can expire, especially upon exposure to air. After opening a new vial, we dispense 1 ml aliquots into microfuge tubes and store at 4 °C. Use within 6 months.

3. Chromophore maturation in mCherryOpt usually takes a few hours [8] but it may take longer if samples are stored at 4 °C. We typically wait overnight for convenience. We do not know if the rate of chromophore maturation will depend upon variables such as the conditions under which the cells were grown or nature of the protein fusion. The cyan fluorescent protein (CFPopt) matures more slowly.

4. Alternatively, overnight cultures can be inoculated directly into TY Thi10 containing various amounts of ATc. But this approach is somewhat inconvenient because ATc concentrations as low as 100 ng/ml can retard growth, so different cultures will be ready for fixation at different times.

Acknowledgments

The work described in this chapter was funded by National Institutes of Health grants GM-083975 to D.S.W., AI-087834 to C.D.E., and the Department of Microbiology at The University of Iowa.

References

1. Tsien RY (1998) The green fluorescent protein. Annu Rev Biochem 67:509–544. doi:10.1146/annurev.biochem.67.1.509

2. Shaner NC, Steinbach PA, Tsien RY (2005) A guide to choosing fluorescent proteins. Nat Methods 2(12):905–909. doi:10.1038/nmeth819

3. Remington SJ (2011) Green fluorescent protein: a perspective. Protein Sci 20(9):1509–1519. doi:10.1002/pro.684

4. Margolin W (2012) The price of tags in protein localization studies. J Bacteriol 194(23):6369–6371. doi:10.1128/JB.01640-12

5. Heim R, Prasher DC, Tsien RY (1994) Wavelength mutations and posttranslational autoxidation of green fluorescent protein. Proc Natl Acad Sci U S A 91(26):12501–12504

6. Buckley AM, Petersen J, Roe AJ, Douce GR, Christie JM (2015) LOV-based reporters for fluorescence imaging. Curr Opin Chem Biol 27:39–45. doi:10.1016/j.cbpa.2015.05.011

7. Drepper T, Huber R, Heck A, Circolone F, Hillmer AK, Buchs J, Jaeger KE (2010) Flavin mononucleotide-based fluorescent reporter proteins outperform green fluorescent protein-like proteins as quantitative in vivo real-time reporters. Appl Environ Microbiol 76(17):5990–5994. doi:10.1128/AEM.00701-10

8. Ransom EM, Ellermeier CD, Weiss DS (2015) Use of mCherry Red fluorescent protein for studies of protein localization and gene expression in *Clostridium difficile*. Appl Environ Microbiol 81(5):1652–1660. doi:10.1128/AEM.03446-14

9. Zhang C, Xing XH, Lou K (2005) Rapid detection of a *gfp*-marked *Enterobacter aerogenes* under anaerobic conditions by aerobic fluorescence recovery. FEMS Microbiol Lett 249(2):211–218. doi:10.1016/j.femsle.2005.05.051

10. Ransom EM, Williams KB, Weiss DS, Ellermeier CD (2014) Identification and characterization of a gene cluster required for proper rod shape, cell division, and pathogenesis in *Clostridium difficile*. J Bacteriol 196(12):2290–2300. doi:10.1128/JB.00038-14

11. Sastalla I, Chim K, Cheung GY, Pomerantsev AP, Leppla SH (2009) Codon-optimized fluorescent proteins designed for expression in low-GC gram-positive bacteria. Appl Environ Microbiol 75(7):2099–2110. doi:10.1128/AEM.02066-08

12. Fagan RP, Fairweather NF (2011) *Clostridium difficile* has two parallel and essential Sec secretion systems. J Biol Chem 286(31):27483–27493. doi:10.1074/jbc.M111.263889

13. Trieu-Cuot P, Arthur M, Courvalin P (1987) Origin, evolution and dissemination of antibiotic resistance genes. Microbiol Sci 4(9):263–266

14. Ausubel FM (2002) Short protocols in molecular biology: a compendium of methods from Current protocols in molecular biology, 5th edn. Wiley, New York

15. Gibson DG (2009) Synthesis of DNA fragments in yeast by one-step assembly of overlapping oligonucleotides. Nucleic Acids Res 37(20):6984–6990. doi:10.1093/nar/gkp687

16. Heap JT, Pennington OJ, Cartman ST, Minton NP (2009) A modular system for *Clostridium* shuttle plasmids. J Microbiol Methods 78(1):79–85. doi:10.1016/j.mimet.2009.05.004

17. Barra-Carrasco J, Olguin-Araneda V, Plaza-Garrido A, Miranda-Cardenas C, Cofre-Araneda G, Pizarro-Guajardo M, Sarker MR, Paredes-Sabja D (2013) The *Clostridium difficile* exosporium cysteine (CdeC)-rich protein is required for exosporium morphogenesis and coat assembly. J Bacteriol 195(17):3863–3875. doi:10.1128/JB.00369-13

18. Pereira FC, Saujet L, Tome AR, Serrano M, Monot M, Couture-Tosi E, Martin-Verstraete I, Dupuy B, Henriques AO (2013) The spore differentiation pathway in the enteric pathogen *Clostridium difficile*. PLoS Genet 9(10):e1003782. doi:10.1371/journal.pgen.1003782

19. Terpe K (2003) Overview of tag protein fusions: from molecular and biochemical fundamentals to commercial systems. Appl Microbiol Biotechnol 60(5):523–533. doi:10.1007/s00253-002-1158-6

Chapter 6

A Fluorescent Reporter for Single Cell Analysis of Gene Expression in *Clostridium difficile*

Carolina Piçarra Cassona, Fátima Pereira, Mónica Serrano, and Adriano O. Henriques

Abstract

Genetically identical cells growing under homogeneous growth conditions often display cell–cell variation in gene expression. This variation stems from noise in gene expression and can be adaptive allowing for division of labor and bet-hedging strategies. In particular, for bacterial pathogens, the expression of phenotypes related to virulence can show cell–cell variation. Therefore, understanding virulence-related gene expression requires knowledge of gene expression patterns at the single cell level. We describe protocols for the use of fluorescence reporters for single cell analysis of gene expression in the human enteric pathogen *Clostridium difficile*, a strict anaerobe. The reporters are based on modified versions of the human DNA repair enzyme O^6-alkylguanine-DNA alkyltransferase, called SNAP-tag and CLIP-tag. SNAP becomes covalently labeled upon reaction with O^6-benzylguanine conjugated to a fluorophore, whereas CLIP is labeled by O^6-benzylcytosine conjugates. SNAP and CLIP labeling is orthogonal allowing for dual labeling in the same cells. SNAP and CLIP cassettes optimized for *C. difficile* can be used for quantitative studies of gene expression at the single cell level. Both the SNAP and CLIP reporters can also be used for studies of protein subcellular localization in *C. difficile*.

Key words Gene expression, Single-cell analysis, SNAP-tag, CLIP-tag, *Clostridium difficile*

1 Introduction

Populations of genetically identical cells growing under uniform conditions may show cell-to-cell heterogeneity in gene expression (reviewed by refs. [1, 2]). Cell–cell variation in gene expression arises because of stochastic fluctuations in the cellular levels of the components of genetic circuits, or noise [3]. Noise is often functional leading to the generation of distinct phenotypes in a population and allowing for division of labor and bet-hedging strategies that facilitate survival of the population in unpredictable environments [1, 2, 4]. Certain genetic circuits can amplify noise, and lead to a type of variation in which subpopulations express a certain gene at high or at low levels, a phenomenon termed bistability

Adam P. Roberts and Peter Mullany (eds.), *Clostridium difficile: Methods and Protocols*, Methods in Molecular Biology, vol. 1476,
DOI 10.1007/978-1-4939-6361-4_6, © Springer Science+Business Media New York 2016

[1, 2]. One example of bistability is seen during exponential growth of *Bacillus subtilis*, in which coexist motile and sessile cells [5]. This heterogeneity is regulated at the level of a protein, σ^D, which directs the transcription of the genes involved in assembly of the flagellum. Increasing the number of sessile cells allows the population to settle and exploit a present favorable location; in contrast, when it is convenient to move to a new place the number of motile cells is increased [5]. Gene expression heterogeneity is also important in developmental decisions, such as competence development or sporulation in *B. subtilis*, or in cell fate determination as during biofilm formation [6–9], and it may be a key factor in promoting evolutionary transitions [3, 10]. Heterogeneity in gene expression is important in bacterial pathogenesis, as phenotypes important to virulence often show heterogeneity. Small subpopulations of antibiotic-tolerant persister cells, have been documented in many bacteria, and are an example of a bet-hedging strategy [4, 11]. In *Salmonella enterica* serovar Typhimurium a slow-growing subpopulation secretes virulence or other factors that promote host colonization by the entire cell population, while a fast-growing population is phenotypically avirulent [12]. Production of virulence factors is costly, and the population is vulnerable to the accumulation of defector mutants that take advantage from the collective action but do not produce virulence factors and therefore do not contribute to it. However, the expression of the avirulent subpopulation slows down the appearance of defector mutants. Hence, bistability in the expression of the virulence genes promotes the evolutionary stability of virulence [12].

The ability of measuring gene expression at the single-cell level using autofluorescent proteins (AFP's) has enabled the characterization of phenotypic heterogeneity in bacterial populations and also detailed studies of the architecture and properties of the underlying genetic circuits [1–3]. AFP's or other reporters for single cell analysis are now indispensible tools in bacterial cell and development biology. Usually the gene coding for the AFP is expressed under the control of a promoter sequence derived from the gene under study, and in this way the spatiotemporal expression of the AFP mimics that of the gene. This methodology has been instrumental in studies of the mechanisms of gene regulation. However the AFP's methodology cannot be applied in strict anaerobes like *Clostridium difficile*, since emission of fluorescence by the GFP chromophore requires cyclization and oxidation of an internal tripeptide motif, and the last step of this reaction, which is autocatalytic, requires oxygen [13]. Nonetheless, CFP_{opt} and $mCherry_{opt}$ were used to localize cell division proteins and as reporters for gene expression in anaerobically grown *C. difficile* [14, 15]. Moreover, a translational fusion to tdTOMATO was used to localize proteins on the surface of the *C. difficile* spores [16]. In these studies fluorescence measurements were done after samples have been exposed to air to enable fluorophore maturation.

Under these conditions unfixed cells lyse and therefore fixed cells were used, preventing live-cell imaging.

To overcome the limitations associated with the use of AFP's in strict anaerobes, new proteins to be used as fluorescent reporters in the absence of oxygen have been developed. Flavin mononucleotide-based (FMN) fluorescent proteins, engineered from the light, oxygen or voltage (LOV) controlled domains of the *B. subtilis* or *Pseudomonas putida* blue-light photoreceptors can be mentioned as a good example [17]. The FMN chromophore provides the LOV domain with an intrinsic green fluorescence when excited with UV/blue light [18]. These proteins were shown to fluoresce in the absence of oxygen, when produced in the facultative anaerobic bacterium *Rhodobacter capsulatus* [17], during hypoxia in the pathogen *Candida albicans* [19, 20] and also when fused to the FtsZ protein in *C. difficile* cells [18]. *C. difficile* FtsZ as well as the secreted protein FliC have been recently localized using the engineered phiLOV domain, more resistant to photobleaching [21]. All of the FMN proteins generated so far emit fluorescence at the same wavelength, which restricts multicolor imaging. Moreover, the wavelength of emission overlaps with the autofluorescence of the *C. difficile* cells ([22]; see below).

Other tools developed to allow fluorescence-based studies in the absence of oxygen consist on protein tags that can be site-specific labeled with chemical probes [23–25] or fluorescent non-natural amino acids [26]. Protein tags are fused to a protein or placed under the command of a promoter of interest, and can be covalently labeled with a small molecule, thereby combining the simplicity of fusion protein expression with the diversity of the molecular probes provided by chemistry. The tetracysteine-tag [27], the Halo-tag [28], and the SNAP-tag [23], are some of these tags. The SNAP-tag is a 20 kDa engineered form of the human repair protein O^6-alkylguanine-DNA alkyltransferase (hAGT) that covalently reacts with O^6-benzylguanine (BG) or O^6-benzyl-4-chloropyrimidine (CP) derivatives, in an irreversible manner [23, 29, 30] (Fig. 1a). Fluorescent BG substrates have a fluorophore conjugated to guanine via a benzyl linker. During the reaction with a substrate, a stable thioether bond is formed between the reactive cysteine of the SNAP-tag (Cys145) that leaves the fluorophore-modified benzyl group attached to the SNAP-tag, while guanine is released (Fig. 1a). SNAP-tag substrates derivatized with different fluorophores were developed [23]. The variety of fluorescent substrates presently commercially available allows detection of the SNAP-tag at emission wavelengths ranging from 437 to 670 nm (www.neb.com), but near-infrared substrates (emission maxima between 700 and 900 nm) for in vivo work have also been described [32]. BG substrates are inert to cells, therefore limiting unspecific labeling, and not toxic; moreover, they allow labeling of the SNAP-tag in any cellular compartment [33]. In addition to labeling with fluorescent probes, SNAP-tagged proteins can be modified with

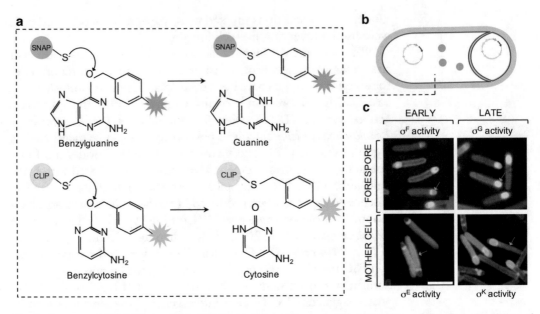

Fig. 1 Use of the SNAP/CLIP-tag in *C. difficile*. (**a**) Schematic representation of the mechanism of reaction of SNAP and CLIP with their substrates. SNAP-tag or CLIP-tag reacts with a fluorophore-modified benzylguanine (SNAP) or benzylcytosine (CLIP) substrate resulting in covalent labeling of the tag and the release of guanine or cytosine. (**b**) A multicopy plasmid carrying the *SNAP-tag* and/or the *CLIP-tag* under the control of the promoter(s) under study is introduced into *C. difficile* by conjugation from *E. coli*. A fluorescent substrate is then added that will label the SNAP (in the example) or CLIP tags. (**c**) Microscopy analysis of cell type-specific gene expression during sporulation of *C. difficile*. Sporulating cells expressing transcriptional *SNAP^Cd* fusions of genes under the control of the four cell type-specific RNA polymerase sigma factors that control sporulation (as indicated) were labeled with the SNAP-Cell TMR-Star substrate (*red*) and the membrane dye MTG (*green*) and imaged by fluorescence microscopy. The MTG labeling allows identification of the sporulation stage (EARLY, before engulfment of the forespore by the larger mother cell is completed; LATE, following engulfment completion). The merged images show the overlap between the signal in the *red* (TMR-Star) and *green* (MTG) channels. The single cell analysis reveals whether the promoters are active in the mother cell or the forespore, and the stage in morphogenesis in which transcription occurs (*see* also ref. 31). Scale bar: 1 μm

affinity ligands such as biotin, or other functional groups and used for pull-downs assays, protein purification, immobilization, protein microarray experiments, for crosslinking experiments to monitor protein-protein interactions inside living cells, among other applications [34–36].

All the applications described above highlight the flexibility of the SNAP-tag. For instance, labeling a SNAP-fusion protein at different time points with different fluorophores allows young and old copies of that same protein to be distinguished [37, 38]. This approach is an elegant alternative to the use of photo-activatable or photo-switchable autofluorescent proteins to track proteins over time. An important application is the measurement of protein half-life in living cells [39]. Additionally, fluorogenic substrates have been described; in these a chemical group attached to the leaving guanine quenches fluorescence from the fluorophore attached to the benzyl moiety [40]. Since the probes only become highly fluorescent upon reaction with (and labeling of) the SNAP-tag, the need for a washing step to eliminate unreacted fluorescent probes, or during sequential labeling is eliminated [40, 41]. Another class of BG substrates has been described in which a fluorophore is partially quenched by the guanine group [40]. However, reaction times of several hours are required to achieve a reasonable signal-to-noise ratio [40]. Recently, near-infrared, membrane permeable fluorogenic substrates for SNAP-tag and CLIP-tag labeling (Sir-SNAP and Sir-CLIP) based on a silicon-rhodamine fluorophore, have been reported [42]. These compounds are bright and photostable and can be used for imaging of cells and tissues, and for live super-resolution microscopy ([41]; www.neb.com). New methods have also been described to improve the properties of commonly used fluorophores [43]. Another recent, highly promising development is the use of a Split-SNAP system to monitor in time and space protein-protein interactions in vivo [44, 45].

Mutagenizing eight amino acids in the SNAP-tag generated the CLIP-tag, which irreversibly reacts with O^2-benzylcytosine (BC) derivatives [35]. Because the SNAP-tag shows high selectivity for BG over BC derivatives, the SNAP-tag and the CLIP-tag can be used for orthogonal labeling of different fusion proteins in the same cell [35] (Fig. 2). Importantly, the similarity of these two protein tags is an advantage when it is of interest to compare the properties of one fusion protein to another.

The SNAP-tag has been mainly used inside and on the surface of mammalian cells. Nevertheless, this technique has also been successfully applied to studies of gene expression and protein localization in yeast and in bacterial cells, including anaerobic bacteria [47–52]. Recently, we have extended the SNAP-tag technology to the strict anaerobe *C. difficile* [31, 53]. Quantitative qRT-PCR and RNAseq are currently the most used techniques for gene expression analysis in *C. difficile*, offering sensitivity, dynamic range, and reproducibility (e.g., [31, 53–58]). As a drawback, these and other lysate-based techniques give an average value for a population, and fail to capture heterogeneity in gene expression across the population. We have used promoter fusions for the SNAP-tag to the analysis of the gene regulatory network that controls spore development in *C. difficile* (Fig. 1b, c). Sporulation takes place in a sporangium partitioned into a larger mother cell and a smaller forespore, which will become the future spore. During the process, genes are expressed in a cell type-specific manner, at different times during the process, and in register with the course of morphogenesis. Sporulation is largely controlled by a cascade of RNA polymerase sigma factors, in the order σ^F, σ^E, σ^G, and σ^K [59–62]. σ^F and σ^E control early stages of development, during engulfment of the forespore by the mother cell, and are replaced following engulfment completion by σ^G and σ^K, respectively. Knowledge of whether genes are expressed in the

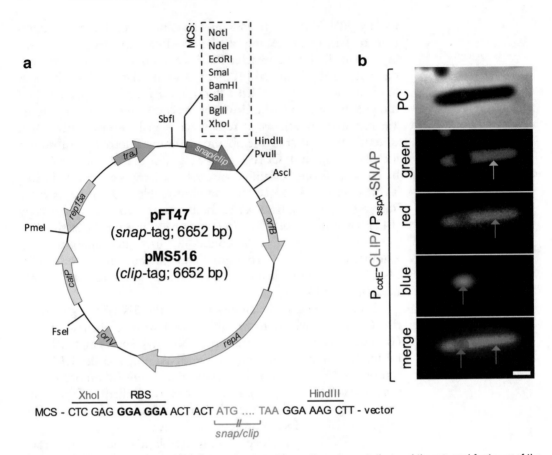

Fig. 2 SNAP/CLIP-tag vectors. (**a**) The figure shows a schematic representation and the general features of the pFT47 and pMS516 vectors. Unique restriction sites (Sbfl, Ascl, Fsel, Pmel) that allow replacement of functional blocks among plasmids of the pMTL80000 series [46] are indicated along the circular plasmid map. A detailed representation of the region between the XhoI and HindIII sites (in *blue*) is shown at the *bottom*. The *SNAP*^{Cd} or *CLIP*^{Cd} genes, preceded by an RBS, were inserted between the XhoI and HindIII sites within the multiple cloning site (MCS) of pMTL84121 (unique sites upstream of XhoI, that are part of the pMTL84121 MCS, are indicated), to yield pFT47 and pMS516, respectively. Both plasmids allow for the construction of transcriptional *SNAP*^{Cd} (pFT47; [31]) or *CLIP*^{Cd} (pMS516; this work) fusions. (**b**) Sporulating cells of *C. difficile* expressing a transcriptional fusion to a forespore-specific promoter (P_{sspA}-*SNAP*^{Cd}) and to a mother cell-specific promoter (P_{cotE}-*CLIP*^{Cd}) were labeled with the CLIP-Cell TMR-Star (*red*) and the SNAP-Cell 360 (*blue*) substrates and imaged by phase contrast (PC) and fluorescence microscopy. The image in the *green channel* shows the auto-fluorescence signal (*green arrow*). This signal is not normally seen in the forespore. The merged image shows the superimposition of the *red* and *blue signals*. Scale bar, 1 μm

mother cell or the forespore and how expression correlates with progress through morphogenesis is essential to understand gene function during spore development. An additional complication with studies of sporulation in *C. difficile* is that in vitro the process is highly asynchronous. Therefore, not only are epistatic relationships based on temporal sampling and lysate-based techniques to measure gene expression difficult to infer, but these techniques also do not provide direct information on the cell type-specificity of gene expression or on how gene expression parallels cellular morphogenesis. However, the combination of studies of gene expression at the single cell level using the SNAP reporter with qRT-PCR and the phenotypic characterization of mutants for regulatory genes proved to be a powerful combination [31, 53, 56]. The cell type-specificity dependencies for transcription and activity in relation to progress through morphology was established for the RNA polymerase sigma factors σ^F, σ^E, σ^G and σ^K [31, 53, 56] (Fig. 1c).

We obtained a synthetic version of the *SNAP26b* gene (New England Biolabs; [23]) codon usage-optimized for expression in *C. difficile* (DNA 2.0, Menlo Park, CA). The synthetic gene cassette, termed *SNAP^{Cd}*, includes a ribosome-binding site (RBS). The synthetic *SNAP^{Cd}* sequence was cloned into pMTL84121 [46] to produce pFT47, allowing transcriptional fusions of regulatory regions of interest to *SNAP^{Cd}* ([31]; Fig. 2a). A fast-labeling version of the SNAP-tag, called SNAP$_f$-tag was described, which differs from the original SNAP26m-tag commercially available from New England Biolabs in ten amino acid substitutions [40]. Plasmid pMS2015 is a pMTL84121 derivative, similar in structure to pFT47, bearing a *C. difficile* codon-usage optimized version of the *SNAP$_f$*-tag (Fig. 2a).

Of the changes introduced into SNAP26m to generate SNAP$_f$, a single amino acid substitution in the context of the CLIP-tag, was sufficient to produce a variant, termed CLIP$_f$, with increasing labeling rates with BC substrates relative to CLIP [40]. Having dual labeling experiments in mind, a synthetic version of the fast-labeling *CLIP$_f$* gene (New England Biolabs; [35]) was obtained with codon usage optimized for *C. difficile*, hereinafter termed *CLIP$_f$^{Cd}*. The *CLIP$_f$^{Cd}* cassette, including a RBS, was cloned into pMTL84121 to create pMS516 (Fig. 2). The complete sequences of the *SNAP^{Cd}*, *SNAP$_f$^{Cd}*, and *CLIP$_f$^{Cd}* synthetic gene cassettes are available for download (http://www.itqb.unl.pt/~aoh/SNAP_CLIP).

The toolbox of plasmids herein described and the following protocols represent the basis for the use of the SNAP/CLIP tags to dissect the cell biology of *C. difficile* at the single cell and population levels (*see* **Note 1**). Although this chapter focuses on the analysis of gene expression at the single cell level, we note that the SNAP^{Cd}-tag has also been used for studies of protein subcellular localization in *C. difficile* ([31, 45, 63]; and unpublished results).

2 Materials

2.1 Culture Media

Brain heart infusion (BHI) medium (Oxoid): Dissolve 37 g BHI in 1 l water; adjust the pH to 7.4 Autoclave (at 120 °C for 30 min).

Sporulation medium (SM): Prepared according to Wilson et al. [64]. Dissolve 90 g Bacto tryptone, 5 g Bacto peptone, 1 g $(NH_4)_2SO_4$ and 1.5 g Tris base in 1 l water; adjust the pH to 7.0. Autoclave (at 120 °C for 30 min).

TY medium: 30 g Bacto tryptone, 20 g yeast extract in 1 l water; adjust the pH to 7.4. Autoclave (at 120 °C for 30 min).

2.2 Fluorescent Dyes

DAPI (Molecular Probes/Invitrogen; *ref.* D1306, 10 mg): dissolve 10 mg of DAPI to in 2 ml of deionized water (ddH$_2$O) to prepare a stock solution (5 mg/ml). For long-term storage the stock solution can be aliquoted and stored at –20 °C. For short-term storage the solution can be kept at 2–6 °C, protected from light.

Mitotracker Green (MTG; Molecular Probes/Invitrogen, *ref.* M-7514; 20 × 54 mg): Dissolve the lyophilized product in DMSO to 1 mg/ml. Store at –20 °C protected from light.

FM4-64 (Molecular Probes/Invitrogen; *ref.* T-13320; 10 × 100 mg): Dissolve the lyophilized product in DMSO to 1 mg/ml. Store at –20 °C protected from light.

2.3 Solutions for Microscopy

Phosphate buffered saline (PBS, 10×): 27 mM KCl, 137 mM NaCl, 43 mM Na$_2$HPO$_4$, 14 mM KH$_2$PO$_4$. Dilute to 1× in sterile ddH$_2$O water before using.

Agarose: 1.7 % agarose (w/v) in ddH$_2$O. Boil and equilibrate at 50 °C before using.

NB: this solution is not intended for agarose gel electrophoresis.

2.4 SNAP and CLIP Substrates

SNAP and CLIP substrates: Dissolve the content of one vial of SNAP/CLIP-tag substrate (from New England Biolabs; see also below) in DMSO to give a solution of 1 mM SNAP/CLIP-tag substrate in DMSO. Mix by vortexing for 10 min until all the SNAP-tag or CLIP-tag substrate is dissolved. Store this stock solution in the dark at 4 °C, or at –20 °C for extended storage. From this stock solution prepare a working solution at 50 µM in DMSO; this solution can be used for 1–2 weeks, stored at 4 °C protected from light (*see* **Note 2**).

A selection of fluorescent substrates for SNAP/CLIP labeling is commercially available with different excitation/emission wavelengths and permeability properties (from *New England Biolabs* or *Cisbio Assays*) (*see* **Notes 3** and **4**). Cell-permeable substrates are suitable for intracellular labeling and are the ones to be used in studies of gene expression. Non-cell-permeable substrates are specific to label extracytoplasmic domains (e.g., as in fusion proteins expressed on the cell surface only), and therefore do not apply to the studies described in this chapter.

2.5 SDS-Polyacrylamide Gels and Electroblotting to Nitrocellulose Membranes

French Press buffer: 10 mM Tris–HCl pH 8.0, 10 mM MgCl$_2$, 0.5 mM EDTA, 0.2 mM NaCl, 1 mM DTT, 10 % glycerol, 1 mM PMSF.

4× *Lower Tris:* 1.5 M Tris-HCl, 0.4 % SDS, pH 8.8.
4× *Upper Tris:* 0.5 M Tris-HCl, 0.4 % SDS, pH 6.8.
Ammonium persulfate (APS): 10 % solution in water.
TEMED: Tetramethylethylenediamine from Sigma (*ref.* T9281).
SDS: 10 % solution in water.

Resolving gel: 1× Lower Tris, 15% acrylamide (from Bio-Rad *ref*. 161-0146), 0.1% SDS, 0.1% APS, 0.05% TEMED.

Stacking gel: 1× Upper Tris, 4.5% acrylamide, 0.1% SDS, 0.1% APS, 0.05% TEMED.

SDS-PAGE running buffer: 25 mM Tris-HCl, 192 mM glycine, 0.1% SDS.

SDS-PAGE loading buffer: 62.5 mM Tris-HCl pH 6.8, 2% SDS, 25% glycerol, 0.02% bromophenol blue.

Staining and fixation solution: 0.3% Coomassie R-250, 50% Ethanol, 10% Acetic Acid.

Destaining solution: 30% ethanol, 10% acetic acid.

Transfer buffer: 25 mM Tris-HCl, 192 mM glycine, 10% ethanol; store at 4 °C.

Blocking solution: 5% low fat powder milk, 1× PBS, 0.1% Tween 20.

Antibody solution: 0.5% low fat powder milk, 1× PBS, 0.1% Tween 20.

PBS-T: 1× PBS, 0.1% Tween 20.

Detection solution: 1 ml luminol enhancer regent, 1 ml stable peroxidase buffer (from Pierce, *ref*. 34080).

X-ray developer: 250 ml X-ray developer stock solution (Kodak, *ref*. 50709330) in 1 l water. Store protected from light.

X-ray fixer: 250 ml X-ray fixer stock solution (Kodak, *ref*. 5071071) in 1 l water. Store protected from light.

2.6 Antibodies

Anti-SNAP-tag Antibody: Polyclonal antibody from New England Biolabs (*ref*. P9310); recommended dilution 1:1000.

Anti-rabbit secondary antibody conjugated to horseradish peroxidase: Antibody from Sigma (*ref*. A9169); recommended dilution 1:10,000.

3 Methods

We routinely grow *C. difficile* anaerobically (5% H_2, 15% CO_2, 80% N_2) at 37 °C in BHI medium, SM medium or TY medium (above). Note that the medium employed depends on the nature of the experiment. For instance, we normally conduct studies of gene expression during sporulation in SM medium where we get better sporulation rates and more synchronized cell populations with respect to the stages of morphogenesis [31]; however, TY medium is a culturing condition in which high levels of toxin production are observed [65].

3.1 SNAP/CLIP Labeling for Microscopy

Validation of the SNAP[Cd]-tag as a transcriptional reporter in *C. difficile* involved showing specific labeling of *C. difficile cells* with a SNAP-tag substrate and the optimization of the SNAP-tag labeling times and of substrate concentration in order to obtain complete labeling of the SNAP-tag [31]. The SNAP[Cd]-tag was used to study the transcription of the genes coding for the four cell type-specific RNA polymerase sigma factors that govern sporulation, as well as their activity, by examining the expression of genes known to be under their control as also shown by qRT-PCR and RNAseq [31, 53, 56]. The early mother cell-specific sigma factor σ^E activates transcription from the *spoIIIA* promoter and expression of a $P_{spoIIIA}$-*SNAP^{Cd}* fusion is detected in the mother cell, as illustrated in Fig. 1 [31]; note the absence of labeling of the forespore with the red SNAP^{Cd} substrate SNAP-Cell TMR-Star. We have also tested the use of *CLIP$_f^{Cd}$* as a reporter in *C. difficile*. Expression of *CLIP$_f^{Cd}$* was placed under the control of an anhydrotetracycline-inducible promoter P*tet* (Fig. 2) [66]. We show that nearly complete labeling of the CLIP$_f^{Cd}$-tag with the CLIP-Cell TMR-Star substrate is achievable (Fig. 3), but we note that labeling of the CLIP-tag is slower than labeling of the SNAP-tag [67]. Furthermore, no background was detected for non-induced cells to which CLIP-Cell TMR-Star was added, or for induced cells to which CLIP-Cell TMR-Star was not added, by either fluorescence microscopy, FACS or the combination of fluoroimaging and immunoblotting with an anti-SNAP antibody (Fig. 3). Dual labeling experiments are possible, for example by introducing divergently oriented transcriptional SNAP^{Cd} or CLIP^{Cd} fusions in one of the plasmids represented in Fig. 2a. We tested this system using two promoters activated during sporulation. One, P_{cotE}, is utilized by σ^K-containing RNA polymerase in the mother cell while the other, P_{sspA}, is utilized by the σ^G form of RNA polymerase in the forespore [31, 53, 56]. As expected, a P_{cotE}-*CLIP^{Cd}* fusion resulted in labeling with CLIP-Cell TMR-Star in the mother cell, whereas expression of a P_{sspA}-*SNAP^{Cd}* fusion resulted in labeling with SNAP-Cell 360 in the forespore (Fig. 2b; however, *see* **Note 5**).

The following protocols describe labeling of either the SNAP^{Cd}- or CLIP^{Cd}-tags, using BG- or BC-based substrates, respectively, in *C. difficile*. Optimization of labeling times and substrate concentrations may be required depending on the promoter under study Fig. 4) or for other clostridial species (*see* **Note 6**).

1. Overnight cultures grown at 37 °C in BHI are used to inoculate SM, TY or BHI medium (at a dilution of 1:200).

2. Approximately 2 h before labeling prepare the number of required eppendorf tubes with 1 μl of the SNAP and/or CLIP substrate at 50 μM and introduce into the anaerobic chamber. Keep these tubes protected from light.

3. At the desired times following inoculation (start with 12 and 24 h samples in SM if sporulation is being studied) collect 200 μl of cells from the cultures to an eppendorf tube already containing 1 μl of the substrate at 50 μM (the final concentration of the SNAP/CLIP substrate will be of 250 nM, see above).

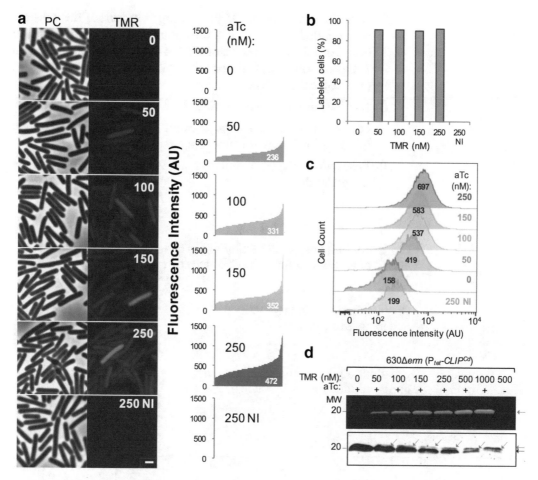

Fig. 3 CLIP labeling of *C. difficile* cells producing CLIP under the control of P$_{tet}$ with different concentrations of TMR-Star substrate. (**a**) Phase contrast (PC) and fluorescence microscopy analysis of cells labeled with the indicated concentrations (nM) of the CLIP substrate TMR-Star. The panels on the *right* show the relative levels of CLIP-TMR-Star fluorescence within individual cells (*n*=150), for the indicated substrate concentrations. Scale bar, 1 µm. (**b**) Percentage of cells showing a fluorescence signal above the background level for each TMR-Star concentration used for labeling. (**c**) Flow cytometry analysis of cells expressing P$_{tet}$-*CLIP^{Cd}* with different concentrations of substrate. The *y*-axis represents cell counts for each concentration; the *x*-axis shows fluorescence intensity in a logarithmic scale (in arbitrary units, AU). (**d**) Fuoroimager scanning (*top*) and immunoblot analysis (*bottom*) of extracts from cells expressing P$_{tet}$-*CLIP^{Cd}* were prepared immediately following labeling with increasing concentrations of TMR-Star (nM; as in **a**–**c**). *Black or red arrows* point to unlabeled or labeled CLIP, respectively. The position of molecular weight markers (in kDa) is shown on the *left side* of the panels

4. Incubate in the dark for 30 min at 37 °C (no shaking required).

5. Remove the samples from the anaerobic chamber (keep the samples protected from light at all times).

6. Centrifuge cells for 2 min, 6000×*g*. Resuspend in 1 ml of 1× PBS. Repeat this step three times for a total of four washes in 1× PBS.

7. If MTG, FM4-64 or DAPI staining is required, the cells are resuspended in 1 ml of PBS containing MTG (10 μg/ml; 0.5 μl of a 1 mg/ml solution), FM4-64 (10 μg/ml; 0.5 μl of a 1 mg/ml solution) [68], or DAPI (1 μl of a 5 mg/ml solution) (*see* **Notes** 7 and **8**).

8. Incubate at room temperature for 2 min, in the dark.

9. Spin again in a microfuge at room temperature (microfuge; $6000 \times g$ for 2 min at room temperature).

10. Resuspend the cell sediment in 10–20 μl of PBS. Do NOT let the pellet dry.

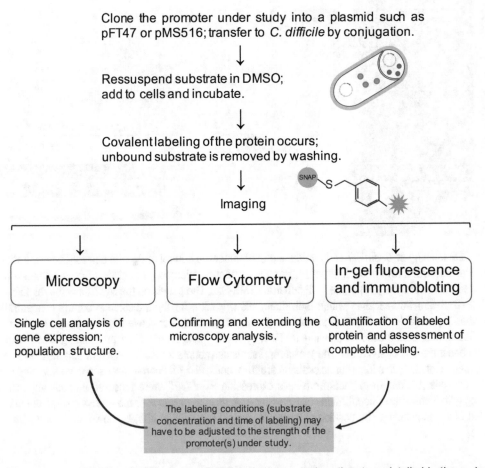

Fig. 4 Flowchart of SNAP[Cd] or CLIP[Cd] labeling. The flowchart summarizes the steps detailed in the protocols presented in this chapter. The microscopy analysis allows the quantification of the percentage of cells in a population in which a specific promoter is active, as well as the quantification of the fluorescence signal. It also allows the identification of the cell type in which the promoter is active (e.g., mother cell/forespore during sporulation; motile cells, etc.). The flow cytometry analysis expands this analysis to a larger population of cells. In gel-fluorescence and immunoblotting permits direct quantification of the SNAP[Cd]/CLIP[Cd] protein and to assess whether labeling was complete or incomplete

11. The cells are mounted on microscope glass slides covered with a thin film of 1.7% agarose. To prepare these slides, place 800 μl of agarose at the center of the glass slide and use a cover slip to spread the agarose solution along the slide. Let it stand at room temperature for about 5 min, so that the agarose polymerizes.

12. Then, apply 2 μl of the cell suspension (from **step 10**), and apply a cover slip.

13. We routinely observe the samples on a Leica DM6000B microscope equipped with a phase-contrast Uplan F1 100× objective plus an additional 1.6× optavar, a CCD Ixon^{EM} camera (Andor Technologies), and phase-contrast optics and standard filters for visualization of GFP or MTG (green), FM4-64 (red), or DAPI (blue).

14. Cells are sequentially imaged by phase contrast first, then in the channel for the SNAP/CLIP substrate, and finally in the channel for the membrane or DNA dye. This order is important to minimize photobleaching.

15. Typical exposure times are as follows (but may require optimization depending on the microscope configuration): 50–100 ms for DAPI; 100 ms for FM4-64; 50 ms for MTG; for the SNAP^{Cd}/CLIP^{Cd} the exposure time will depend on the strength of the promoter under study.

16. Images are acquired and analyzed using the *Metamorph* software suite version 5.8 (Universal Imaging). For quantification of the SNAP^{Cd} signal resulting from transcriptional fusions, define 6×6 pixel regions in the desired cell and calculate the average pixel intensity. This number is corrected by subtracting the average pixel intensity determined for the background; small fluctuations of fluorescence among different fields are corrected by normalizing to the average pixel intensity obtained for the intrinsic autofluorescence of *C. difficile* cells.

3.2 SNAP/CLIP Labeling for Flow Cytometry Analysis

Flow cytometric analysis to quantify the population expressing the reporter genes allows a statistical assessment of the expression level in individual cells within a heterogeneous population (*see* Subheading 1).

1. Grow the cells and label as indicated in Subheading 3.1 (**steps 1–6**).

2. Cells were diluted 1:10 in PBS and directly measured on an LSR Fortessa SORP flow cytometer (BD Biosciences, CA, USA) operating a solid-state laser at 561 nm. For each sample, at least 80,000 events are analyzed. Fluorescence is collected using a 590/20 nm bandpass filter. Data is acquired using FACSDiva v6.2 software and further analyzed using the FlowJo v10.0.8 software.

3.3 SNAP/CLIP-Tag Fusions Detected by In-Gel Fluorescence

The reaction of the substrates with the SNAP/CLIP-tag is irreversible and quantitative, and thus suited for the detection and quantification of labeled protein via in-gel fluorescence scanning following SDS-PAGE.

1. Grow the cells as indicated in Subheading 3.1.

2. Approximately 2 h before labeling prepare the number of required 15 ml tubes with 1.25 μl of the SNAP/CLIP substrate at 1 mM and introduce into the chamber. Protect these tubes from light.

3. At the desired times following inoculation (start with 12 and 24 h samples) collect 5 ml of cells from the cultures to a 15 ml tube already containing the substrate (**step 2**; the final concentration of the substrate will be 250 nM).

4. Incubate in the dark for 30 min at 37 °C.

5. Remove the samples from the anaerobic chamber (always keep the samples protected from light).

6. Collect the cells by centrifugation ($4000 \times g$ for 5 min at 4 °C) and wash twice with the same volume of PBS as the culture; if needed the pellet can be frozen at this point at –80 °C until further use.

7. Resuspend the pellet in 1 ml French Press buffer and lyse the cells using a French pressure cell at 18,000 lb/in.[2]

8. Determine the concentration of solubilized protein in the extract, using for example the Bio-Rad protein assay (*ref.* 500-0006). Apply 10–30 μg of total protein to a 15% SDS-PAGE gels.

9. To prepare the resolving gel mix 7.5 ml of Lower tris, 11.3 ml of acrylamide mixture, and 10.5 ml water. Add 300 μl of SDS, 300 μl of ammonium persulfate, and 15 μl of TEMED, and cast gel within a 7.25 cm × 10 cm × 1.5 mm gel cassette. Allow space for stacking the gel and gently overlay with isobutanol or water. Prepare the stacking gel by mixing 2.5 ml of Upper tris, 1.1 ml of acrylamide mixture, and 6 ml water. Add 100 μl of SDS, 100 μl of ammonium persulfate, and 10 μl of TEMED. Insert a 10-well gel comb immediately without introducing air bubbles.

10. For SDS-PAGE add loading buffer to the samples, mix, and then load onto gel (DO NOT boil or heat the samples).

11. Run the gel at 40 mA until the Bromophenol blue dye (present in the loading buffer) reaches the end of the gel (approximately 90 min).

12. After electrophoresis, scan the gel directly on a fluoroimager scanner at the appropriate wavelength depending on the substrate used (e.g., Fuji TLA-5100 fluoroimager). Signal intensities can be quantified using freely available software such as *ImageJ* (http://imagej.nih.gov/ij/).

13. The gels can then be fixed and stained with Coomassie R250. Transfer the gel to a plastic box and cover with staining and fixation solution for 30 min. Wash with running water and transfer to Destaining solution and incubate overnight with gentle shaking. Alternatively, the gels can be subject to immunoblot analysis.

3.4 Western Blot Analysis

After electrophoresis and scan the gel can be subject to immunoblot analysis using anti-SNAP-tag antibody. Fluorimager analysis combined with immunoblot experiments is important to assess complete labeling of the all the SNAP^{Cd}/CLIP^{Cd} produced. This analysis is only possible due to the slower migration of the SNAP^{Cd}/CLIP^{Cd} protein when covalently attached to the fluorescent substrate on SDS-PAGE gels. Only when all SNAP^{Cd}/CLIP^{Cd}-tag are labeled, can the SNAP^{Cd}/CLIP^{Cd} can be used as a quantitative reporter for analysis of gene expression at the single cell level in *C. difficile*. If labeling is incomplete, two bands will be detected by immunoblotting, and only the slower migrating species will be detected by fluoroimaging (Fig. 3). The efficiency of labeling can be estimated from the relative intensities of the labeled and unlabeled bands. Samples should be analyzed before and after labeling with the fluorescent substrate so that the position of unlabeled in the gel SNAP^{Cd}/CLIP^{Cd} can be identified by immunoblotting. A lane with a sample prepared from a strain that does not produce SNAP^{Cd}/CLIP^{Cd} should be included, as well as a lane in which the reporter is produced but was not labeled with the substrate. The labeling conditions (time and substrate concentration) my have to be adjusted to the specific promoter under study (Fig. 4).

1. After electrophoresis transfer the gel to a plastic box containing 30 ml of transfer buffer.

2. Soak sponges, blot paper and a 0.45 μm nitrocellulose membrane (Bio-Rad cat. 162-0090) in transfer buffer.

3. Assemble the blot apparatus as follows (be sure no air bubbles are trapped between the different layers): cathode (black) side down, sponge, blot paper, gel. Membrane, blot paper, sponge, anode (clear) side up.

4. Insert the assembled cassette into the electrode (black to black, clear to red). Also insert a magnetic bar and the cooling unit (ice block). Fill the Trans-Blot apparatus with cold Transfer buffer.

5. Operate on top of a magnetic stirrer, applying 100 V for 60 min.

6. Disassemble unit and transfer the membrane to a clean plastic box containing 50 ml of blocking solution (always keep the side containing the transferred proteins up!). Incubate for 60 min at room temperature with orbital agitation (200 rpm).

7. Remove blocking solution and add 10 ml of primary antibody solution (10 µl of anti-SNAP-tag polyclonal antibody diluted 1:1000 in antibody solution). Incubate overnight at 4 °C.

8. Discard the solution and wash the membrane twice for 10 min in PBS-T with agitation.

9. Add 10 ml of secondary antibody solution (1 µl anti-Rabbit IgG peroxidase conjugated antibody, 1:10,000 dilution). Incubate at room temperature for 30 min with gentle agitation.

10. Discard the solution and wash three times with PBS-T at room temperature with agitation. Do not discard the last wash solution so that the membrane does not dry before the detection solution is applied.

11. Prepare detection solution. Cut a piece of a polypropylene bag to the size of the interior of the exposure cassette.

12. Soak the membrane in detection solution for 5 min. Use gloves all the time and handle membrane with forceps!

13. Place the membrane inside the polypropylene bag, in the exposure cassette.

14. Place the Hyperfilm (Amersham Hyperfilm ECL from GE Healthcare) on top of the membrane. Do not reposition the film! Close the Hyperfilm box to prevent exposure to light.

15. Close the cassette and wait for 15–60 s. Use longer periods of exposure this result is not satisfactory.

16. While waiting, fill three containers with X-ray developer, X-ray fixer and water.

17. Take out the Hyperfilm from the cassette and place it in the X-ray developer for 2–3 min. Rinse in water and place it for 2–3 min in X-ray fixer. Rinse in water. Let it dry on air.

4   Notes

1. pFT47 and pMS516 are replicative plasmids in *C. difficile*, coding for chloramphenicol resistance, as it is the easiest way to transfer the reporter fusions to *C. difficile* [69]. The resulting plasmids are introduced into *C. difficile* by conjugation from *E. coli*. Problems with gene dosage effects may be resolved by introducing the transcriptional SNAP^{Cd}/CLIP^{Cd} fusion in single copy at the *pyrE* locus using Allele Coupled Exchange (ACE; [70]). This involves cloning of the transcriptional fusion on a *pyrE* integrational plasmid, and introduction of the resulting construct *in trans* at the *pyrE* locus [70]. Several fusions can be introduced at the *pyrE* locus by successive rounds of selection for PyrE$^+$ and counter-selection for PyrE$^-$ cells in the presence of uracil and fluoroorotic acid as described [70].

2. Always keep the SNAP/CLIP substrate solutions and the labeled samples protected from light.

3. Of the different SNAP/CLIP-tag cell-permeable substrates that we have tested the TMR-Star fluorophore, whose emission peak is the furthermost from the wavelength at which *C. difficile* cells show autofluorescence [21], was the one that produced the highest signal-to-noise ratio. However, recently described near-infrared substrates may perform even better ([41]; www.neb.com; see also above). The efficiency of labeling SNAP/CLIP-tag in vivo will depend on the cell permeability of each substrate, so different substrates may work better with specific strains.

4. The excitation/emission wavelengths for different $SNAP^{Cd}$/$CLIP^{Cd}$ substrates are available (www.neb.com; [71]); the choice of the BG- or BC-based substrate for $SNAP^{Cd}$/$CLIP^{Cd}$ labeling will dictate the filter used for fluorescence microscopy and the settings used for flow cytometry analysis.

5. The SNAP-tag shows a 1000-fold preference for a BG-fluorescein substrate over a BC-fluorescein substrate; conversely CLIP-tag shows a 100-fold preference for BC-fluorescein over BG-fluorescein [35]. However, we observed that production of $SNAP^{Cd}$ in the forespore from very strong promoters, results in some labeling with the CLIP-Cell TMR-Star substrate. The reason for this nonspecific labeling is presently unclear. It may be related to some feature of the forespore, because production of $SNAP^{Cd}$ in exponentially growing cells from the fully induced P_{tet} promoter did not result in labeling by CLIP-Cell TMR-Star. We note that a cleavable BC-S-S-Alexa 488 probe was reported to show some reactivity with SNAP fusion proteins [72]. To minimize the nonspecific labeling of the SNAP-tag by CLIP-tag substrates (if this is an issue in a specific experiment), cells could be labeled first with the BG substrate and then with the BC substrate. We observed no residual activity of the CLIP-tag for BG substrates. Also, if information on promoter strength is available, a precaution in dual labeling experiments may be to express $SNAP^{Cd}$ from the weaker of the two promoters under study.

6. We have not tested the SNAP/CLIP-tag in other *Clostridium* species. Our plasmids pFT47 and pMS516 contain the unique restriction sites (SbfI, AscI, FseI, PmeI) that allow replacement of functional blocks among plasmids of the pMTL80000 series (*see* Fig. 2) and therefore may be used to create combinations of components suitable for use in other *Clostridium* species [46].

7. Imaging the cells in the green channel can be useful, as the green autofluorescence provides a marker for the cytoplasm.

8. Even though *C. difficile* cells show strong green autofluorescence, the use of the MTG dye to label membranes is possible because labeling with the dye generates a signal far stronger than the autofluorescence (Fig. 1c). The use of an alternative membrane dye, such as FM4-64 that emits red fluorescence is possible depending on the SNAP^{Cd} or CLIP^{Cd} substrate being used.

Acknowledgements

The authors would like to thank Rui Gardner from the Gulbenkian Institute of Science, Flow Cytometry Facility, for technical support during the Flow Cytometry experiments and Ivan Côrrea (New England Biolabs) for critical reading of the manuscript and many helpful suggestions. This work was supported by the European Union Marie Sklodowska Curie Innovative Training Networks (ITN), "Clospore", (contract number 642068) to AOH and by programme IF (IF/00268/2013/CP1173/CT0006) from Fundação para a Ciência e a Tecnologia (FCT) to MS; CC is the recipient of a PhD fellowship (PD/BD/52212/2013) from the FCT; FP was the recipient of doctoral fellowship from the FCT (SFRH/BD/45459/08).

References

1. Dubnau D, Losick R (2006) Bistability in bacteria. Mol Microbiol 61(3):564–572. doi:10.1111/j.1365-2958.2006.05249.x

2. Veening JW, Smits WK, Kuipers OP (2008) Bistability, epigenetics, and bet-hedging in bacteria. Annu Rev Microbiol 62:193–210. doi:10.1146/annurev.micro.62.081307.163002

3. Eldar A, Elowitz MB (2010) Functional roles for noise in genetic circuits. Nature 467(7312):167–173. doi:10.1038/nature09326, PubMed PMID: 20829787, PubMed Central PMCID: PMC4100692

4. Stewart MK, Cookson BT (2012) Non-genetic diversity shapes infectious capacity and host resistance. Trends Microbiol 20(10):461–466. doi:10.1016/j.tim.2012.07.003, PubMed PMID: 22889945, PubMed Central PMCID: PMC3704078

5. Kearns DB, Losick R (2005) Cell population heterogeneity during growth of *Bacillus subtilis*. Genes Dev 19(24):3083–3094. doi:10.1101/gad.1373905, PubMed PMID: 16357223, PubMed Central PMCID: PMC1315410

6. Cairns LS, Hobley L, Stanley-Wall NR (2014) Biofilm formation by *Bacillus subtilis*: new insights into regulatory strategies and assembly mechanisms. Mol Microbiol 93(4):587–598. doi:10.1111/mmi.12697, PubMed PMID: 24988880, PubMed Central PMCID: PMC4238804

7. Vlamakis H, Chai Y, Beauregard P, Losick R, Kolter R (2013) Sticking together: building a biofilm the *Bacillus subtilis* way. Nat Rev Microbiol 11(3):157–168. doi:10.1038/nrmicro2960, PubMed PMID: 23353768, PubMed Central PMCID: PMC3936787

8. Chastanet A, Losick R (2011) Just-in-time control of SpoOA synthesis in *Bacillus subtilis* by multiple regulatory mechanisms. J Bacteriol 193(22):6366–6374. doi:10.1128/JB.06057-11, PubMed PMID: 21949067, PubMed Central PMCID: PMC3209201

9. Maamar H, Raj A, Dubnau D (2007) Noise in gene expression determines cell fate in *Bacillus subtilis*. Science 317(5837):526–529. doi:10.1126/science.1140818, PubMed PMID: 17569828, PubMed Central PMCID: PMC3828679

10. Eldar A, Chary VK, Xenopoulos P, Fontes ME, Loson OC, Dworkin J et al (2009) Partial penetrance facilitates developmental evolution in bacteria. Nature 460(7254):510–514. doi:10.1038/nature08150, PubMed PMID: 19578359, PubMed Central PMCID: PMC2716064

11. Allison KR, Brynildsen MP, Collins JJ (2011) Heterogeneous bacterial persisters and engineering approaches to eliminate them. Curr Opin Microbiol 14(5):593–598. doi:10.1016/j.mib.2011.09.002, PubMed PMID: 21937262, PubMed Central PMCID: PMC3196368

12. Diard M, Garcia V, Maier L, Remus-Emsermann MN, Regoes RR, Ackermann M et al (2013) Stabilization of cooperative virulence by the expression of an avirulent phenotype. Nature 494(7437):353–356. doi:10.1038/nature11913

13. Reid BG, Flynn GC (1997) Chromophore formation in green fluorescent protein. Biochemistry 36(22):6786–6791. doi:10.1021/bi970281w

14. Ransom EM, Ellermeier CD, Weiss DS (2015) Use of mCherry Red fluorescent protein for studies of protein localization and gene expression in *Clostridium difficile*. Appl Environ Microbiol 81(5):1652–1660. doi:10.1128/AEM.03446-14, PubMed PMID: 25527559, PubMed Central PMCID: PMC4325159

15. Ransom EM, Williams KB, Weiss DS, Ellermeier CD (2014) Identification and characterization of a gene cluster required for proper rod shape, cell division, and pathogenesis in *Clostridium difficile*. J Bacteriol 196(12):2290–2300. doi:10.1128/JB.00038-14, PubMed PMID: 24727226, PubMed Central PMCID: PMC4054185

16. Pizarro-Guajardo M, Olguin-Araneda V, Barra-Carrasco J, Brito-Silva C, Sarker MR, Paredes-Sabja D (2014) Characterization of the collagen-like exosporium protein, BclA1, of *Clostridium difficile* spores. Anaerobe 25:18–30. doi:10.1016/j.anaerobe.2013.11.003

17. Drepper T, Eggert T, Circolone F, Heck A, Krauss U, Guterl JK et al (2007) Reporter proteins for in vivo fluorescence without oxygen. Nat Biotechnol 25(4):443–445. doi:10.1038/nbt1293

18. Buckley AM, Petersen J, Roe AJ, Douce GR, Christie JM (2015) LOV-based reporters for fluorescence imaging. Curr Opin Chem Biol 27:39–45. doi:10.1016/j.cbpa.2015.05.011

19. Ernst JF, Tielker D (2009) Responses to hypoxia in fungal pathogens. Cell Microbiol 11(2):183–190. doi:10.1111/j.1462-5822.2008.01259.x

20. Tielker D, Eichhof I, Jaeger KE, Ernst JF (2009) Flavin mononucleotide-based fluorescent protein as an oxygen-independent reporter in *Candida albicans* and *Saccharomyces cerevisiae*. Eukaryot Cell 8(6):913–915. doi:10.1128/EC.00394-08, PubMed PMID:

19377038, PubMed Central PMCID: PMC2698303

21. Buckley AM, Jukes C, Candlish D, Irvine JJ, Spencer J, Fagan RP, Roe AJ, Christie JM, Fairweather NF, Douce GR (2016) Lighting up clostridium difficile: reporting gene expression using fluorescent LOV domains. Scientific Rep 6:23463. doi:10.1038/srep23463

22. George G, Richards RJ (1979) Preliminary studies on the isolation, separation and identification of pulmonary-lavage proteins from the rabbit [proceedings]. Biochem Soc Trans 7(6):1285–1287, Epub 1979/12/01

23. Keppler A, Gendreizig S, Gronemeyer T, Pick H, Vogel H, Johnsson K (2003) A general method for the covalent labeling of fusion proteins with small molecules in vivo. Nat Biotechnol 21(1):86–89. doi:10.1038/nbt765

24. Johnsson N, Johnsson K (2007) Chemical tools for biomolecular imaging. ACS Chem Biol 2(1):31–38. doi:10.1021/cb6003977

25. Hinner MJ, Johnsson K (2010) How to obtain labeled proteins and what to do with them. Curr Opin Biotechnol 21(6):766–776. doi:10.1016/j.copbio.2010.09.011

26. Liu CC, Schultz PG (2010) Adding new chemistries to the genetic code. Annu Rev Biochem 79:413–444. doi:10.1146/annurev.biochem.052308.105824

27. Hoffmann C, Gaietta G, Zurn A, Adams SR, Terrillon S, Ellisman MH et al (2010) Fluorescent labeling of tetracysteine-tagged proteins in intact cells. Nat Protoc 5(10):1666–1677. doi:10.1038/nprot.2010.129, PubMed PMID: 20885379, PubMed Central PMCID: PMC3086663

28. Los GV, Encell LP, McDougall MG, Hartzell DD, Karassina N, Zimprich C et al (2008) HaloTag: a novel protein labeling technology for cell imaging and protein analysis. ACS Chem Biol 3(6):373–382. doi:10.1021/cb800025k

29. Keppler A, Kindermann M, Gendreizig S, Pick H, Vogel H, Johnsson K (2004) Labeling of fusion proteins of O⁶-alkylguanine-DNA alkyltransferase with small molecules in vivo and in vitro. Methods 32(4):437–444. doi:10.1016/j.ymeth.2003.10.007

30. Gronemeyer T, Chidley C, Juillerat A, Heinis C, Johnsson K (2006) Directed evolution of O⁶-alkylguanine-DNA alkyltransferase for applications in protein labeling. Protein Eng Des Sel 19(7):309–316. doi:10.1093/protein/gzl014

31. Pereira FC, Saujet L, Tome AR, Serrano M, Monot M, Couture-Tosi E et al (2013) The

spore differentiation pathway in the enteric pathogen *Clostridium difficile*. PLoS Genet 9(10):e1003782. doi:10.1371/journal.pgen.1003782. Epub 2013/10/08. PGENETICS-D-13-00285 [pii]. PubMed PMID: 24098139; PubMed Central PMCID: PMC3789829

32. Gong H, Kovar JL, Baker B, Zhang A, Cheung L, Draney DR et al (2012) Near-infrared fluorescence imaging of mammalian cells and xenograft tumors with SNAP-tag. PLoS One 7(3):e34003. doi:10.1371/journal.pone.0034003, PubMed PMID: 22479502, PubMed Central PMCID: PMC3316518

33. Keppler A, Pick H, Arrivoli C, Vogel H, Johnsson K (2004) Labeling of fusion proteins with synthetic fluorophores in live cells. Proc Natl Acad Sci U S A 101(27):9955–9959. doi:10.1073/pnas.0401923101, PubMed PMID: 15226507, PubMed Central PMCID: PMC454197

34. Lemercier G, Gendreizig S, Kindermann M, Johnsson K (2007) Inducing and sensing protein–protein interactions in living cells by selective cross-linking. Angew Chem Int Ed Engl 46(23):4281–4284. doi:10.1002/anie.200700408

35. Gautier A, Juillerat A, Heinis C, Correa IR Jr, Kindermann M, Beaufils F et al (2008) An engineered protein tag for multiprotein labeling in living cells. Chem Biol 15(2):128–136. doi:10.1016/j.chembiol.2008.01.007

36. Kindermann M, Sielaff I, Johnsson K (2004) Synthesis and characterization of bifunctional probes for the specific labeling of fusion proteins. Bioorg Med Chem Lett 14(11):2725–2728. doi:10.1016/j.bmcl.2004.03.078

37. Vivero-Pol L, George N, Krumm H, Johnsson K, Johnsson N (2005) Multicolor imaging of cell surface proteins. J Am Chem Soc 127(37):12770–12771. doi:10.1021/ja0533850

38. Jansen LE, Black BE, Foltz DR, Cleveland DW (2007) Propagation of centromeric chromatin requires exit from mitosis. J Cell Biol 176(6):795–805. doi:10.1083/jcb.200701066, PubMed PMID: 17339380, PubMed Central PMCID: PMC2064054

39. Bojkowska K, Santoni de Sio F, Barde I, Offner S, Verp S, Heinis C et al (2011) Measuring in vivo protein half-life. Chem Biol 18(6):805–815. doi:10.1016/j.chembiol.2011.03.014

40. Sun X, Zhang A, Baker B, Sun L, Howard A, Buswell J et al (2011) Development of SNAP-tag fluorogenic probes for wash-free fluorescence imaging. Chembiochem 12(14):2217–2226. doi:10.1002/cbic.201100173, PubMed PMID:

21793150, PubMed Central PMCID: PMC3213346

41. Stohr K, Siegberg D, Ehrhard T, Lymperopoulos K, Oz S, Schulmeister S et al (2010) Quenched substrates for live-cell labeling of SNAP-tagged fusion proteins with improved fluorescent background. Anal Chem 82(19):8186–8193. doi:10.1021/ac101521y

42. Lukinavicius G, Umezawa K, Olivier N, Honigmann A, Yang G, Plass T et al (2013) A near-infrared fluorophore for live-cell super-resolution microscopy of cellular proteins. Nat Chem 5(2):132–139. doi:10.1038/nchem.1546

43. Grimm JB, English BP, Chen J, Slaughter JP, Zhang Z, Revyakin A et al (2015) A general method to improve fluorophores for live-cell and single-molecule microscopy. Nat Methods 12(3):244–250. doi:10.1038/nmeth.3256, PubMed PMID: 25599551; PubMed Central PMCID: PMC4344395

44. Mie M, Naoki T, Uchida K, Kobatake E (2012) Development of a split SNAP-tag protein complementation assay for visualization of protein-protein interactions in living cells. Analyst 137(20):4760–4765. doi:10.1039/c2an35762c

45. Serrano M, Crawshaw AD, Dembek M, Monteiro JM, Pereira FC, de Pinho MG et al (2016) The SpoIIQ-SpoIIIAH complex of Clostridium difficile controls forespore engulfment and late stages of gene expression and spore morphogenesis. Mol Microbiol 100(1):204–228. doi:10.1111/mmi.13311

46. Heap JT, Pennington OJ, Cartman ST, Minton NP (2009) A modular system for Clostridium shuttle plasmids. J Microbiol Methods 78(1):79–85. doi:10.1016/j.mimet.2009.05.004

47. Donovan C, Bramkamp M (2009) Characterization and subcellular localization of a bacterial flotillin homologue. Microbiology 155(Pt 6):1786–1799. doi:10.1099/mic.0.025312-0

48. Regoes A, Hehl AB (2005) SNAP-tag mediated live cell labeling as an alternative to GFP in anaerobic organisms. Biotechniques 39(6):809–810, 12

49. Martincova E, Voleman L, Najdrova V, De Napoli M, Eshar S, Gualdron M et al (2012) Live imaging of mitosomes and hydrogenosomes by HaloTag technology. PLoS One 7(4):e36314. doi:10.1371/journal.pone.0036314, PubMed PMID: 22558433, PubMed Central PMCID: PMC3338651

50. Nicolle O, Rouillon A, Guyodo H, Tamanai-Shacoori Z, Chandad F, Meuric V et al (2010) Development of SNAP-tag-mediated live cell

labeling as an alternative to GFP in *Porphyromonas gingivalis*. FEMS Immunol Med Microbiol 59(3):357–363. doi:10.1111/j.1574-695X.2010.00681.x

51. Stagge F, Mitronova GY, Belov VN, Wurm CA, Jakobs S (2013) SNAP-, CLIP- and Halo-tag labelling of budding yeast cells. PLoS One 8(10):e78745. doi:10.1371/journal.pone.0078745, PubMed PMID: 24205303, PubMed Central PMCID: PMC3808294

52. Sateriale A, Roy NH, Huston CD (2013) SNAP-tag technology optimized for use in *Entamoeba histolytica*. PLoS One 8(12):e83997. doi:10.1371/journal.pone.0083997, PubMed PMID: 24391864, PubMed Central PMCID: PMC3877135

53. Saujet L, Pereira FC, Serrano M, Soutourina O, Monot M, Shelyakin PV et al (2013) Genome-wide analysis of cell type-specific gene expression during spore formation in Clostridium difficile. PLoS Genet 9(10): e1003756

54. Soutourina OA, Monot M, Boudry P, Saujet L, Pichon C, Sismeiro O et al (2013) Genome-wide identification of regulatory RNAs in the human pathogen Clostridium difficile. PLoS Genet 9(5):e1003493. doi:10.1371/journal.pgen.1003493, PubMed PMID: 23675309, PubMed Central PMCID: PMC3649979

55. Janoir C, Deneve C, Bouttier S, Barbut F, Hoys S, Caleechum L et al (2013) Adaptive strategies and pathogenesis of Clostridium difficile from in vivo transcriptomics. Infect Immun 81(10):3757–3769. doi:10.1128/IAI.00515-13, PubMed PMID: 23897605, PubMed Central PMCID: PMC3811758

56. Fimlaid KA, Bond JP, Schutz KC, Putnam EE, Leung JM, Lawley TD et al (2013) Global analysis of the sporulation pathway of *Clostridium difficile*. PLoS Genet 9(8):e1003660. doi:10.1371/journal.pgen.1003660, PubMed PMID: 23950727, PubMed Central PMCID: PMC3738446

57. Saujet L, Monot M, Dupuy B, Soutourina O, Martin-Verstraete I (2011) The key sigma factor of transition phase, SigH, controls sporulation, metabolism, and virulence factor expression in *Clostridium difficile*. J Bacteriol 193(13):3186–3196. doi:10.1128/JB.00272-11, PubMed PMID: 21572003, PubMed Central PMCID: PMC3133256

58. El Meouche I, Peltier J, Monot M, Soutourina O, Pestel-Caron M, Dupuy B et al (2013) Characterization of the SigD regulon of *C. difficile* and its positive control of toxin production through the regulation of *tcdR*. PLoS One 8(12):e83748. doi:10.1371/journal.pone.0083748, PubMed PMID: 24358307, PubMed Central PMCID: PMC3865298

59. Saujet L, Pereira FC, Henriques AO, Martin-Verstraete I (2014) The regulatory network controlling spore formation in *Clostridium difficile*. FEMS Microbiol Lett 358(1):1–10. doi:10.1111/1574-6968.12540

60. Hilbert DW, Piggot PJ (2004) Compartmentalization of gene expression during *Bacillus subtilis* spore formation. Microbiol Mol Biol Rev 68(2):234–262. doi:10.1128/MMBR.68.2.234-262.2004, PubMed PMID: 15187183, PubMed Central PMCID: PMC419919

61. Fimlaid KA, Shen A (2015) Diverse mechanisms regulate sporulation sigma factor activity in the Firmicutes. Curr Opin Microbiol 24:88–95. doi:10.1016/j.mib.2015.01.006

62. Al-Hinai MA, Jones SW, Papoutsakis ET (2015) The Clostridium sporulation programs: diversity and preservation of endospore differentiation. Microbiol Mol Biol Rev 79(1):19–37. doi:10.1128/MMBR.00025-14

63. Fimlaid KA, Jensen O, Donnelly ML, Siegrist MS, Shen A (2015) Regulation of *Clostridium difficile* spore formation by the SpoIIQ and SpoIIIA proteins. PLoS Genet 11(10):e1005562. doi:10.1371/journal.pgen.1005562, PubMed PMID: 26465937, PubMed Central PMCID: PMC4605598

64. Wilson KH, Kennedy MJ, Fekety FR (1982) Use of sodium taurocholate to enhance spore recovery on a medium selective for *Clostridium difficile*. J Clin Microbiol 15(3):443–446, PubMed PMID: 7076817, PubMed Central PMCID: PMC272115

65. Garnier T, Cole ST (1986) Characterization of a bacteriocinogenic plasmid from Clostridium perfringens and molecular genetic analysis of the bacteriocin-encoding gene. J Bacteriol 168(3):1189–1196, PubMed PMID: 2877971, PubMed Central PMCID: PMC213621

66. Fagan RP, Fairweather NF (2011) *Clostridium difficile* has two parallel and essential Sec secretion systems. J Biol Chem 286(31):27483–27493. doi:10.1074/jbc.M111.263889, PubMed PMID: 21659510, PubMed Central PMCID: PMC3149341

67. Hanek A, Corrêa IR Jr (2011) Chemical modification of proteins in living cells, Methods in protein chemistry. DE GRUYTER, Berlin, pp 197–218

68. Pogliano J, Osborne N, Sharp MD, Abanes-De Mello A, Perez A, Sun YL et al (1999) A vital stain for studying membrane dynamics in bacteria: a novel mechanism controlling septation during *Bacillus subtilis* sporulation. Mol Microbiol 31(4):1149–1159, PubMed PMID: 10096082, PubMed Central PMCID: PMC2885269

69. Heap JT, Kuehne SA, Ehsaan M, Cartman ST, Cooksley CM, Scott JC et al (2010) The ClosTron: mutagenesis in *Clostridium* refined and streamlined. J Microbiol Methods 80(1):49–55. doi:10.1016/j.mimet.2009.10.018, Epub 2009/11/07. S0167-7012(09)00350-9 [pii]

70. Ng YK, Ehsaan M, Philip S, Collery MM, Janoir C, Collignon A et al (2013) Expanding the repertoire of gene tools for precise manipulation of the *Clostridium difficile* genome: allelic exchange using *pyrE* alleles. PLoS One 8(2):e56051. doi:10.1371/journal.pone.0056051, PubMed PMID: 23405251, PubMed Central PMCID: PMC3566075

71. Lukinavicius G, Reymond L, Johnsson K (2015) Fluorescent labeling of SNAP-tagged proteins in cells. Methods Mol Biol 1266:107–118. doi:10.1007/978-1-4939-2272-7_7

72. Cole NB (2013) Site-specific protein labeling with SNAP-tags. Curr Protoc Protein Sci. 73:Unit 30 1. doi:10.1002/0471140864.ps3001s73. PubMed PMID: 24510614; PubMed Central PMCID: PMC3920298

Chapter 7

Clostridium difficile Adhesins

Séverine Péchiné, Cécile Denève-Larrazet, and Anne Collignon

Abstract

Clostridium difficile is responsible for a large spectrum of intestinal diseases ranging from mild diarrhea to fatal colitis depending on the one hand on the strain virulence and on the other on the host. The pathogenesis of *C. difficile* infection could be seen as a three-step process that takes place after disruption of the digestive microbiota by antibiotics: (1) contamination by and germination of spores; (2) multiplication of vegetative cells in the colonic niche using colonization factors; (3) production of the two toxins TcdA and TcdB and for some strains an additional toxin, the binary toxin CDT. Several studies have been performed to characterize the bacterial factors involved in the colonization step and particularly adhesins.

Here, we describe first the methods used to study *C. difficile* adherence in vitro to epithelial cells and in vivo in animal model intestinal tract, and second the methods used to demonstrate the adhesive properties of surface proteins using Cwp66, GroEL, and FbpA as examples.

Key words *Clostridium difficile*, Adherence, Surface proteins, Adhesins, Intestinal colonization

1 Introduction

Clostridium difficile is a gram-positive anaerobic spore-forming enteropathogen responsible for post-antibiotic diarrhea and pseudomembranous colitis. The pathophysiology of *C. difficile* infections (CDI) could be seen as a three-step process: (1) germination of spores, the infectious form causing CDI; (2) multiplication of *C. difficile* vegetative cells and colonization in the colonic niche thanks to colonization factors; (3) production of the two toxins TcdA and TcdB and for some strains an additional toxin, the binary toxin CDT [1, 2].

Colonization is clearly an essential process in CDI, and *C. difficile* produces many surface proteins, which may contribute to colonization [1, 3]. Many studies have described the in vitro adherence of *C. difficile* to epithelial cells. *C. difficile* has been shown to adhere to human colonic enterocyte-like Caco-2 cells and mucus-secreting HT29 cells [4]. Adherence can be visualized by microscopy at the surface of Caco-2 cells, but also at the periphery of the cells. Cerquetti et al., observed a dramatic increase of adherent

Adam P. Roberts and Peter Mullany (eds.), *Clostridium difficile: Methods and Protocols*, Methods in Molecular Biology, vol. 1476,
DOI 10.1007/978-1-4939-6361-4_7, © Springer Science+Business Media New York 2016

bacteria after treatment of confluent monolayers of Caco-2 cells with EGTA, which disrupts the intercellular junctions and makes the basolateral cell surface accessible to bacteria [5]. *C. difficile* can also adhere to other epithelial cell lines such as Hela cells and Vero cells and adherence is mediated by proteinaceous components recognizing specific receptors [6, 7]. Adherence of *C. difficile* to Vero cells under anaerobic conditions is growth phase dependent, reaching a maximum in stationary phase, and is increased by a high sodium concentration in the growth medium, an acidic pH and iron starvation. In addition, the adherence is increased by heat shock in aerobiosis [8]. In animal models, *C. difficile* appears to be associated with the intestinal mucosa [9, 10].

Several surface proteins have been identified in *C. difficile*. The *C. difficile* cell wall proteins (CWPs) are encoded by genes located on a cluster of 37 kb carrying several paralogs, which display the same organization in two domains, one anchoring domain containing three copies of the cell wall binding domain (Pfam 04122), and a second domain with variable properties [11, 12]. Among these CWPs, the two components of the S-layer (LMW-SLP and HMW-SLP) [13, 14] and the Cwp66 protein [7, 8, 15] have been shown to have adhesin properties and could be implicated as colonization factors.

Other surface proteins with adhesin properties are likely involved in the colonization process: the fibronectin binding protein FbpA [16, 17], the heat shock protein GroEL [18, 19], the flagellar proteins FliC (flagellin) and FliD (flagellar cap protein) [20, 21], the collagen binding protein CbpA [22], and the lipoprotein CD0873 [23] recently characterized.

This chapter describes first the methods used to study *C. difficile* adherence in vitro to epithelial cells and in vivo in animal model intestinal tract, second the methods used to demonstrate the adhesive properties of surface proteins using Cwp66, GroEL, and Fbp68 as examples.

The localization of these proteins was studied by cell fractionation and immunoblot using specific antibodies [24] and by immunoelectron microscopy as well. Their role in adherence to epithelial cells was demonstrated by adherence inhibition assays of *C. difficile* to cells with specific antibodies and/or recombinant proteins. For FbpA, adherence properties were compared between the mutant and the wild type strains. Far-immuno dot-blotting demonstrated that FbpA binds fibronectin, fibrinogen, and also vitronectin. Indirect immunofluorescence assay and ELISA demonstrated that *C. difficile* binds both soluble and immobilized fibronectin.

2 Materials

2.1 Bacterial Culture Media

1. Brain Heart Infusion (BHI) broth or agar (Difco) 0.2% (w/v) yeast extract, pH 7.0.

2. Tryptone–Glucose–Yeast (TGY) infusion broth (Difco).

3. Columbia agar, 5 % defibrinated horse blood.

4. Selective supplement: 25 mg/L D-cycloserine, and 8 mg/L cefoxitin (Oxoid supplement).

2.2 In Vitro Adhesion and Inhibition Adhesion Assays

1. Cell cultures: Caco-2 TC7 and Vero cells.

2. Dulbecco's Modified Eagle Medium (DMEM) (25 mM glucose) (Invitrogen/Gibco) supplemented with heat-inactivated (30 min, 56 °C) fetal bovine serum (FBS) (Invitrogen/Gibco), 1 % L-glutamine 200 mM, and 1 % non essential amino acids (Invitrogen/Gibco).

3. Trypsin 0.025 % (Invitrogen/Gibco).

4. Dulbecco's phosphate buffer saline (Invitrogen/Gibco).

5. PBS: 10 mM phosphate buffer—150 mM NaCl pH 7.2.

6. Tissue-culture plates (6 or 24 wells), flasks (Falcon or TPP).

7. TNT + 5 % skimmed milk.

8. Specific antibodies.

9. Recombinant proteins.

2.3 In Vivo Adhesion Assay

1. 6–12 Weeks germfree mice (C3H/HeN or BALB/c Charles River laboratories, or CNRS Orléans, France).

2. Germfree and gnotobiotic rodent facilities. Sterile isolators and transfer devices (plastic isolator, DPTE transfer device, La Calhène, France).

3. Diet: sterilized by irradiation, vacuum packed, RO3-40 (SAFE, France).

4. Autoclave and sterilization apparatus (Sterilizator FPS92A, JCE Biotechnology, France).

5. Sterilizing liquid agent: Soproper (Peracetic acid 3.5 % and hydrogen peroxyde) (Air Liquide Seppic, France).

2.4 Immunoelectron Microscopy

1. Formvar coated nickel grids (Sigma).

2. Specific antibodies (appropriate dilution in PBS with 1 % BSA).

3. 10 nm diameter colloidal gold particle-labeled Protein-A (Sigma).

4. 3 % glutaraldehyde.

5. 0.5 % phosphotungstic acid.

6. Transmission electron microscope (TEM).

2.5 Far-Immuno Dot Blotting

1. Fibronectin (Roche), fibrinogen (Sigma), collagen type VI (Sigma), vitronectin (Sigma), and BSA as negative control (Sigma).

2. Nitrocellulose or PVDF membrane (Millipore).

3. TNT: 10 mM Tris–HCl (pH 8), 150 mM NaCl, Tween 20 0.05 %.

4. Blocking buffer: 5 % skimmed milk in TNT.

5. Rabbit anti-rFbpA antibody.

6. Goat anti-rabbit IgG-alkaline phosphatase conjugate (Sigma).

7. NBT-BCIP (Sigma).

2.6 Indirect Immunofluorescence

1. Glass microscope slides.

2. Anti-fibronectin rabbit antibody (Sigma).

3. Fluorescein isothiocyanate (FITC)-conjugated mouse anti-rabbit IgG antibody (Immunotech).

4. Epifluorescence microscope (Leitz Aristoplan coupled to an Image Analyzer Visiolab 1000 Biocom).

2.7 Enzyme-Linked Immunosorbent Assay (ELISA)

1. Human fibronectin (Sigma).

2. ELISA coating buffer: 0.05 M sodium carbonate buffer pH 9.5.

3. Washing buffer: 1× PBS supplemented with 0.05 % tween (PBS-T) (Sigma).

4. Blocking buffer: 1 % BSA in PBS pH 7.2.

5. Primary rabbit antibodies to *C. difficile* or proteins of interest.

6. Detection labeled antibodies: alkaline phosphatase-labeled goat anti-rabbit IgG (Sigma).

7. Substrate: *p*-nitrophenyl phosphate (Sigma).

8. Stop solution: 3 N NaOH.

9. 96-well plates (Nunc or TPP).

10. ELISA plate reader (Model Anthos HTII, Anthos Labtec Instruments).

2.8 C. difficile Strains

The strains were grown under anaerobic conditions at 37 °C in TGY or BHI broth (Difco), and Colombia agar containing L-cysteine HCl (0.05 %) supplemented with horse blood (5 %).

C. difficile selective supplement can be added to make the medium selective: 25 mg/L D-cycloserine, and 8 mg/L cefoxitin (supplement Oxoid).

3 Methods

3.1 In Vitro Adhesion and Inhibition Adhesion Assays

3.1.1 Cell Lines: Caco-2 TC7, Vero Cells

1. Cell lines were routinely grown at 37 °C in 5 % (for Vero cells) or 10 % CO_2 (for Caco-2 TC7 cells) in DMEM (25 mM glucose) supplemented with heat-inactivated (30 min 56 °C) FBS (15 % (v/v) for Caco-2 TC7 and 10 % for Vero cells), 1 % glutamine, and 1 % nonessential amino acids (only for Caco-2 TC7 cells). The culture medium is daily changed (*see* **Notes 1** and **2**).

2. When cell monolayer is confluent, rinse them twice by 5 mL of sterile PBS. Then, add trypsin 0.025 % (0.5 mL for T25 flask or 1 mL for T75 flask). Incubate for 10–15 min at 37 °C until cell detachment (*see* **Note 3**).

3. Stop the reaction by adding cell culture medium + FBS, which neutralizes trypsin (4.5 mL for T25 flask or 9 mL for T75 flask). Homogenize the suspension by pipetting.

4. Enumerate cells under sterile conditions. Take 100–200 µL of cell suspension and add an equal volume of Trypan Blue. Mix by gentle pipetting. Use a clean hemocytometer to count the number of viable cells (seen as bright cells; nonviable cells are stained blue) (*see* **Note 4**).

5. Seed the cells at a concentration of 10^5 cells/well (0.5 mL) directly in 24-well tissue-culture plates for enumeration by culture or on glass coverslips placed into the wells for enumeration by microscopy.

6. Incubate for 24 h at 37 °C in CO_2 atmosphere (*see* **Note 5**).

3.1.2 In Vitro Adherence Assay

1. Culture *C. difficile* strains (wild type or mutants) in TGY or BHI broth in an anaerobic chamber (CO_2 5 %, H_2 5 %, N_2 90 %) at 37 °C overnight.

2. Harvest the bacteria by centrifugation ($3500 \times g$ for 10 min) and wash *C. difficile* cells twice in PBS in anaerobiosis. Resuspend the bacterial pellet for microscopic counting, adjust bacterial culture to 10^7–10^8 bacteria/mL in cell culture medium without FBS and essential amino acids or in PBS.

3. Prepare the cell culture by washing twice in sterile PBS, then add 0.5 mL of cell culture medium without FBS per well.

4. Add 0.5 mL of the bacterial suspension to each well of cells and incubate for 1 h at 37 °C. Incubation of *C. difficile* cells with the culture cells can be done in anaerobiosis during 1 h or after heat shock (48 or 60 °C for 20 min) in 10 % CO_2 atmosphere.

5. Eliminate non adherent bacteria by five washings in PBS pH 7.2 (1 mL/well).

6. Fix with methanol 70 % for 15 min and stain the cells and adherent bacteria with May-Grünwald-Giemsa or Gram's stain.

7. Enumeration by microscopy. Count the number of adherent bacteria per cell on a light microscope at a magnification of 1000× (*see* **Note 6**).

8. Enumeration by culture: remove the adherent bacteria by adding 0.5 mL of saponine 1 % per well or by adding 1 mL of cold water followed by an incubation on ice for 1 h. Perform serial dilutions and plate on BHI or Columbia agar plates with 5 % blood. Count CFU after 48 h of incubation in anaerobiosis. Express the number of CFU/cell (*see* **Note 7**).

3.1.3 In Vitro Adherence Inhibition Assays

Inhibition by Specific Antibodies

1. Pellet the culture and wash *C. difficile* cells twice in PBS in anaerobiosis. Adjust bacterial culture to 10^7–10^8 bacteria/mL. Possibility to perform a heat shock at 48 or 60 °C for 20 min.

2. Incubate the bacteria for 30 min to 1 h at 37 °C in anaerobiosis with antibodies against *C. difficile* protein of interest (1:10, 1:100, 1:500, 1:1000 dilutions in TNT + 5 % skimmed milk) (*see* **Note 8**).

3. Add 0.5 mL of the bacterial suspension on cells and incubate for 1 h at 37 °C in anaerobiosis.

4. Eliminate non adherent bacteria by five washings in PBS.

5. Fix the cells, stain and count adherent bacteria (*see* **Note 9**).

Inhibition by Recombinant Proteins

1. Pre-incubate washed culture cells for 15 min at 37 °C in CO_2 atmosphere with 10, 50 and 100 µg/mL of protein in DMEM (0.5 mL).

2. Add 0.5 mL of the bacterial suspension (10^7–10^8 bacteria/mL) to cells and incubate for 1 h at 37 °C in anaerobiosis.

3. Proceed as described above.

3.2 In Vivo Adherence with a Monoxenic C. difficile Mouse Model

1. Challenge axenic mice by intra-gastric (i.g.) administration of 0.5 mL of a 24 h *C. difficile* culture in TGY broth (10^8 CFU/mL) [25].

2. A few days (depending on the virulence of the strain) after *C. difficile* challenge, sacrifice the mice and transfer them in an anaerobic chamber.

3. Remove the entire caecum of each mouse, rinse by gentle shaking eight times in PBS pH 7.2 and weigh it.

4. Crush each caecum with an Ultra-Turrax apparatus (T25-Janke & Kunkel, IKA-Labortechnik, Germany) for 1 min at 8000 to 24 000 rpm rpm and dilute in TGY broth to obtain a concentration of 10 mg/mL.

5. Make serial dilutions and plate them in duplicate on Columbia agar 5 % horse blood. After 48 h of incubation in anaerobiosis, count the characteristic colonies.

3.3 Immunoelectron Microscopy to Visualize the Surface Localization of a Protein of Interest

1. Wash 24 h cultures of *C. difficile*, harvest bacteria by centrifugation and resuspend in PBS to obtain a dense bacterial suspension.

2. Place a single drop of the bacterial suspension onto Formvar coated nickel grids, wait for 5 min and remove excess moisture by absorption (*see* **Note 10**).

3. Invert the grids onto drops (25 µL) of PBS with BSA 1 % for 30 min.

4. Incubate the grids for 1 h onto drops of appropriate dilution of anti-protein antibodies (in PBS + BSA 1 %).

5. Perform three washings in PBS. Then, incubate the grids for 1 h onto drops of 1:20 dilution of 10 nm diameter colloidal gold particle-labeled Protein-A.

6. Wash the grids three times in PBS.

7. Fix with PBS with glutaraldehyde 3%.

8. Wash three times with water (Milli-Q grade water) and stain with 0.5% phosphotungstic acid.

9. Observe by transmission electron microscopy (TEM).

3.4 Binding of FbpA to Extracellular Matrix Proteins by Far-Immuno Dot-Blotting

1. Put onto a nitrocellulose membrane 10 μg of fibronectin, fibrinogen, collagen type VI, vitronectin, and BSA as negative control and air-dry.

2. Incubate the membrane for 1 h at 37 °C in blocking buffer (5% skimmed milk in TNT).

3. Incubate the membrane in 10 mL of the same buffer containing 10 μg of rFbpA.

4. After four washings, reveal rFbpA binding by adding rabbit anti-rFbpA antibody (1:2500).

5. After four washings, detect with goat anti-rabbit IgG-alkaline phosphatase conjugate (1:2500 dilution).

6. Reveal with NBT-BCIP as substrate as recommended by the supplier.

3.5 C. difficile Binding to Soluble Fibronectin by Indirect Immunofluorescence

1. Prepare an overnight culture of *C. difficile* (wild type strain or mutant).

2. Harvest bacteria by centrifugation and wash twice with PBS pH 7.2.

3. Incubate bacteria for 2 h in 10 mL of a solution of 0.5 μg/mL of fibronectin in PBS in anaerobiosis.

4. Harvest bacteria by centrifugation and wash three times with PBS pH 7.2.

5. Place a drop of culture onto a glass microscope slide and dry.

6. Immerse the slide in a solution of rabbit anti-fibronectin monoclonal antibody (1:2500 dilution in PBS pH 7.2). Incubate for 1 h at room temperature (*see* **Note 11**).

7. Wash the slide three times with PBS pH 7.2 for 15 min.

8. Incubate for 30 min with fluorescein isothiocyanate (FITC)-conjugated mouse anti-rabbit IgG antibody (Immunotech; 1:160 dilution in PBS).

9. After three washings, dry the slide and examine the specimens with epifluorescence microscope (Leitz Aristoplan coupled to an Image Analyzer Visiolab 1000 Biocom).

3.6 C. difficile Binding to Immobilized Fibronectin by ELISA

1. Coat purified human fibronectin (Sigma) on 96-well microtiter plates by adding 100 μL of the protein solution (10 μg/mL in 0.05 M sodium carbonate buffer) to each well and incubate plates for 1 h at 37 °C.

2. Wash the wells three times with PBS-Tween 20 0.1 % (PBS-T), then add 200 μL of blocking buffer per well and incubate for 2 h at 37 °C.

3. Wash the wells three times with PBS-T before use.

4. Prepare a *C. difficile* culture of the wild type strain or the mutants (late stationary phase) and harvest by centrifugation for 10 min at $5000 \times g$.

5. Wash the bacterial pellet with PBS and resuspend in PBS at 10^7 CFU/mL and then perform a twofold serial dilution.

6. Apply the different bacterial dilutions to the fibronectin-coated assay plates (100 μL/well) and incubate at 37 °C for 30 min (*see* **Note 12**).

7. Remove unbound bacteria with five washings in PBS.

8. Reveal with a 1:2500 dilution of a rabbit anti-serum against *C. difficile*. Incubate for 30 min at 37 °C.

9. Wash the plates three times with PBS.

10. Reveal with 1:2500 dilution of alkaline phosphatase-labeled goat anti-rabbit IgG. Incubate for 30 min at 37 °C.

11. Eliminate the unbound anti-rabbit IgG by three washings.

12. Reveal by addition of 200 μL of *p*-nitrophenyl phosphate substrate/well (1 mg/mL dissolved in 0.1 M carbonate buffer (pH 9.6) with 1 mM $MgCl_2$) for 15 min at room temperature.

13. Stop the reaction by the addition of 50 μL of 3 N NaOH.

14. Measure the absorbance at 405 nm in an ELISA plate reader (*see* **Notes 13** and **14**).

4   Notes

1. For maintenance purposes, cells were passaged weekly using 0.025 % trypsin in Ca^{2+} Mg^{2+}-free PBS containing EDTA 0.53 mM. After enumeration, cell suspensions are added at appropriated concentrations to culture flasks.

2. To prevent bacterial contamination, 200 U of penicillin per mL and 40 mg of streptomycin per mL can be added. However, these antibiotics can inhibit only partially bacterial growth and mask a contamination.

3. Avoid long incubation in trypsin, just enough time for cells to detach.

4. Trypan blue is toxic and is a potential carcinogen. Protective clothing, gloves, and face/eye protection should be worn.

5. Caco-2 TC7 cells were used between the 20 and 60th cell passage. Differentiated monolayers were obtained 15 days after seeding. Compared to Caco-2, Caco-2 TC7 cells do not form dome.

6. After staining, use a needle to pick up the coverslip and stick it on the microscope glass slide (cells facing the glass side).

7. The experiments are made in triplicate in three independent experiments to perform statistical analyses. The adhesion index is given as the mean number of adherent bacteria per cell $\pm$ SD. Three wells are used to count the number of cultured cells in order to express the results as CFU per cell. Briefly, detach the cells with 200 μL of trypsin 0.025 % during 10 min and add 300 μL of DMEM. Scratch the cells and homogenize for subsequent enumeration.

8. The positive adherence controls consist of bacterial adhesion with a 1:10 dilution of pre-immune serum in PBS or with PBS alone.

9. The results of the inhibition assays were compared to the positive controls (considered as a percentage of adhesion of 100 %) and expressed as a percentage of relative adherence.

10. The drops of the different materials are deposited on a Parafilm and the grids are inverted onto material drops.

11. Controls were carried out similarly: rabbit anti-*C. difficile* antibody was used as a positive control; the primary antibody omitted or bacteria incubated without fibronectin with antiserum raised against fibronectin were used as negative controls.

12. The experimental part with *C. difficile* is carried out in anaerobic conditions.

13. Wells without bacteria or without the first or second antibodies served as negative controls. The adhesion index is given by the average A_{405} of triplicate test wells of three different assays.

14. Fibronectin adherence inhibition assays. Incubate 10^7 bacteria with different dilutions (1:100, 1:500, 1:1000) of anti-FbpA in PBS for 30 min before binding to immobilized fibronectin on ELISA plates as described. Positive control: adhesion in presence of a 1:500 dilution of pre-immune serum; negative control: adhesion to wells without bacteria.

Acknowledgments

The authors thank the researchers and Ph.D. students of the unit EA4043 UBaPS for developing some of the methods described in this chapter.

References

1. Deneve C, Janoir C, Poilane I, Fantinato C, Collignon A (2009) New trends in *Clostridium difficile* virulence and pathogenesis. Int J Antimicrob Agents 33(Suppl 1):S24–S28. doi:10.1016/S0924-8579(09)70012-3, S0924-8579(09)70012-3 (pii)

2. Kuehne SA, Collery MM, Kelly ML, Cartman ST, Cockayne A, Minton NP (2014) Importance of toxin A, toxin B, and CDT in virulence of an epidemic *Clostridium difficile* strain. J Infect Dis 209(1):83–86. doi:10.1093/infdis/jit426, jit426 (pii)

3. Vedantam G, Clark A, Chu M, McQuade R, Mallozzi M, Viswanathan VK (2012) *Clostridium difficile* infection: toxins and non-toxin virulence factors, and their contributions to disease establishment and host response. Gut Microbes 3(2):121–134. doi:10.4161/gmic.19399, 19399 (pii)

4. Eveillard M, Fourel V, Barc MC, Kerneis S, Coconnier MH, Karjalainen T, Bourlioux P, Servin AL (1993) Identification and characterization of adhesive factors of *Clostridium difficile* involved in adhesion to human colonic enterocyte-like Caco-2 and mucus-secreting HT29 cells in culture. Mol Microbiol 7(3):371–381

5. Cerquetti M, Serafino A, Sebastianelli A, Mastrantonio P (2002) Binding of *Clostridium difficile* to Caco-2 epithelial cell line and to extracellular matrix proteins. FEMS Immunol Med Microbiol 32(3):211–218. doi:10.1016/S0928824401003017

6. Karjalainen T, Barc MC, Collignon A, Trolle S, Boureau H, Cotte-Laffitte J, Bourlioux P (1994) Cloning of a genetic determinant from *Clostridium difficile* involved in adherence to tissue culture cells and mucus. Infect Immun 62(10):4347–4355

7. Karjalainen T, Waligora-Dupriet AJ, Cerquetti M, Spigaglia P, Maggioni A, Mauri P, Mastrantonio P (2001) Molecular and genomic analysis of genes encoding surface-anchored proteins from *Clostridium difficile*. Infect Immun 69(5):3442–3446. doi:10.1128/IAI.69.5.3442-3446.2001

8. Waligora AJ, Barc MC, Bourlioux P, Collignon A, Karjalainen T (1999) *Clostridium difficile* cell attachment is modified by environmental factors. Appl Environ Microbiol 65(9):4234–4238

9. Gomez-Trevino M, Boureau H, Karjalainen T, Bourlioux P (1996) *Clostridium difficile* adherence to mucus: results of an in vivo and ex vivo assay. Microb Ecol Health Dis 9:329–334

10. Tasteyre A, Barc MC, Collignon A, Boureau H, Karjalainen T (2001) Role of FliC and FliD flagellar proteins of *Clostridium difficile* in adherence and gut colonization. Infect

Immun 69(12):7937–7940. doi:10.1128/IAI.69.12.7937-7940.2001

11. Savariau-Lacomme MP, Lebarbier C, Karjalainen T, Collignon A, Janoir C (2003) Transcription and analysis of polymorphism in a cluster of genes encoding surface-associated proteins of *Clostridium difficile*. J Bacteriol 185(15):4461–4470

12. Fagan RP, Janoir C, Collignon A, Mastrantonio P, Poxton IR, Fairweather NF (2011) A proposed nomenclature for cell wall proteins of *Clostridium difficile*. J Med Microbiol 60(Pt 8):1225–1228. doi:10.1099/jmm.0.028472-0, jmm.0.028472-0 (pii)

13. Calabi E, Ward S, Wren B, Paxton T, Panico M, Morris H, Dell A, Dougan G, Fairweather N (2001) Molecular characterization of the surface layer proteins from *Clostridium difficile*. Mol Microbiol 40(5):1187–1199, doi:mmi2461 (pii)

14. Calabi E, Calabi F, Phillips AD, Fairweather NF (2002) Binding of *Clostridium difficile* surface layer proteins to gastrointestinal tissues. Infect Immun 70(10):5770–5778

15. Waligora AJ, Hennequin C, Mullany P, Bourlioux P, Collignon A, Karjalainen T (2001) Characterization of a cell surface protein of *Clostridium difficile* with adhesive properties. Infect Immun 69(4):2144–2153. doi:10.1128/IAI.69.4.2144-2153.2001

16. Hennequin C, Janoir C, Barc MC, Collignon A, Karjalainen T (2003) Identification and characterization of a fibronectin-binding protein from *Clostridium difficile*. Microbiology 149(Pt 10):2779–2787

17. Barketi-Klai A, Hoys S, Lambert-Bordes S, Collignon A, Kansau I (2011) Role of fibronectin-binding protein A in *Clostridium difficile* intestinal colonization. J Med Microbiol 60(Pt 8):1155–1161. doi:10.1099/jmm.0.029553-0, jmm.0.029553-0 (pii)

18. Hennequin C, Collignon A, Karjalainen T (2001) Analysis of expression of GroEL (Hsp60) of *Clostridium difficile* in response to stress. Microb Pathog 31(5):255–260. doi:10.1006/mpat.2001.0468, S0882-4010(01)90468-1 (pii)

19. Hennequin C, Porcheray F, Waligora-Dupriet A, Collignon A, Barc M, Bourlioux P, Karjalainen T (2001) GroEL (Hsp60) of *Clostridium difficile* is involved in cell adherence. Microbiology 147(Pt 1):87–96

20. Tasteyre A, Barc MC, Karjalainen T, Dodson P, Hyde S, Bourlioux P, Borriello P (2000) A *Clostridium difficile* gene encoding flagellin. Microbiology 146(Pt 4):957–966

21. Tasteyre A, Karjalainen T, Avesani V, Delmee M, Collignon A, Bourlioux P, Barc MC (2001)

Molecular characterization of fliD gene encoding flagellar cap and its expression among *Clostridium difficile* isolates from different serogroups. J Clin Microbiol 39(3):1178–1183. doi:10.1128/JCM.39.3.1178-1183.2001

22. Tulli L, Marchi S, Petracca R, Shaw HA, Fairweather NF, Scarselli M, Soriani M, Leuzzi R (2013) CbpA: a novel surface exposed adhesin of *Clostridium difficile* targeting human collagen. Cell Microbiol 15(10):1674–1687. doi:10.1111/cmi.12139

23. Kovacs-Simon A, Leuzzi R, Kasendra M, Minton N, Titball RW, Michell SL (2014) Lipoprotein CD0873 is a novel adhesin of *Clostridium difficile*. J Infect Dis 210(2):274–284. doi:10.1093/infdis/jiu070, jiu070 (pii)

24. Fagan R, Fairweather N (2010) Dissecting the cell surface. Methods Mol Biol 646:117–134. doi:10.1007/978-1-60327-365-7_8

25. Collignon A (2010) Methods for working with the mouse model. Methods Mol Biol 646:229–237. doi:10.1007/978-1-60327-365-7_15

Chapter 8

Intestinal Epithelial Cell Response to *Clostridium difficile* Flagella

Jameel Batah and Imad Kansau

Abstract

Clostridium difficile is the bacterium responsible for most antibiotic-associated diarrhea in North America and Europe. This bacterium, which colonizes the gut of humans and animals, produces toxins that are known to contribute directly to damage of the gut. It is known that bacterial flagella are involved in intestinal lesions through the inflammatory host response. The *C. difficile* flagellin recognizes TLR5 and consequently activates the NF-κB and the MAPK signaling pathways which elicit the synthesis of pro-inflammatory cytokines. Increasing interest on the role of *C. difficile* flagella in eliciting this cell response was recently developed and the development of tools to study cell response triggered by *C. difficile* flagella will improve our understanding of the pathogenesis of *C. difficile*.

Key words *Clostridium difficile* flagella, Flagellin FliC, TLR5 signaling, NF-κB, MAPK, Innate immune response

1 Introduction

Clostridium difficile has become the most common enteropathogen responsible for intestinal nosocomial post-antibiotic infections in developed countries [1–3]. Even if toxins explain some of the lesions observed during *C. difficile* infection [4–8], other factors appear to play important roles in the intestinal mucosal injury. Such factors could contribute to the genesis of mucosal damage through the induction and/or amplification of the inflammatory response of the host. We have focused our interest on *C. difficile* flagella which, apart their role in mobility, could play a role in pathogenesis through abnormal stimulation of the immune response of the host cell via the innate immune response Toll-like receptor 5 (TLR5) [9–13]. Indeed, bacterial flagellins, like others pathogen-associated molecular patterns (PAMPs), are specifically recognized by pattern-recognition receptor (PRR) TLR5 which is expressed at the basolateral pole of intestinal epithelial cells. This TLR5-flagellin interaction elicits the TLR5-related signaling

Adam P. Roberts and Peter Mullany (eds.), *Clostridium difficile: Methods and Protocols*, Methods in Molecular Biology, vol. 1476, DOI 10.1007/978-1-4939-6361-4_8, © Springer Science+Business Media New York 2016

pathways involving mitogen-activated protein kinases (MAPKs) and nuclear factor-kappa B (NF-κB), which are responsible for the secretion of pro-inflammatory cytokines (including the interleukins IL-1β, IL-6, and IL-8) and for initiating an immune response against these pathogens [9, 10].

Our understanding of the role of the *C. difficile* flagella in eliciting this cell response begins to grow. We can analyze the TLR5 signaling elicited by *C. difficile* FliC (the structural subunit of the flagellar filament) in vitro using the human epithelial Caco-2 cell model.

2   Materials

2.1 Purification of C. difficile Recombinant Flagellin

1. *Escherichia coli* strain Bl21 with plasmid pET28 *fliC*-his tag.

2. Luria–Bertani (LB) broth supplemented with 50 mg/ml kanamycin.

3. 1 M isopropyl-β-D-thiogalactopyranoside (IPTG) solution.

4. Protease inhibitors (Sigma P-8465).

5. Bacterial lysing buffer: 25 mM Tris–HCl, pH 8, 300 mM NaCl, 1 mg/ml lysozyme, 500 μl protease inhibitors. Lysozyme and the protease inhibitors are added extemporaneously (*see* **Note 1**).

6. Equilibration buffer: 50 mM sodium dihydrogen phosphate dihydrate (NaH_2PO_4), 8 M urea, 300 mM NaCl.

7. Elution buffer: 45 mM sodium dihydrogen phosphate dihydrate (NaH_2PO_4), 8 M urea, 270 mM NaCl, 150 mM imidazole.

8. His-Select Nickel Affinity Gel (Clontech or equivalent).

9. PBS.

10. Slide-A-Lyzer Dialysis Cassette G2® (Thermo Scientific), 10,000 MW cutoff or equivalent dialysis membrane.

2.2 Cell Culture

1. Caco-2 (ATCC, HTB-37) human colon carcinoma cells.

2. Dulbecco's Modified Eagle Medium with GlutaMAX-I (DMEM) (Invitrogen/Gibco) supplemented with 10% fetal bovine serum (Invitrogen/Gibco), 1% L glutamine 200 mM (Invitrogen/Gibco), and 1 % MEM nonessential amino acid solution (Invitrogen/Gibco).

3. Trypsin–EDTA solution (0.025% trypsin, 0.01% EDTA) (Invitrogen/Gibco).

4. D-PBS, Dulbecco's phosphate buffered saline (Invitrogen/Gibco).

5. 0.4% trypan blue solution.

6. TNFα (Sigma).

7. Purified anti-human TLR5-IgA antibody and human IgA2 control (which targets *E. coli* β-galactosidase) (Invivogen).

2.3 Protein Extraction from Cell Cultures

1. PAGE solution (5×): 313 mM Tris–HCl pH 6.8, 20 % (w/v) SDS.
2. Bromophenol blue solution (5×): PAGE solution 1×, 50 % (v/v) glycerol, 5 % (w/v) bromophenol blue.
3. 100 mM sodium fluoride (NaF) solution (10×).
4. 250 mM NaPPi solution (10×). Store frozen in <1 ml aliquots.
5. 100 mM sodium vanadate (Na$_3$VO$_4$) solution (100×).
6. 100 mM EDTA solution pH 8 (20×) (*see* **Note 2**).
7. Sterile PBS-vanadate solution containing PBS, 0.5 mM EDTA, 1 mM NaF, 10 mM hydrogen peroxide (H$_2$O$_2$), 0.1 mM Na$_3$VO$_4$ (*see* **Note 3**).
8. Lysing buffer containing PAGE solution 1×, 186 mM β-Mercaptoethanol, bromophenol blue solution 1×, NaF solution 1×, NaPPi solution 1×, Na$_3$VO$_4$ solution 1× (final concentration: 62.6 mM Tris–HCl pH 6.8, 4 % (w/v) SDS, 186 mM β-Mercaptoethanol, 1 % (w/v) bromophenol blue, 10 mM NaF, 25 mM NaPPi, 1 mM Na$_3$VO$_4$ (*see* **Note 4**).

2.4 SDS PAGE

1. Resolving gel buffer: 1.5 M Tris–HCl, pH 8.8, 0.4 % (w/v) SDS.
2. Stacking gel buffer: 0.5 M Tris–HCl, pH 6.8, 0.4 % (w/v) SDS.
3. 10 % SDS (w/v) solution.
4. 40 % acrylamide/bis-acrylamide (19:1) solution (*see* **Note 5**).
5. N,N,N',N'-tetramethylethylenediamine (TEMED).
6. Ammonium persulfate (APS) (10 %). Store frozen in small aliquots (<200 μl). The number of freeze–thaw cycles should be minimized.
7. Isopropanol.
8. Running buffer (10×): 250 mM Tris base, 1.92 M glycine, 1 % (w/v) SDS. Dilute to 1× with H$_2$O before use.
9. Protein marker broad range (New England Biolabs®, Fermentans® or equivalent).
10. Coomassie stain: 0.25 % (w/v) Coomassie brilliant blue R-250, 45 % (v/v) methanol, 10 % (v/v) acetic acid.
11. Coomassie destain: 45 % (v/v) methanol, 10 % (v/v) acetic acid.
12. Acetic acid (10 %).

2.5 Western Immunoblotting

1. Amersham Hybond P polyvinylidene difluoride (PVDF) membrane (GE Healthcare).
2. Whatman® 3MM blotting paper.
3. Ethanol 90 %, methanol.
4. Transfer buffer (10×): 0.2 M Tris-base, pH 9.4, 1.5 M glycine. Dilute to 1× with H$_2$O and 20 % (v/v) ethanol before use.
5. TBS buffer 10×: 0.5 M Tris–HCl pH 7.5, 1.5 M NaCl.

6. Ponceau S stain: 0.5% (w/v) Ponceau S, 1% (v/v) acetic acid.

7. Washing buffer: TBS 1×, 0.1% (v/v) Tween 20.

8. Blocking buffer: TBS 1×, 0.1% (v/v) Tween 20, 5% nonfat milk.

9. Antibody dilution solution: TBS 1×, 0.1% (v/v) Tween 20, 3% (w/v) bovine serum albumin (BSA).

10. Specific antibodies rose against the protein of interest: anti-ERK1/2, anti-JNK, anti-p38, and anti-IκBα, anti-NF-κB p65, anti-phosphorylated (anti-p)ERK1/2, anti-pJNK, anti-pMAPKAPK-2 (Cell Signaling Technology), or anti-actin (Millipore).

11. HRP-linked secondary antibodies recognizing the species used to raise antibodies above (Cell Signaling Technology).

12. Chemiluminescence detection ECL Plus kit (Millipore).

13. CCD (charge-coupled device) camera imaging device or phosphorimager for chemiluminescence detection (*see* **Note 6**), e.g., Fusion FX® (Vilber Lourmat) and image analysis software, e.g., Fusion-CAPT software® (Vilber Lourmat).

14. Stripping solution: Tris–HCl 62.5 mM pH 6.8, 100 mM β-mercaptoethanol, 2% (w/v) SDS.

2.6 ELISA

1. Quantibody® Human Inflammation Array 1 (RayBiotech), for quantitative measurement of ten human cytokines.

2. Benchtop rocker or orbital rocker.

3. Laser scanner for fluorescence detection.

4. Aluminum foil.

5. Ultrapure water (type 1, e.g., Milli-Q®).

6. 1.5 ml Polypropylene microcentrifuge tubes.

3   Methods

3.1 Purification of C. difficile Recombinant Flagellin

In order to purify the FliC flagellin of the *C. difficile* R20291 strain, the following procedure described previously can be used [14].

In order to attach a His tag to the N-terminal position of the FliC protein, two oligonucleotide primers, CCCCTGGGATCCAT GAGAGTTAATACAAATGTAAGTGC and CCGGGAATTCC TATCCTAATAATTGTAAAACTCC, incorporating *Bam*HI and *Eco*RI sites respectively, were used to amplify by PCR the full-length coding region of the *fliC* gene of strain R20291. The resulting 895 bp DNA product was digested with *Bam*HI and *Eco*RI, purified and cloned into the corresponding sites of pET-28a(+). The nucleotide sequence of the junction between vector and insert was confirmed by sequencing analysis. The ligation product was transformed first into *E. coli* Top10 and then into *E. coli* BL21. Subsequent protein purification is performed by denaturing single-step affinity chromatography employing a His-Select Nickel Affinity Gel. This method was optimized for the highly precipitant *C. difficile* flagellin.

1. A 20 ml overnight liquid culture of the *E. coli* strain Bl21 harboring the plasmid pET28 *fliC*-his tag is prepared in LB broth supplemented with 50 mg/ml kanamycin.

2. Transfer the overnight *E. coli* culture to 2 l LB broth supplemented with 50 mg/ml kanamycin. Incubate at 37 °C with shaking at 180 rpm for about 2.5 h to 3 h, until an OD_{600} of 0.8–1.2.

3. Add 2 ml of 1 M IPTG solution and incubate at 37 °C with shaking at 180 rpm for 3 h.

4. Harvest cells by centrifugation at $3350 \times g$ for 15 min at 4 °C.

5. Discard the supernatant. The bacterial pellet can be frozen at −80 °C until lysis.

6. Bacterial lysis is obtained by adding 50 ml lysis buffer. Incubate with gentle agitation at 4 °C for 1 h.

7. To obtain complete bacterial lysis, three cycles of freeze–thaw at −80 °C, followed by 3–4 cycles of 45 s sonication are performed (*see* **Note 7**).

8. Centrifuge at $10,000 \times g$ at 4 °C for 40 min. Discard supernatant. Pellet can be frozen until use.

9. Resuspend the pellet in 10 ml equilibration buffer and incubate at room temperature for 1 h to achieve FliC solubilization.

10. Centrifuge at $10,000 \times g$ at room temperature for 40 min (*see* **Note 8**). Carefully remove the supernatant containing recombinant protein and filter into a clean tube.

11. Prepare the metal affinity resin for batch/gravity-flow column purification: thoroughly resuspend the resin. Wash 2 ml resin with 4 ml ultrapure water and centrifuge at $270 \times g$ for 1 min to pellet the resin. Remove and discard the supernatant. Add 6 ml of equilibration buffer and mix briefly to pre-equilibrate the resin. Recentrifuge at $270 \times g$ for 1 min to pellet the resin. Discard the supernatant.

12. Apply the sample to the resin and incubate with gently agitation on a platform shaker at room temperature for 1 h to allow the his-tagged FliC protein to bind the resin.

13. Transfer the resin to a 2 ml gravity-flow column with an end-cap in place, and allow the resin to settle out of suspension. Remove the end-cap and allow the liquid to drain until it reaches the top of the resin bed, making sure no air bubbles are trapped in the resin bed.

14. Wash the resin three times with 7 ml equilibration buffer, to obtain an eluate with an OD_{280} close to 0.

15. Elute the his-tagged FliC protein by adding 3 ml elution buffer to the column. Collect the eluate in 500 μl fractions.

16. Use spectrophotometric and SDS-PAGE analysis to determine which fractions contain the majority of the his-tagged FliC. The *C. difficile* his-tagged FliC apparent molecular weight is 36 kDa.

17. To remove urea from eluate, pool the fractions containing the highest concentration of protein and dialyze overnight in 1 l PBS, on Slide-A-Lyzer Dialysis Cassette G2 (10,000 MW cutoff). Replace the PBS and dialyse again for 3 h.

18. Protein quantification can be obtained using a Bradford protein assay or a standard bovine serum albumin range on SDS-PAGE and Coomassie blue stain (*see* Subheading 3.5 below).

3.2 Cell Culture

1. Caco-2 human colon carcinoma cells are grown in Dulbecco's Modified Eagle Medium (DMEM) supplemented with 10% fetal calf serum (FCS), 1% L-glutamine, and 1% nonessential amino acids. Cultures are maintained at 37 °C in 10% CO_2. When cell monolayer is confluent they are briefly rinsed with PBS and detached using 2 ml of trypsin–EDTA for 5 min (*see* **Note 9**).

2. Fresh growth medium (containing FCS which neutralizes trypsin) is added until 10 ml, gently pipetted to break up clumps and centrifuged at $1000 \times g$ for 5 min.

3. Ensure to complete removal of supernatant. Cell pellet is resuspended in fresh culture medium.

4. Cell quantification: under sterile conditions remove 100–200 μl of cell suspension and add an equal volume of trypan blue (dilution factor 2) (*see* **Note 10**). Mix by gentle pipetting. Use a clean hemocytometer to count the number of viable cells (seen as bright cells; nonviable cells are stained blue). Ideally >100 cells should be counted in order to increase the accuracy of the cell count.

5. The concentration of cells is calculated and cell suspensions at appropriated concentrations are added to culture flasks (150,000 cells/25 cm² flasks), 24-well plates (100,000 cells/well), or 96-well plates (50,000 cells/well) and incubated at 37 °C (*see* **Note 11**).

3.3 Stimulation of Caco-2 Cells with FliC

1. Confluent Caco-2 monolayers grown in 24-well plates to 3 days post-confluence are FCS depleted for a minimum of 4 h before signaling experiments.

2. Monolayers are incubated with 5–6 μg/ml recombinant *C. difficile* FliC for 1 h or with 2.5 μg TNFα for 15 min.

3. For TLR5 inhibition, Caco-2 cells are grown in 96-well plates:

    (a) Prepare a Caco-2 cell suspension at 500,000 cells/ml.

(b) Add 100 μl of cell suspension per well and then incubate for 48 h after the seeding at 37 °C, 10% CO_2.

(c) Add 100 μl of anti-hTLR5 IgA or Control IgA2 dilution (5 μg/ml final).

(d) Incubate for 1 h at 37 °C, 10% CO_2.

(e) Add 5–6 μg/ml recombinant FliC. Incubate for 1 h at 37 °C, 10% CO_2.

3.4 Protein Extraction from Cell Cultures

1. Supernatant is removed and stocked at –80 °C (for ELISA) and monolayers are immediately washed with PBS-vanadate (pre-warmed at 37 °C) (*see* **Note 12**).

2. PBS-vanadate is removed and plate is placed at –80 °C for at least 15 min (*see* **Note 13**).

3. 300 μl of lysing buffer are added. Complete homogenization by passing solution through syringe and needle (ten times) is necessary to ensure complete cell lysis and DNA breaking.

4. Boil cell lysates 5 min at 100 °C. The cell lysates can be analyzed by gel electrophoresis.

3.5 SDS PAGE

The method for denaturing polyacrylamide gel electrophoresis of proteins used here is based on the method of Laemmli using the Bio-Rad Mini-Protean 3 gel system. This system is readily adaptable for use with other systems. Proteins are denatured and reduced in SDS and β-mercaptoethanol and separated on the basis of their size rather than charge as they migrate through a polyacrylamide gel towards the anode. The discontinuous gel is prepared using different buffers at different pH to first focus the separating proteins into narrow bands and then separate them according to their size.

1. Assemble the gel casting system using clean, dry glass plates according to the manufacturer's instructions.

2. Prepare the acrylamide gel solutions as indicated in Tables 1 and 2. Both resolving gel and stacking gel solutions can be prepared simultaneously without adding APS and TEMED to avoid gel polymerization.

3. Just before pouring the gel, add APS and TEMED to the resolving gel solution mix gently and add approximately 4 ml of the solution between the glass plates to cover ¾ of the plates. Overlay gently 0.5–1 ml of isopropanol on top of the resolving gel solution to allow a straight edge to the top of the gel and avoid contact with oxygen which slows down polymerization. Allow to polymerize for approximately 30 min (at room temperature). The remaining resolving gel solution can be used as a control of the polymerization state of the gel.

4. Once the resolving gel has polymerized, pour off the isopropanol and allow drying briefly.

Table 1
Mix for 12% resolving gel, for two gels

Reagents	Volume
Bis-acrylamide 40%	5 ml
Resolving gel buffer	4.2 ml
APS 10%	70 μl
TEMED	35 μl
Ultrapure H_2O	7.5 ml

Table 2
Mix for 5% SDS-PAGE stacking gel, for two gels

Reagents	Volume
Bis-acrylamide 40%	850 μl
Stacking gel buffer pH 6.8	1.7 ml
APS 10%	35 μl
TEMED	25 μl
Ultrapure H_2O	4.2 ml

5. Finish the stacking gel solution by adding APS and TEMED and mix gently. Pour the solution on top of the resolving gel, filling all of the space between the glass plates, and gently insert the desired comb according to the desired number of lines. Allow to polymerize for approximately 30 min.

6. Prepare the running buffer 1× (approximately 450 ml for two gels using the Bio-Rad Mini-Protean 3 system) by dilution of the 10× stock solution.

7. Boil cell lysates 5 min at 100 °C. Cell lysates from whole cells require boiling prior to electrophoresis to complete denaturing of proteins.

8. After polymerization of the stacking gel gently remove the comb and rinse the wells with running buffer. Assemble the gel running system and fill the upper and lower gel compartments with running buffer.

9. Load 10 μl of sample per well. Reserve one well for the protein size marker. Add an equal volume of 1× lysing buffer to any empty wells to prevent samples spreading horizontally into the empty lanes during electrophoresis.

10. Connect the gel running apparatus to a power supply and run at 80 V for 10 min to allow protein stacking, and then at 200 V until the bromophenol blue dye front has reached the bottom of the resolving gel (approximately 30 min for a 12 % gel).

11. Disassemble the running apparatus and the glass plates and carefully remove the gel for staining or for Western immunoblotting (*see* Subheading 3.6 below).

12. For blue staining, place the gel in a suitably sized glass or plastic container and completely cover with Coomassie stain solution. Incubate at room temperature with gentle agitation for at least 2 h.

13. Remove the stain solution and completely cover the stained gel with Coomassie destain solution. Incubate at room temperature with gentle agitation at least 1 h. Repeat several times with fresh destain solution until the background staining has reached an adequate level of transparency.

3.6 Western Immunoblotting

The following protocol is optimized for the transfer of a wide size range of proteins and gives generally lower background and high sensitivity. It has been optimized for use with a Bio-Rad Mini Trans-Blot® Cell transfer system but should be readily applicable for use with any tank transfer apparatus. It is also possible to perform a semi-wet or wet electrotransfer using standard methods and then continue with the rapid detection protocol.

1. Separation of protein samples is performed on a denaturing gel (SDS-PAGE) as described above (see Subheading 3.5).

2. After carefully remove the gel from the glass plates, equilibrate in the transfer buffer at room temperature for 5 min. Cut a piece of PVDF membrane and two pieces of blotting paper to the size of the gel to be transferred. Wet PVDF membrane briefly in methanol, incubate in ultrapure water for 2 min and then equilibrate with paper blotting and fiber pad in the transfer buffer for 5 min.

3. Assemble the gel sandwich: place the cassette, with the gray side down, and place one prewetted fiber pad on the gray side of the cassette. Place a sheet of filter paper on the fiber pad and then the equilibrated gel on the filter paper. Place the prewetted membrane on the gel and gently roll a pipette over the transfer stack to remove any air bubbles. Complete the gel sandwich by placing a piece of prewetted filter paper on the membrane and finally the second prewetted fiber pad. Close the cassette being careful not to move the gel and filter paper sandwich.

4. Place the cassette in the bath module. This transfer system is designed for two cassettes. Place the frozen cooling unit in tank (the cooling unit should be stored at –20 °C until ready to use). Fill the tank with transfer buffer. It is important to shake the buffer by a stir bar to help maintain even buffer temperature and ion distribution in the tank.

5. Connect to a power supply and run at 350 mA for 1 h (suitable for the transfer of two mini-gels).

6. At the end of the transfer, disassemble the blotting sandwich and remove the membrane.

7. Remove the membrane from the transfer system to a clean plastic dish. Efficiency of transfer can be evaluated by Ponceau S staining. Pour over enough Ponceau S stain to cover the membrane and incubate at room temperature for 2–5 min. Remove the stain solution and wash the membrane with ultra-pure water. Successive washing is necessary until the background staining is removed. However, residual red stain will not affect any of the subsequent steps.

8. Primary antibody is appropriated diluted in Antibody dilution solution. For optimal results, specific anti-MAPK (phosphorylated or not) and anti-NF-κB antibodies should be diluted respectively at 1/2000 and 1/1000. Anti-actin antibody is diluted at 1/30,000. About 5 ml of diluted primary antibody is sufficient to cover two membranes in a heat-sealed plastic pouch. Incubation overnight with gentle agitation at 4 °C reduces background. Incubation at room temperature for 1 h is possible.

9. Pour the primary antibody away and wash the membrane three times with washing buffer. Washing should be performed with gentle agitation for 10 min each time.

10. The secondary HRP-conjugated antibody is prepared as described above at 1/2000. Add to the membrane and incubate with gentle agitation for 30 min–1 h.

11. Pour the secondary antibody away and wash the membrane as before with washing buffer and leave the membrane in washing buffer following the final wash.

12. Prepare sufficient (1 ml per membrane) chemiluminescence detection ECL substrate to cover the membrane. Remove the membrane from the washing buffer, drain briefly on absorbent paper, place on a clean dry surface and pipette the substrate carefully onto the membrane, ensuring the entire surface of the membrane is covered. Incubate for 2 min at room temperature, drain briefly and completely wrap in cling film to prevent the membrane drying out.

13. Chemiluminescence signals can be detected using either an X-ray film or luminescence imager such as the Fusion FX. Densitometrical analysis can be performed with Fusion-CAPT software or ImageJ software. The density of the bands is measured and ratio phosphorylated/non phosphorylated protein (or actin) is calculated. The ratio of samples can be reported to the negative control.

3.7 ELISA-Based Quantitative Array

Cytokines play an important role in innate immunity by mediating interaction between different cell types and cellular responses to environmental conditions. The traditional method for cytokine detection and quantification is the enzyme-linked immunosorbent assay (ELISA) in which target protein is immobilized to a solid support and then complexed with an antibody that is linked to an enzyme. Detection of the resulting enzyme complex can then be visualized using a substrate that produces a detectable signal. We use the Quantibody® array, a multiplexed sandwich ELISA-based quantitative array to accurately determine the concentration of multiple cytokines simultaneously (IL-1α, IL-1β, IL-4, IL-6, IL-8, IL-10, IL-13, MCP-1, IFNγ, and TNFα).

It combines the advantages of the high detection sensitivity and specificity of ELISA and the high throughput of arrays. Like a traditional sandwich-based ELISA, it uses a pair of cytokine specific antibodies for detection onto a glass support. A biotin-labeled detection second antibody is used and the cytokine-antibody-biotin complex can be visualized using the streptavidin-conjugated Cy3 equivalent dye through a laser scanner.

1. Before use, completely air dry the glass slide and reconstitute the lyophilized standard within 1–2 h. Cytokine Standard dilutions are prepared enough for making two standard curves.

2. Reconstitution of the lyophilized Cytokine Standard Mix is obtained by adding 500 μl Sample Diluent. Gentle mix. The cytokine standard mix contains different concentrations for each antigen included (as indicated in manufacturer protocol).

3. Perform six serial dilutions by adding 100 μl Cytokine Standard Mix to a microcentrifuge tube containing 200 μl Sample Diluent and so on. Sample Diluent is used as negative control. For best results, include a set of standards in each slide.

4. To block slides add 100 μl Sample Diluent into each well and incubate at room temperature for 30 min.

5. Remove buffer from each well and add 100 μl Cytokine Standard dilutions or samples to each well. Incubate at room temperature for 1–2 h (or overnight at 4 °C). For higher signals, longer incubation time is recommended. 50 μl of original or diluted supernatant can be used. Cover the incubation chamber with adhesive film during incubation.

6. For washing, dilute 20× Wash Buffer I with H_2O. Wash five times (5 min each) with 150 μl of 1× Wash Buffer I at room temperature with gentle rocking. Completely remove wash buffer in each wash step.

7. Dilute 20× Wash Buffer II with H_2O. Decant the Wash Buffer I and wash two times (5 min each) with 150 μl of 1× Wash Buffer II at room temperature with gentle rocking. Completely remove wash buffer in each wash step (*see* **Note 14**).

8. Add 80 μl Biotinylated Antibody Cocktail (reconstituted with 1.4 ml of Sample Diluent) to each well. Incubate at room temperature for 1–2 h. For higher signals, longer incubation time is preferable.

9. Wash five times (5 min each) with 150 μl of 1× Wash Buffer I and then two times with 150 μl of 1× Wash Buffer II at room temperature with gentle rocking. Completely remove wash buffer in each wash step.

10. Reconstitute Cy3 Equivalent Dye-Streptavidin: after briefly spinning down, add 1.4 ml of Sample Diluent to Cy3 equivalent dye-conjugated streptavidin tube and mix gently.

11. Add 80 μl of Cy3 equivalent dye-conjugated streptavidin to each well and incubate in dark room (or cover the chamber with aluminum foil) to avoid exposure to light. Incubate at room temperature for 1 h.

12. Wash as in **step 6**.

13. Carefully remove the slide from the chamber device. Submerge the slide in a 1× Wash Buffer I bath (about 20 ml), and then gently shake at room temperature for 15 min. Replace Wash Buffer I by 1× Wash Buffer II and gently shake at room temperature for 5 min.

14. Gently aspirate and remove water droplets completely without touching the array.

15. Fluorescence detection: the signals can be visualized using a laser scanner equipped with a green channel for Cy3 wavelength (*see* **Note 15**).

16. Data extraction can be obtained using the GAL file which is specific for this array along with the microarray analysis software (GenePix, ScanArray Express, ArrayVision, MicroVigene, etc.). GAL files can be found at: www.RayBiotech.com/Gal-Files. html. Copy and paste data into the QAnalyzer Tool specific for this kind of array (catalog number: QAH-INF-1-SW). Additional information can be found in the manufacturer's protocol.

4   Notes

1. The lysozyme and protease inhibitors should be added immediately before use in order to preserve stability. Lysozyme helps to fully disrupt bacterial walls, and thus to extract high molecular weight proteins (>40 kDa).

2. Adjust pH to 8 to obtain fully dissolved EDTA.

3. Sodium fluoride (NaF) and sodium vanadate (Na_3VO_4) are added to prevent the dephosphorylation of post-transduction-modified proteins involved in cell signaling.

4. The lysing buffer should be prepared immediately before use in order to preserve stability. Nevertheless, stock solutions of some constituents can be prepared at stable concentrations as indicated.

5. The Acrylamide:Bis-Acrylamide 19:1 ratio (5 % cross-linker concentration), is recommended for low and mean molecular weight protein separation. Polyacrylamide is toxic and is a potential carcinogen. Protective gloves should be worn.

6. The chemiluminescence reaction emits light at 425 nm which can be captured with X-ray film, CCD camera imaging devices and phosphorimagers. Although X-ray film is useful to confirm the presence of target proteins and provides qualitative and semiquantitative data, CCD cameras offer the advantages of qualitative analysis, higher sensitivity, greater resolution, instant image manipulation and a larger dynamic range than film. When X-ray films are used, it is often necessary to expose several films for different time periods to obtain the proper balance between signal and background. This is difficult to accomplish since the process cannot be observed and stopped when the desired end-point is reached. If the film is underexposed, the signal will not be visible and if it is overexposed, the signal may be lost in the background or separate bands may become blurred together.

7. The sonication should be performed on ice to prevent warming. Breaks of 1 min after each sonication cycle must be scheduled. The medium must not remain viscous but opalescent.

8. Centrifugation at 4 °C elicits urea precipitation.

9. Longer incubation in trypsin–EDTA will lead to increased proteolytic cleavage, consequently cells will take longer to recover; therefore, avoid long incubation time in trypsin–EDTA, just enough time for cells to detach.

10. Trypan Blue is toxic and is a potential carcinogen. Protective clothing, gloves and face/eye protection should be worn.

11. At these concentrations, cell monolayers can be used at 3–5 days post-confluence. At this stage, no complete polarization (including functional tight junction) is achieved but TLR5 is expressed at the apical cell pole.

12. Adding preheated PBS-vanadate prevent cellular cold stress during experiments and consequently MAPKs activation.

13. Cells without medium can be stocked at –80 °C until following experiments.

14. Incomplete removal of the washing buffer II in each wash step may cause "dark spots", the background signals higher than the spots.

15. It is important that the signal from the well containing the highest standard concentration takes the highest possible reading, yet remains unsaturated. Since different cytokine are detected, the signal intensity varies greatly in the same array, so using multiple scans, with a higher PMT for low-signal cytokines, and a low PMT for high-signal cytokines is highly recommended.

References

1. Barbut F, Jones G, Eckert C (2011) Epidemiology and control of Clostridium difficile infections in healthcare settings: an update. Curr Opin Infect Dis 24(4):370–376

2. Bauer MP, Notermans DW, van Benthem BH, Brazier JS, Wilcox MH, Rupnik M, Monnet DL, van Dissel JT, Kuijper EJ (2011) Clostridium difficile infection in Europe: a hospital-based survey. Lancet 377(9759):63–73

3. Cohen SH, Gerding DN, Johnson S, Kelly CP, Loo VG, McDonald LC, Pepin J, Wilcox MH (2010) Clinical practice guidelines for Clostridium difficile infection in adults: 2010 update by the society for healthcare epidemiology of America (SHEA) and the infectious diseases society of America (IDSA). Infect Control Hosp Epidemiol 31(5): 431–455

4. Genth H, Dreger SC, Huelsenbeck J, Just I (2008) Clostridium difficile toxins: more than mere inhibitors of Rho proteins. Int J Biochem Cell Biol 40(4):592–597

5. Just I, Selzer J, von Eichel-Streiber C, Aktories K (1995) The low molecular mass GTP-binding protein Rho is affected by toxin A from Clostridium difficile. J Clin Invest 95(3):1026–1031

6. Just I, Selzer J, Wilm M, von Eichel-Streiber C, Mann M, Aktories K (1995) Glucosylation of Rho proteins by Clostridium difficile toxin B. Nature 375(6531):500–503

7. Kuehne SA, Cartman ST, Heap JT, Kelly ML, Cockayne A, Minton NP (2010) The role of toxin A and toxin B in Clostridium difficile infection. Nature 467(7316):711-713

8. Lyras D, O'Connor JR, Howarth PM, Sambol SP, Carter GP, Phumoonna T, Poon R, Adams V, Vedantam G, Johnson S, Gerding DN, Rood JI (2009) Toxin B is essential for virulence of Clostridium difficile. Nature 458(7242):1176–1179

9. Gewirtz AT, Navas TA, Lyons S, Godowski PJ, Madara JL (2001) Cutting edge: bacterial flagellin activates basolaterally expressed TLR5 to induce epithelial proinflammatory gene expression. J Immunol 167(4):1882–1885

10. Prince A (2006) Flagellar activation of epithelial signaling. Am J Respir Cell Mol Biol 34(5):548–551

11. Sierro F, Dubois B, Coste A, Kaiserlian D, Kraehenbuhl JP, Sirard JC (2001) Flagellin stimulation of intestinal epithelial cells triggers CCL20-mediated migration of dendritic cells. Proc Natl Acad Sci U S A 98(24):13722–13727

12. Yoshino Y, Kitazawa T, Ikeda M, Tatsuno K, Yanagimoto S, Okugawa S, Yotsuyanagi H, Ota Y (2013) Clostridium difficile flagellin stimulates toll-like receptor 5, and toxin B promotes flagellin-induced chemokine production via TLR5. Life Sci 92(3):211–217

13. Batah J, Denève-Larrazet C, Jolivot PA, Kuehne S, Collignon A, Marvaud JC, Kansau I (2016) Clostridium difficile flagella predominantly activate TLR5-linked NF-κB pathway in epithelial cells. Anaerobe 38:116–124

14. Tasteyre A, Barc MC, Karjalainen T, Dodson P, Hyde S, Bourlioux P, Borriello P (2000) A Clostridium difficile gene encoding flagellin. Microbiology 146(Pt 4):957–966

Chapter 9

Isolating and Purifying *Clostridium difficile* Spores

Adrianne N. Edwards and Shonna M. McBride

Abstract

The ability for the obligate anaerobe, *Clostridium difficile* to form a metabolically dormant spore is critical for the survival of this organism outside of the host. This spore form is resistant to a myriad of environmental stresses, including heat, desiccation, and exposure to disinfectants and antimicrobials. These intrinsic properties of spores allow *C. difficile* to survive long-term in an oxygenated environment, to be easily transmitted from host-to-host, and to persist within the host following antibiotic treatment. Because of the importance of the spore form to the *C. difficile* life cycle and treatment and prevention of *C. difficile* infection (CDI), the isolation and purification of spores are necessary to study the mechanisms of sporulation and germination, investigate spore properties and resistances, and for use in animal models of CDI. Here we provide basic protocols, in vitro growth conditions, and additional considerations for purifying *C. difficile* spores for a variety of downstream applications.

Key words *Clostridium difficile*, Sporulation, Endospore, Anaerobe, Anaerobic chamber, Antibiotic-associated diarrhea

1 Introduction

Clostridium difficile is a significant gastrointestinal pathogen of humans and other animals and is the primary agent of antibiotic-associated diarrhea. *C. difficile* infection (CDI) is responsible for billions of dollars in healthcare costs and causes greater than 14,000 deaths annually in the USA alone [1, 2]. *C. difficile* has been recently named an urgent public health threat by the US Centers for Disease Control and Prevention [1]. This anaerobic organism survives outside of its host by forming a metabolically inactive spore. Spore formation is a complex process in which a vegetative cell forms a dormant structure that protects *C. difficile* from exposure to oxygen, heat, disinfectants and desiccation and provides inherent resistance to antibiotics and other antimicrobials. Once ingested by the host, the spore germinates in the presence of bile salts [3], producing the vegetative form of the bacterium. The vegetative cell reproduces and secretes toxins, which cause disease symptoms. As the vegetative cells transit through the gastrointestinal

Adam P. Roberts and Peter Mullany (eds.), *Clostridium difficile: Methods and Protocols*, Methods in Molecular Biology, vol. 1476,
DOI 10.1007/978-1-4939-6361-4_9, © Springer Science+Business Media New York 2016

tract, unknown host and intracellular signals spur sporulation. Once shed from the host in feces, *C. difficile* spores can survive in the environment for long periods of time and are an enormous obstacle in preventing CDI in short-term and long-term healthcare facilities.

Because *C. difficile* spores are the infectious form of the organism, they are used to study infection in animal models of CDI [4–6] and to perform molecular biological experiments to discover sporulation and germination characteristics, resistances, and susceptibilities [7–9]. The emergence of the epidemic 027 ribotype strain [10] has underscored the need for further studies on spore properties and the development of antimicrobials that directly target the *C. difficile* spore.

Here, we describe how to elucidate the best conditions to optimize the production of *C. difficile* spores in vitro. We provide protocols that allow for the isolation of *C. difficile* spores and for further spore preparation purification, necessary for some downstream applications, of spore preparations. These protocols rely on the intrinsic heat, cold, and chemical resistances of *C. difficile* spores to kill vegetative cells and separate these and other debris from the spores. Finally, conditions and additional considerations for the use and long-term storage of *C. difficile* spores are discussed. Propagation and purification of *C. difficile* spores is relatively simple as long as a strict anaerobic environment is provided during *C. difficile* growth and spore formation.

2   Materials

For reliable growth of *C. difficile*, is it critical to pre-reduce all liquid and solid media in the anaerobic chamber for at least 2 h before use. Handle all materials with appropriate aseptic technique to prevent contamination from other prevalent spore forming species (e.g., *Clostridium perfringens*).

2.1   Culture Media

1. Brain heart infusion supplement (BHIS) medium: Dissolve 37 g brain heart infusion extract (BD Difco) and 5 g yeast extract (BD Difco) in 800 ml dH_2O. Bring to 1 L with dH_2O. Autoclave for 30 min and store at room temperature. Add 15 g agar per liter before autoclaving for 1.5 % (w/v) agar plates.

2. BHIS medium supplemented with 0.1 % taurocholate: Prepare medium as described above and autoclave. To prevent the growth of contaminating *Mycoplasma* species on the surface of plates containing taurocholate (which is a cholesterol derivative [11]), add 10 ml of 10 % taurocholate to 1 L BHIS when the autoclaved medium reaches ~60–65 °C. Incubate medium with 0.1 % taurocholate for 20 min as the medium cools, before pouring plates.

3. 70:30 Sporulation Medium ([12]; *see* **Note 1**): Dissolve 63 g Bacto peptone (BD Difco), 3.5 g proteose peptone (BD Difco), 0.7 g ammonium sulfate $((NH_4)_2SO_4)$, 1.06 g Tris base, 11.1 g brain heart infusion extract (BD Difco), and 1.5 g yeast extract (BD Difco) in 800 ml dH_2O. Bring to 1 L with dH_2O. Autoclave for 30 min; once medium is cool to touch, add 3 ml 10 % (w/v) cysteine (dissolve 0.4 g cysteine in 4 ml dH_2O and filter-sterilize with a 0.45 μm filter; *see* **Note 2**). Add 15 g agar per liter before autoclaving for 1.5 % (w/v) agar plates; use 35 ml per plate for consistent sporulation results. Important: 70:30 sporulation medium provides the best conditions for efficient *C. difficile* sporulation if used fresh (within a week; *see* **Note 3**).

2.2 Media Supplements

1. Taurocholate: To induce germination of *C. difficile* spores, 0.1 % (w/v) taurocholate must be supplemented in BHIS medium [13, 14]. Prepare a stock solution of 10 % (w/v) taurocholate (1 g taurocholate dissolved in 10 ml dH_2O) and filter-sterilize with a 0.22 μm filter. Store at room temperature.

2. Fructose: To prevent high rates of sporulation of *C. difficile* in overnight cultures (unpublished data, Edwards and McBride), 0.2 % (w/v) fructose may be added to BHIS medium. Prepare a stock solution of 20 % (w/v) d-fructose (2 g fructose dissolved in 10 ml dH_2O) and filter-sterilize with a 0.45 μm filter. Store at room temperature.

3. Antibiotic supplements: The use of antibiotics can influence spore formation in *C. difficile* [15]; however, antibiotic supplements are necessary for maintaining plasmids. Using the lowest concentration of antibiotic necessary for stable plasmid maintenance is strongly recommended (e.g., use a final concentration of 2 μg/ml thiamphenicol [15] instead of the commonly used 10–15 μg/ml thiamphenicol [16, 17]).

2.3 Solutions for C. difficile Spore Stocks

1. 10× phosphate buffered saline (PBS) Stock Solution: Dissolve 25.6 g $Na_2HPO_4 \cdot 7H_2O$, 80 g NaCl, 2 g KCl, and 2 g KH_2PO_4 in 800 ml dH_2O. Bring to 1 L. Autoclave for 30 min and store at room temperature.

2. 1× PBS: Dilute 10× PBS Stock Solution 1:10 (100 ml 10× PBS into 900 ml dH_2O). Sterilize by autoclaving for 30 min or using a 0.45 μm vacuum filter. Store at room temperature.

3. 1× PBS + 1 % (w/v) BSA: Dissolve 10 g bovine serum albumin (BSA) into 1 L 1× PBS. Sterilize only by using a 0.45 μm vacuum filter as BSA denatures and precipitates in high heat and pressure. Store at room temperature.

2.4 Additional Reagents

1. 95 % ethanol.

2. 0.7 % (w/v) agarose: Dissolve 0.7 g agarose in 100 ml of dH_2O and heat by stir plate or microwave to fully solubilize agarose.

The agarose solution can be stored as a solid at room temperature and be reheated for subsequent use or as a liquid at 60 °C for long-term storage.

3. 50% (w/v) sucrose: Dissolve 50 g in 100 ml dH$_2$O. Filter-sterilize.

3 Methods

One of the more vital considerations to remember when working with *C. difficile* spores is that their hydrophobic and anionic properties allow them to adhere to many surfaces, including pipet tips and polypropylene. When working with spore stocks, it is important to pipet up and down several times, especially when making dilutions, to ensure as few spores as possible are left behind. The use of polypropylene materials, such as conical tubes, is sufficient when working with high concentrations of spore stocks (greater than 10^7 colony forming units (CFU)/ml) for a short period of time; however, for long-term storage of high concentration spore stocks and when diluting spores to a concentration of 10^6 CFU/ml or less, the use of glass [15] or Teflon-coated tubes [18] is highly recommended to prevent loss and obtain reproducible spore counts. Finally, the use of 1% BSA in final spore preparations decreases clumping of spores, prevents loss, and facilitates accurate enumeration [15].

While it is not necessary to use phase-contrast microscopy to track sporulation, as described in Subheading 3.1, the use of this method is a reliable and efficient way to determine the progress of sporulation without removing the plates from the anaerobic chamber and interrupting an experiment. This technique allows for the accurate enumeration of sporulation efficiency in various conditions and at different time points before embarking on the more time-consuming spore isolation and purification protocol.

3.1 Growth and Sporulation Efficiency of *C. difficile* on Various Media

This protocol describes the general methods needed for determining the best sporulation conditions in preparation for isolating and purifying spore stocks. Methods for general cultivation of *C. difficile* and anaerobic chamber maintenance can be found elsewhere [19, 20].

1. Streak strain(s) from glycerol stock(s) onto BHIS medium agar plates and incubate overnight at 37 °C.

2. Inoculate 10 ml BHIS supplemented with 0.1% taurocholate and 0.2% fructose from a single colony using a sterile inoculating loop (*see* **Note 4**). Incubate overnight at 37 °C.

3. In the morning, while the overnight culture is still in active growth (OD$_{600}$ < 1.0; again, *see* **Note 4**), backdilute the cells to

an OD_{600} of 0.5 with BHIS. Spread 250 μl of culture onto a fresh, pre-reduced 70:30 agar plate and incubate anaerobically at 37 °C for a minimum of 24 h.

4. After a minimum of 24 h, take a small sample from the plate with a sterile inoculating loop and resuspend in 500 μl BHIS in a microcentrifuge tube. Remove sample(s) from the anaerobic chamber (*see* **Note 5**).

5. Centrifuge the cells at $16,100 \times g$ for 30 s at room temperature and decant the supernatant. Resuspend the cells in 10–50 μl BHIS.

6. Prepare a microscope slide by applying a small amount (<0.5 ml) of 0.7% agarose in the center of slide (*see* **Note 6**). Allow to solidify for ~2 min.

7. Apply 5 μl of resuspended culture to the agarose pad and carefully place a coverslip over the sample.

8. Observe cells by phase-contrast microscopy (*see* **Note 7**). Mature spores will appear phase bright while vegetative cells and prespores will appear phase dark and phase gray (partially refractile), respectively (Fig. 1). Ensure that the field of view contains only a single layer of cells, as overlapping vegetative cells may falsely appear phase bright.

9. To determine the sporulation efficiency, enumerate the number of phase bright spores and phase dark vegetative cells and use the equation detailed below:

$$\text{Sporulation efficiency} \left(\% \right) = \frac{\text{Spores}}{\text{Vegetative cells} + \text{Spores}} \times 100$$

Count at least 1000 cells to obtain an accurate representation of the population.

10. This protocol can be performed and repeated on different types of medium and at multiple time points to determine the best conditions for sporulation for the strain or mutant of interest (Fig. 1; *see* **Note 8**).

3.2 Isolation of C. difficile Spores from Solid Medium

This method relies on the intrinsic alcohol and heat resistance of *C. difficile* spores to kill vegetative cells present in the spore stock. Importantly, this protocol does not remove lysed or killed vegetative cells or debris; however, this is not necessary for many downstream applications, including most animal studies [15].

1. Once the optimal sporulation conditions are determined for the *C. difficile* strain(s) of interest (Subheading 3.1), inoculate 3–10 fresh agar plates with an actively growing overnight culture, as outlined in Subheading 3.1, and incubate for the appropriate amount of time.

| Strain: | 630 | R20291 | 5325 | VPI 10463 |
| Ribotype: | 012 | 027 | 078 | 087 |

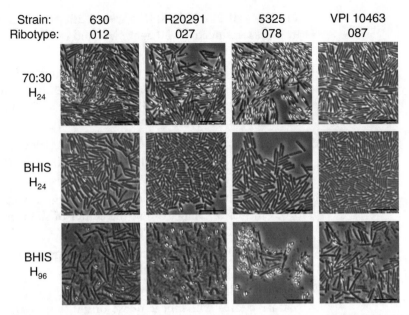

Fig. 1 Phase-contrast micrographs of *C. difficile* strains 630 [32, 33], R20291 [34], 5325 (ATCC BAA-1875), and VPI 10463 (ATCC 43255) grown on 70:30 sporulation medium agar plates or BHIS agar plates for the indicated amount of time (h). All strains were obtained from the ATCC except R20291, which was a gift from Linc Sonenshein. Images were corrected for exposure differences, which were applied uniformly across each image

2. At the appropriate time point(s), verify spore formation via phase-contrast microscopy as detailed above.

3. Remove plates from the anaerobic chamber. Scrape off the entire bacterial lawn using a sterile inoculating loop and resuspend in 10 ml 1× PBS. Vortex well to thoroughly resuspend the cells.

4. Centrifuge the cells at $8000 \times g$ for 10 min at room temperature.

5. Decant the supernatant and thoroughly resuspend the cell pellet in 10 ml 1× PBS.

6. Add 10 ml of 95 % ethanol to the resuspended cell pellet, vortex well and incubate at room temperature for 1 h.

7. Centrifuge the cells at $8000 \times g$ for 10 min at room temperature.

8. Decant the supernatant and resuspend in 20 ml 1× PBS. Wash twice more in 20 ml 1× PBS to ensure complete removal of residual ethanol.

9. Resuspend the cell pellet in 10 ml 1× PBS + 1 % BSA after final wash.

10. Heat spore stock to 70 °C for 20 min (*see* **Note 9**). Allow spore stock to cool to room temperature. Time permitting, immediately enumerate the spore stock (*see* Subheading 3.4).

3.3 Purification of
C. difficile Spores

Some downstream applications, including spore germination and outgrowth studies [7, 9], require pure spore stocks in which the spores are physically separated from vegetative cells, lysed mother cells, and other debris. This protocol describes a slightly different purification method than described in Subheading 3.2, and utilizes a density gradient centrifugation step to obtain free *C. difficile* spores [7, 9, 21].

1. Propagate spores as described in Subheading 3.1 to achieve the highest sporulation efficiency possible. At the appropriate time point(s), verify spore formation via phase-contrast microscopy as detailed above.

2. Remove plates from the chamber and resuspend cells from one-half of a plate in 1 ml sterile, ice-cold dH_2O. Repeat for the remaining half.

3. Centrifuge at $16,100 \times g$ for 2 min at 4 °C. Carefully remove supernatant and resuspend in 1 ml sterile, ice-cold dH_2O. Wash with sterile, ice-cold dH_2O two more times.

4. Incubate the spore preparation at –20 °C for 48 h to facilitate the lysis of mother cells and subsequent release of mature endospores.

5. After incubation, centrifuge at $16,100 \times g$ for 2 min at 4 °C, decant the supernatant and resuspend the spore preparation with 1 ml sterile, ice-cold dH_2O. Repeat for a total of five washes in sterile, ice-cold dH_2O as described in **step 3**.

6. After the final wash, combine both cell pellets in 3 ml sterile, ice-cold dH_2O.

7. Apply the entire 3 ml spore preparation slowly to the top of a 10 ml 50 % sucrose gradient in a 15 ml polypropylene conical tube.

8. Centrifuge in a swinging bucket rotor at $4000 \times g$ for 20 min at 4 °C. The vegetative cells and debris will collect at the interface and throughout the gradient, while the spores move through the gradient and form a pellet at the bottom of the centrifuge.

9. Remove the cell debris at the interface, then remove the rest of the solution, leaving the spore pellet.

10. Resuspend the spore pellet in 1 ml of sterile dH_2O. Centrifuge at $16,100 \times g$ for 2 min at room temperature, decant the supernatant and resuspend the spore preparation in 1 ml sterile dH_2O.

11. Repeat **step 10** for a total of five washes in sterile dH_2O and three washes in 1× PBS + 1 % BSA.

12. Resuspend the final spore preparation in 1 ml of 1× PBS + 1 % BSA and quantify as described in Subheading 3.4.

3.4 Enumeration of Initial Spore Stock and Serial Dilutions

To determine the number of viable spores per ml for the spore preparation, a range of serial dilutions of the primary, highly concentrated spore stock are plated and enumerated. The range of serial dilutions required to achieve accurate enumeration of a spore stock depends on the sporulation efficiency of the strain, the type and number of agar plates used for spore propagation, and the length of time the plates are incubated before beginning spore isolation and purification. *Remember*: when making serial dilutions of spores, vortex each dilution well and pipet up and down multiple times to reduce the retention of spores on tube walls and in pipet tips.

1. Pre-reduce the same number of BHIS supplemented with 0.1% taurocholate agar plates as the number of serial dilutions performed.

2. Vortex the spore stock vigorously for 15 s.

3. Prepare a series of tenfold dilutions in 1× PBS + 1% BSA. Dilute 100 μl of the spore stock into 900 μl 1× PBS + 1% BSA (which results in the 10^{-1} dilution). Dilute 100 μl of the 10^{-1} dilution into 900 μl 1× PBS + 1% BSA (which results in the 10^{-2} dilution). Continue until the appropriate dilutions have been made (*see* **Note 10** for an example).

4. Heat the dilutions to 55 °C for 20 min. *Important*: If you are performing these dilutions immediately after **step 10** in Subheading 3.2, the dilutions do not have to be reheated. However, a small proportion of spores become "inactivated" over time, and reheating the spore stocks immediately before plating assists in in vitro germination and provides more accurate representation of spores.

5. Cycle the reheated, serial dilutions into the anaerobic chamber. Apply 100 μl of each serial dilution onto individual pre-reduced BHIS supplemented with 0.1% taurocholate agar plates and evenly spread the dilution onto the surface of the plate using a sterile inoculating loop.

6. Incubate plates at 37 °C for at least 24 h to allow spore germination and sufficient growth of a colony.

7. Remove plates from chamber. For most accurate enumeration, use a plate that has between 30 and 300 colonies with few to no overlapping or clustered colonies (*see* **Note 11**).

8. Calculate the number of spores per ml of spore stock using the following equation:

$$\frac{CFU}{ml} = \frac{\text{Number of colonies} \left(CFU\right)}{\text{Dilution factor} \times \text{Volume plated} \left(ml\right)}$$

9. Finally, one last concern with the high concentration spore stocks is the presence of contaminants. Optionally, a small

amount of the spore stock (50–100 μl) may be plated onto (1) a BHIS agar plate and incubated aerobically and (2) a pre-reduced BHIS agar plate and incubated anaerobically to ensure no growth of non-*C. difficile* bacteria occurs. It is important to note here that a small number of *C. difficile* spores will germinate in the absence of taurocholate, so it is possible to see some *C. difficile* colonies on the BHIS agar plate incubated anaerobically. This will vary based on the strain of *C. difficile* used.

3.5 Preparation of Final Working Spore Stocks

To create a working spore stock, the original spore preparation needs to be diluted to the desired concentration. The working spore stock concentration will vary depending upon the downstream application (e.g., germination studies, spore outgrowth inhibition concentration (OIC) assays, and animal studies all use a wide range of spore concentrations [3, 7, 9, 15, 22–24]).

1. Calculate the dilution required to achieve the needed working spore stock concentration using the following equation (solve for X):

$$\text{Original stock concentration}\left(\frac{\text{CFU}}{\text{ml}}\right) \times X \text{ ml original stock}$$

$$= \text{Desired working stock concentration}\left(\frac{\text{CFU}}{\text{ml}}\right) \times \text{Total volume of working stock required}$$

Of note: it will likely be necessary to perform a few dilutions before making the final dilution of the final working spore stock.

2. Perform all dilutions using 1× PBS + 1% BSA as the diluent. Store the final working spore stock in glass or Teflon-coated tubes, as mentioned above, at room temperature. The shelf-life of spores varies by strain and stock, and should be retested if more than 2 weeks old. Remember to always reheat the spore stock to 55 °C for 20 min before replating.

4 Notes

1. 70:30 sporulation medium is a mixture of 70% SMC medium [14, 25] and 30% BHIS medium and was specifically developed to enhance and reliably determine the sporulation frequency of *C. difficile* [12].

2. A stock solution of 10% cysteine must be prepared fresh as cysteine will precipitate when stored at room temperature or cooler.

3. At H_{24} (24 h after plates are inoculated with an actively growing *C. difficile* culture), sporulation efficiency is ~30% for most strains tested when grown on 70:30 sporulation medium agar

plates (Fig. 1; unpublished data, Edwards and McBride), which is similar to previously observed sporulation frequencies on 70:30 sporulation plates for similar strains [12]. For unknown reasons, the sporulation efficiency significantly decreases after 70:30 sporulation medium is a week old. To obtain consistent results, we suggest using plates that are no more than 3 days old.

4. We achieve the most reliable and reproducible results in a variety of molecular biological assays by starting with *C. difficile* cultures that are in exponential phase. Oftentimes, overnight cultures of *C. difficile* will have already reached stationary phase after 12–16 h of growth. To combat this, we immediately dilute our initial, already-inoculated overnight culture 1:500 into another test tube with 10 ml BHIS supplemented with 0.1 % taurocholate and 0.2 % fructose. This results in two overnight cultures: the original culture and a 1:500 dilution of the original culture.

5. Because the protocol from this point is performed outside of the chamber, the use of pre-reduced BHIS medium is not important in this step. However, if the final time point has been reached or the plates will no longer be needed, the plates can be removed from the chamber, and this step may be performed in aerobic conditions.

6. The use of a thin agarose pad (0.7–1.0 % agarose) immobilizes the bacteria for microscopy. We caution against the use of higher percentages of agarose as this decreases the amount of visible light that can be seen through the sample.

7. Phase-contrast microscopy allows the observation of the later stages of sporulation (Stage IV+) in endospore-forming bacteria [26, 27] and is a frequently used technique to observe and quantitate sporulation frequencies in *C. difficile* [12, 15, 28–31]. Although this technique requires special equipment, it is easy to perform, does not require special dyes, sample fixation or preparation and is relatively inexpensive beyond the initial cost of the equipment. For the most accurate results, 100× magnification with oil immersion is needed.

8. Some strains do not always grow or sporulate well on 70:30 sporulation medium. Spores for these strains can instead be propagated on BHIS or TY agar plates. To increase the production and recovery of spores on these richer media, incubate plates for 4–5 days before harvesting.

9. To ensure that the 10 ml volume of spores is thoroughly heated to 70 °C, we have found it easier to divide the spores into 10–1 ml aliquots in microcentrifuge tubes and heat the spore preparation using a benchtop heat block. Once this step is completed, the aliquots are then recombined into a fresh conical tube.

10. When initially enumerating a new spore stock, we typically plate 100 µl of 10^{-4}, 10^{-5} and 10^{-6} dilutions of the original spore stock. With most strains, we easily obtain spore stocks of 1×10^8 CFU/ml from three to four 70:30 sporulation medium agar plates incubated for 48–72 h. For example, with a spore stock of this concentration, we obtain approximately 100 CFU on a BHIS supplemented with 0.1 % taurocholate agar plate inoculated with 100 µl of a 10^{-5} dilution.

11. Before removing plates from the chamber, ensure that all of the colonies are large enough to be accurately counted. If not, allow colonies to grow longer in the anaerobic chamber. While counting, we find placing the plate on top of a light source and using a digital colony counter allows the accurate enumeration of smaller and clustered colonies and reduces user error.

References

1. CDC (2013) Antibiotic resistance threats in the United States. In: Control CfD (ed) http://www.cdc.gov/features/Antibiotic ResistanceThreats/2013

2. Dubberke ER, Olsen MA (2012) Burden of *Clostridium difficile* on the healthcare system. Clin Infect Dis 55(Suppl 2):S88–S92, PMCID: 3388018

3. Sorg JA, Sonenshein AL (2008) Bile salts and glycine as cogerminants for Clostridium difficile spores. J Bacteriol 190(7):2505–2512, PMCID: 2293200

4. Chen X, Katchar K, Goldsmith JD, Nanthakumar N, Cheknis A, Gerding DN, Kelly CP (2008) A mouse model of Clostridium difficile-associated disease. Gastroenterology 135(6):1984–1992

5. Goulding D, Thompson H, Emerson J, Fairweather NF, Dougan G, Douce GR (2009) Distinctive profiles of infection and pathology in hamsters infected with Clostridium difficile strains 630 and B1. Infect Immun 77(12):5478–5485, PMCID: 2786451

6. Douce G, Goulding D (2010) Refinement of the hamster model of Clostridium difficile disease. Methods Mol Biol 646:215–227

7. Sorg JA, Sonenshein AL (2010) Inhibiting the initiation of Clostridium difficile spore germination using analogs of chenodeoxycholic acid, a bile acid. J Bacteriol 192(19):4983–4990, PMCID: 2944524

8. Francis MB, Allen CA, Shrestha R, Sorg JA (2013) Bile acid recognition by the Clostridium difficile germinant receptor, CspC, is important for establishing infection. PLoS Pathog 9(5):e1003356, PMCID: 3649964

9. Liu R, Suarez JM, Weisblum B, Gellman SH, McBride SM (2014) Synthetic polymers active against Clostridium difficile vegetative cell growth and spore outgrowth. J Am Chem Soc. PMCID: 4210120

10. Kuijper EJ, Coignard B, Tull P (2006) Emergence of Clostridium difficile-associated disease in North America and Europe. Clin Microbiol Infect 12(Suppl 6):2–18

11. Berg JM, Tymoczko JL, Stryer L, Stryer L (2002) Biochemistry, 5th edn. W.H. Freeman, New York

12. Putnam EE, Nock AM, Lawley TD, Shen A (2013) SpoIVA and SipL are Clostridium difficile spore morphogenetic proteins. J Bacteriol 195(6):1214–1225

13. George WL, Sutter VL, Citron D, Finegold SM (1979) Selective and differential medium for isolation of Clostridium difficile. J Clin Microbiol 9(2):214–219, PMCID: 272994

14. Wilson KH, Kennedy MJ, Fekety FR (1982) Use of sodium taurocholate to enhance spore recovery on a medium selective for Clostridium difficile. J Clin Microbiol 15(3):443–446, PMCID: 272115

15. Edwards AN, Nawrocki KL, McBride SM (2014) Conserved oligopeptide permeases modulate sporulation initiation in Clostridium difficile. Infect Immun 82(10):4276–4291

16. Bouillaut L, McBride SM, Sorg JA (2011) Genetic manipulation of Clostridium difficile. Curr Protoc Microbiol; Chapter 9: Unit 9A 2. PMCID: 3615975

17. Kuehne SA, Heap JT, Cooksley CM, Cartman ST, Minton NP (2011) ClosTron-mediated engineering of Clostridium. Methods Mol Biol 765:389–407

18. Francis MB, Sorg JA (2013) Virulence studies of Clostridium difficile. Bio-protocol 3(24):e1002

19. Edwards AN, Suarez JM, McBride SM (2013) Culturing and maintaining Clostridium difficile in an anaerobic environment. J Vis Exp (79)

20. Sorg JA, Dineen SS (2009) Laboratory maintenance of Clostridium difficile. Curr Protoc Microbiol; Chapter 9: Unit 9A.1

21. Lawley TD, Croucher NJ, Yu L, Clare S, Sebaihia M, Goulding D, Pickard DJ, Parkhill J, Choudhary J, Dougan G (2009) Proteomic and genomic characterization of highly infectious Clostridium difficile 630 spores. J Bacteriol 191(17):5377–5386, PMCID: 2725610

22. Sorg JA, Sonenshein AL (2009) Chenodeoxycholate is an inhibitor of Clostridium difficile spore germination. J Bacteriol 191(3):1115–1117

23. Francis MB, Allen CA, Sorg JA (2015) Spore cortex hydrolysis precedes DPA release during Clostridium difficile spore germination. J Bacteriol 197(14):2276–2283

24. Paredes-Sabja D, Bond C, Carman RJ, Setlow P, Sarker MR (2008) Germination of spores of Clostridium difficile strains, including isolates from a hospital outbreak of Clostridium difficile-associated disease (CDAD). Microbiology 154(Pt 8):2241–2250

25. Permpoonpattana P, Tolls EH, Nadem R, Tan S, Brisson A, Cutting SM (2011) Surface layers of Clostridium difficile endospores. J Bacteriol 193(23):6461–6470, PMCID: 3232898

26. Hashimoto T, Black SH, Gerhardt P (1960) Development of fine structure, thermostability, and dipicolinate during sporogenesis in a bacillus. Can J Microbiol 6:203–212

27. Hitchins AD, Kahn AJ, Slepecky RA (1968) Interference contrast and phase contrast microscopy of sporulation and germination of Bacillus megaterium. J Bacteriol 96(5):1811–1817, PMCID: 315245

28. Burns DA, Minton NP (2011) Sporulation studies in Clostridium difficile. J Microbiol Methods 87(2):133–138

29. Pereira FC, Saujet L, Tome AR, Serrano M, Monot M, Couture-Tosi E, Martin-Verstraete I, Dupuy B, Henriques AO (2013) The spore differentiation pathway in the enteric pathogen Clostridium difficile. PLoS Genet 9(10):e1003782, PMCID: 3789829

30. Fimlaid KA, Bond JP, Schutz KC, Putnam EE, Leung JM, Lawley TD, Shen A (2013) Global analysis of the sporulation pathway of Clostridium difficile. PLoS Genet 9(8):e1003660, PMCID: 3738446

31. Saujet L, Pereira FC, Serrano M, Soutourina O, Monot M, Shelyakin PV, Gelfand MS, Dupuy B, Henriques AO, Martin-Verstraete I (2013) Genome-wide analysis of cell type-specific gene transcription during spore formation in Clostridium difficile. PLoS Genet 9(10):e1003756, PMCID: 3789822

32. Sebaihia M, Wren BW, Mullany P, Fairweather NF, Minton N, Stabler R, Thomson NR, Roberts AP, Cerdeno-Tarraga AM, Wang H, Holden MT, Wright A, Churcher C, Quail MA, Baker S, Bason N, Brooks K, Chillingworth T, Cronin A, Davis P, Dowd L, Fraser A, Feltwell T, Hance Z, Holroyd S, Jagels K, Moule S, Mungall K, Price C, Rabbinowitsch E, Sharp S, Simmonds M, Stevens K, Unwin L, Whithead S, Dupuy B, Dougan G, Barrell B, Parkhill J (2006) The multidrug-resistant human pathogen Clostridium difficile has a highly mobile, mosaic genome. Nat Genet 38(7):779–786

33. Monot M, Boursaux-Eude C, Thibonnier M, Vallenet D, Moszer I, Medigue C, Martin-Verstraete I, Dupuy B (2011) Reannotation of the genome sequence of Clostridium difficile strain 630. J Med Microbiol 60(Pt 8):1193–1199

34. Stabler RA, He M, Dawson L, Martin M, Valiente E, Corton C, Lawley TD, Sebaihia M, Quail MA, Rose G, Gerding DN, Gibert M, Popoff MR, Parkhill J, Dougan G, Wren BW (2009) Comparative genome and phenotypic analysis of Clostridium difficile 027 strains provides insight into the evolution of a hypervirulent bacterium. Genome Biol 10(9):R102, PMCID: 2768977

Chapter 10

Inducing and Quantifying *Clostridium difficile* Spore Formation

Aimee Shen, Kelly A. Fimlaid, and Keyan Pishdadian

Abstract

The Gram-positive nosocomial pathogen *Clostridium difficile* induces sporulation during growth in the gastrointestinal tract. Sporulation is necessary for this obligate anaerobe to form metabolically dormant spores that can resist antibiotic treatment, survive exit from the mammalian host, and transmit *C. difficile* infections. In this chapter, we describe a method for inducing *C. difficile* sporulation in vitro. This method can be used to study sporulation and maximize spore purification yields for a number of *C. difficile* strain backgrounds. We also describe procedures for visualizing spore formation using phase-contrast microscopy and for quantifying the efficiency of sporulation using heat resistance as a measure of functional spore formation.

Key words Sporulation, Spore, Phase-contrast microscopy, Induction

1 Introduction

The Gram-positive spore-former *Clostridium difficile* is a leading cause of health care-associated infections around the world and a primary cause of antibiotic-associated diarrhea [1]. In order for *C. difficile* to cause infection, its metabolically dormant spore-form must germinate in the gastrointestinal tract and outgrow to form toxin-producing vegetative cells [2]. Since the vegetative form of *C. difficile* cannot tolerate extended exposure to oxygen [3], *C. difficile* must form spores prior to exiting the host [4]. Spore formation is thus essential for *C. difficile* survival outside of the host as well as for disease transmission. In order to study the developmental processes of spore formation and germination, a method for efficiently inducing sporulation in a genetically tractable *C. difficile* strain background is essential. In addition, a method for quantifying functional spore formation is critical for identifying factors that affect spore formation and/or germination [4].

This report describes a method for strongly inducing *C. difficile* sporulation in vitro [5] and measuring heat-resistant spore

Adam P. Roberts and Peter Mullany (eds.), *Clostridium difficile: Methods and Protocols*, Methods in Molecular Biology, vol. 1476,
DOI 10.1007/978-1-4939-6361-4_10, © Springer Science+Business Media New York 2016

formation [6]. While this method is frequently used to measure sporulation efficiency, it is important to note that heat-resistant spore formation reflects the ability of C. *difficile* to not only form spores but also to germinate those spores (typically in response to the bile salt germinant taurocholate [7]). Heat-resistance defects can result from defects at any stage of (1) spore assembly, including but not limited to, the initiation of sporulation to the assembly of coat [5, 6, 8, 9], and (2) germination, including but not limited to, germinant sensing and cortex hydrolysis [10, 11]. Certain mutations can also enhance heat-resistant spore formation [12].

The sporulation induction method described here can also be used to obtain samples for Western blot analysis [5], RNA isolation [6], and spore purification [10]; a detailed procedure for purifying spores is described in Chapter XX. While alternative methods for inducing sporulation in broth culture exist and are particularly well suited for kinetic analyses and fluorescence microscopy analyses of sporulation [8, 9, 13], this method does not work as well for all C. *difficile* strains. In addition to using this method to induce sporulation in the genetically tractable JIR8094 strain [14], a derivative of strain 630 [15], we have also used this method of sporulation induction to obtain high yields of the non-toxigenic strains ATCC 43601 [16] and ATCC 43593 [16], and in unpublished work, the virulent clinical isolates M120 [17], M68 [18], 630 (including Δerm variants, Fig. 1, [19, 20]), and R20291 (Fig. 1 [21]).

2 Materials

2.1 Reagents

1. Bacto Peptone (Becton Dickinson BBL/Difco, Franklin Lakes, NJ).

2. Protease Peptone (Becton Dickinson BBL/Difco, Franklin Lakes, NJ).

3. Brain Heart Infusion Broth (Becton Dickinson BBL/Difco, Franklin Lakes, NJ).

4. Ammonium sulfate (NH$_4$SO$_4$, Fisher Bioreagents Waltham, MA).

5. Tris Base (Fisher Bioreagents, Waltham, MA).

6. Brain Heart Infusion Broth (BHI, Thermo Scientific Remel, Waltham, MA).

7. Yeast Extract (Fisher Bioreagents, Pittsburgh, PA).

8. Agar (Fisher Bioreagents, Pittsburgh, PA).

9. l-cysteine (Acros Organics, Thermo Fisher Scientific, Waltham, MA).

10. Taurocholate (TA, Alfa Aesar, Ward Hill, MA).

11. Phosphate buffered saline (PBS, Fisher Bioreagents, Waltham, MA).

12. Thiamphenicol (if strain is carrying exogenous plasmid for complementation studies, Acros Organics, ThermoFisher Scientific, Waltham, MA).

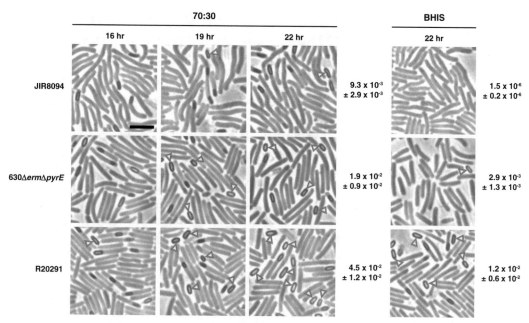

Fig. 1 Effect of media composition on the sporulation of commonly used *C. difficile* strains. Three genetically tractable strains [4, 14, 19, 28] were analyzed for spore formation on BHIS [22] and 70:30 [5] media plates using phase-contrast microscopy at the indicated time points; heat-resistant spore formation was assayed after 22 h growth. R20291 exhibits a higher level of sporulation relative to 630 and JIR8094 when grown on BHIS media plates alone. As a result, growth of R20291 on BHIS(TA) plates for overnight cultures may lead to carryover of spores in the inoculum used to initiate sporulation on 70:30 plates. Since this elevated rate of sporulation may complicate measurements of heat-resistant spore formation using the plate-based method described here, it may be necessary to use the broth-based method for inducing sporulation to allow for more accurate quantification of sporulation induction. Using a lower inoculum to induce sporulation of R20291 would minimize the contribution of preexisting spores to measurements of sporulation efficiency. In contrast, JIR8094 sporulates poorly when grown on BHIS plates but can be induced to sporulate at significantly higher levels when grown on 70:30 as previously shown [5], highlighting the importance of sporulation media on spore formation. Regardless, sporulation induction on 70:30 plates increased heat-resistant spore production in 630Δ*erm*Δ*pyrE* and R20291 strains by ~7-fold and ~4-fold, respectively. The heat resistance reported (H.R.) shown represents the average of three biological replicates; the associated standard deviations are shown. *Red arrows* demarcate mature, phase-bright spores. Scale bars represent 5 μm

13. Sterile, disposable 10 μL inoculating loops (Nunc, Thermo Fisher Scientific, Waltham, MA).

14. 96-well sterile U-bottom plates (Corning, Corning, NY).

15. Glass slides (25 mm × 75 mm × 1.0 mm, Thermo Fisher Scientific, Waltham, MA).

16. Glass coverslips (25 mm × 50 mm × 0.18 mm, Thermo Fisher Scientific, Waltham, MA).

17. Kimwipes (21.33 × 11.17 cm, Kimberly-Clark, Milton, NH).

18. 0.1–10 μL filter tips (USA Scientific, Orlando, FL).

19. 10–40 μL filter tips (USA Scientific, Orlando, FL).

20. 10–300 μL filter tips (USA Scientific, Orlando, FL).

21. 100–1000 μL filter tips (USA Scientific, Orlando, FL).

22. Permanent markers (multiple colors ideally, Sharpie).

2.2 Media

1. 70:30 media.
   - To make 1 L of media, add 63 g Bacto Peptone, 3.5 g Protease Peptone, 0.7 g NH_4SO_4, 1.6 g Tris Base, 11.1 g Brain Heart Infusion Broth, 1.5 g Yeast Extract, 15 g Agar to a 2 L Erlenmeyer flask. Add 1 L of milliQ water (*see* **Note 1**) and autoclave for 30–40 min. Cool to 55 °C and add 3 mL 10 % (w/v) Cysteine. Mix thoroughly and pour plates thick (*see* **Notes 2** and **3**).

2. BHIS(TA) plates.
   - To make 1 L of media, add 37 g of Brain Heart Infusion Broth, 5 g of yeast extract, 15 g agar to a 2 L Erlenmeyer flask. Add 1 L of milliQ water (*see* **Note 1**) and autoclave for 30–40 min. Cool to 55 °C and add 10 mL 10 % (w/v) Cysteine and 10 mL of 10 % (w/v) taurocholate (*see* **Notes 2** and **4**). Mix thoroughly and pour plates.

2.3 Equipment

1. Microscope with 100× objective for phase-contrast microscopy.

2. Water baths or heat blocks for stably heating the sample to 60 °C.

3. Multichannel pipettes (0.5–10 μL, 1–100 μL, and 10–200 μL).

3 Methods

3.1 Inducing Sporulation

<u>Day 1</u>

1. Pre-dry and pre-reduce BHIS(TA) plates (1 per strain) at least 3 h in advance of streaking out strains.

2. Streak out strains to be used in sporulation assay from frozen stocks onto BHIS(TA) plates [22] (*see* **Note 5**).

3. Grow strains anaerobically for 20–28 h (*see* **Note 6**).

4. Pre-dry and pre-reduce 70:30 plates needed to induce sporulation (e.g., 1 plate per strain being tested for heat resistance assay, *see* **Notes 7** and **8**).

<u>Day 2</u>

1. Using a 10 μL inoculating loop, scrape up 1/5 loopful of colonies from the BHIS(TA) plate (*see* **Note 9**).

2. Inoculate the loopful down the center of the plate using tight "squiggles" to try and spread the initial inoculum down the center of the plate.

3. Use the loop to spread the inoculum across the entire plate using back-and-forth motions to reach every edge of the plate. This inoculation step represents the 0 h time point of the sporulation assay (*see* **Notes 10** and **11**).

4. Incubate the plates anaerobically for at least 12 h. Sporulation is maximal ~20–24 h ([8], Fig. 1, *see* **Note 12**). Samples for RNA isolation, Western blotting, and microscopy analyses can be taken at a variety of time points that should be empirically determined (*see* **Note 13**).

5. Pre-dry and pre-reduce BHIS(TA) plates (*see* **Note 14**) that will be used to measure heat-resistant spore formation.

6. If performing a heat-resistance assay, label the following sets of 1.5 mL microcentrifuge tubes to pre-reduce in the chamber overnight. Each set comprises the number of strains tested in the sporulation assay.

   (a) *Set 1*: Add 750 µL PBS to these tubes (labeled 1, 2, 3, etc. with black marker). These tubes will be used to harvest samples in the chamber for phase contrast microscopy and Western blotting.

   (b) *Set 2*: Add 600 µL PBS to these tubes (labeled 1-N in blue marker) for measuring the number of viable cells and spores in the "Untreated" sample.

   (c) *Set 3*: Label these tubes 1-N in red marker (they remain empty). These will become the "Heat-treated" samples for measuring the number of viable spores in the sample.

Day 3

Phase contrast microscopy (see **Note 15***)*

1. At the time point desired (at least 12 h after sporulation has been induced), harvest half of the 70:30 plate lawn into the tubes for "Set 1" using a 10 µL inoculating loop. Shake the loop vigorously to remove the cells from the loop (or twirl the loop).

2. Remove the samples for "Set 1" from the chamber.

3. Pellet the cells at maximum speed for 3–5 min.

4. Remove the supernatant, and thoroughly resuspend the pellet in 100 µL PBS (*see* **Note 16**).

5. Optional: harvest samples for Western blotting by transferring 50 µL of cells into tubes and processing as described by Adams et al. ([10], *see* **Note 17**).

6. Remove 7 µL of the sample and pipet it onto a glass slide in a continuous line.

7. Cover the sample with a cover slip (*see* **Note 18**).

8. Fold a Kimwipes lengthwise into fourths. Place the Kimwipes on top of the slide and apply even pressure onto the coverslip using your palm or a microcentrifuge rack (*see* **Note 19**).

9. Analyze the sample using phase-contrast microscopy (Fig. 2, *see* **Note 20**). Image enough fields of view to enumerate ~500 cells/sample (*see* **Note 21**).

3.2 Quantifying Sporulation Using Heat Resistance

<u>Day 3</u>

1. Prepare two 96-well plates for performing 1:10 serial dilutions of the "Untreated" and "Heat-treated" samples (*see* **Note 22**).

   - For each "Untreated" sample, use a multichannel pipette to add 90 μL PBS to 7 wells, for 10^{-1} and 10^{-7} dilutions.

   - For each "Heat-treated" sample, leave the first well empty, and use a multichannel pipette to add 90 μL PBS to the six rows below, for undiluted and 10^{-6} dilutions. Mark the top of the plate with a red sharpie to indicate that the samples will be heat treated.

2. Preheat a heat block or water bath to 60 °C (ensure that it is at temperature before beginning the assay, *see* **Note 23**).

3. At the time point desired for measuring heat resistance, harvest the remaining half of the plate into the "Set 2" tubes using a 10 μL inoculating loop. Shake the loop vigorously to remove the cells from the loop (or twirl the loop, *see* **Note 24**).

4. Pipet the mixture several times to ensure an even suspension and then transfer 300 μL of the sample into the empty "Set 3" tubes.

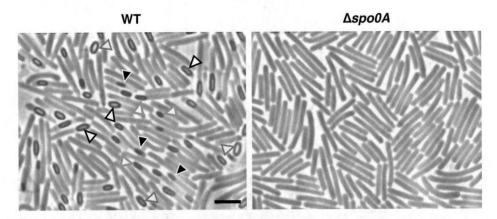

Fig. 2 Phase-contrast microscopy analyses comparing sporulating 630Δ*erm*Δ*pyrE* [28] relative to a Δ*spo0A*Δ*erm*Δ*pyrE* mutant incapable of initiating sporulation after 24 h of growth on 70:30 media. *Black arrows* indicate immature phase-dark forespores; *blue arrows* demarcate phase-dark forespores that appear to have completed engulfment as indicated by the phase-dark outline surrounding the forespore; *white arrows* indicate phase-bright forespores; and *red arrows* demarcate mature, phase-bright spores. Scale bars represent 5 μm

5. Remove the "Untreated" and "Heat-treated" samples from the chamber.

6. Place the "Heat-treated" sample into the 60 °C heat block and incubate for 30–40 min. Invert the "Heat-treated" sample every 10 min during this incubation to ensure even heating.

7. Meanwhile, briefly vortex the "Untreated" sample then add 10 μL of the "Untreated" cell suspension into 90 μL of PBS in the first row of the 96-well plate (*see* **Note 25**).

8. Make six additional 1:10 serial dilutions of the "Untreated" samples: use the 1–100 μL multichannel pipette to transfer 10 μL of the sample into the next well containing 90 μL of PBS, and use the 10–200 μL multichannel pipette to mix the sample between dilutions (*see* **Note 26**).

9. Transfer the "Untreated" sample dilutions into the chamber. This plate will contain 10^{-1} to 10^{-7} dilutions of the "Untreated" sample.

10. Plate 4.5 μL of the 10^{-2} to 10^{-7} dilutions in triplicate onto the BHIS(TA) plates on the "Untreated" side of the plate (*see* **Note 27**).

11. Following heat treatment, briefly vortex the "Heat-treated" sample and transfer 100 μL into the empty well in the 96-well "Heat treated" plate.

12. Make six additional 1:10 serial dilutions of the "Heat-treated" sample: use the 1–100 μL multichannel pipette to transfer 10 μL of the sample into the next well containing 90 μL of PBS, and use the 10–300 μL multichannel pipette to mix the sample between dilutions. The plate will contain the undiluted sample.

13. Plate 4.5 μL of the undiluted to 10^{-6} dilutions in triplicate onto the BHIS(TA) plates on the "Heat-treated" side of the plate (*see* **Note 28**).

Day 4

1. After 20–22 h after plating the "Untreated" and "Heat-treated" samples, count the numbers of colony forming units (CFUs) for the lowest dilution in which colonies are visible (*see* **Note 29**).

2. For a given replicate, determine the ratio of heat-resistant spores by dividing the CFUs for the "Heat-treated" sample by the CFUs for the "Untreated" sample (*see* **Note 30** and Table 1).

3. Determine the average ratio of "Heat-treated" CFUs: "Untreated" CFUs for each replicate performed (*see* Table 1).

4. To determine the sporulation efficiency of a strain relative to a reference strain, divide the average ratio of "Heat-treated"

Table 1

Example calculation of heat-resistant spore formation for 630ΔermΔpyrE as shown in Fig. 1 after 22 h of growth on 70:30 plates

630ΔermΔpyrE	Treatment	Dil.	1	2	3	Avg	Cell count	Ratio of spores
Replicate 1	Untreated	10^{-7}	4	3	4	3.67	3.7×10^7	1.1×10^{-2}
Replicate 2	Untreated	10^{-7}	5	4	7	5.33	5.3×10^7	2.8×10^{-2}
Replicate 3	Untreated	10^{-7}	4	4	3	3.67	3.7×10^7	1.7×10^{-2}
Replicate 1	Heat	10^{-5}	5	5	2	4.00	4.0×10^5	*Average H.R.*
Replicate 2	Heat	10^{-5}	9	19	17	15.00	1.5×10^6	(avg) 1.9×10^{-2}
Replicate 3	Heat	10^{-5}	7	9	3	6.33	6.3×10^5	(stdev) 0.9×10^{-2}

Replicates represent three independent biological replicates, i.e., cultures derived from three separate 70:30 plates. The "Heat-treated" samples were incubated at 60 °C for 30 min. The counts for the 4.5 μL spots plated in triplicate (1–3) are given for the indicated dilution (Dil.). The ratio of heat-resistant spores was determined by dividing the average (Avg) cell count for the "Heat"-treated sample of a given replicate by the average cell count of the equivalent "Untreated" sample. Average heat resistance (H.R.) represents the mean of the ratio of heat-resistant spores for the three biological replicates. Stdev represents the standard deviation of the sample.

CFUs:"Untreated" CFUs for a given strain by the average ratio of "Heat-treated" CFUs:"Untreated" CFUs measured for the reference strain.

4   Notes

1. Please note that we do not account for the change in volume caused by the media components.

2. 10% (w/v) cysteine: For 1 L of media, dissolve 1.1 g of l-cysteine in 11 mL water. Warm to 55 °C, and filter-sterilize. Add 3.5 mL of solution to 1 L of 70:30 media; 10 mL of solution to 1 L of BHIS(TA) media.

3. The thickness of the plate can affect the sporulation efficiency of a given strain. If the plates are too thin, sporulation is likely to be reduced (Fig. 3). At least 30 mL of media should be added per plate.

4. 10% (w/v) taurocholate: For 1 L of media, dissolve 1.1 g of taurocholate in 11 mL water. Warm to 55 °C then filter-sterilize. Add 10 mL of solution to 1 L of BHIS(TA) media.

5. A *spo0A* mutant is a critical control for testing heat-resistant spore formation to ensure that the heat treatment kills all vegetative cells ([23], Fig. 2). Alternatively, a strain that cannot produce heat-resistant spores due to a different sporulation defect can be used instead of a *spo0A* mutant [6, 25].

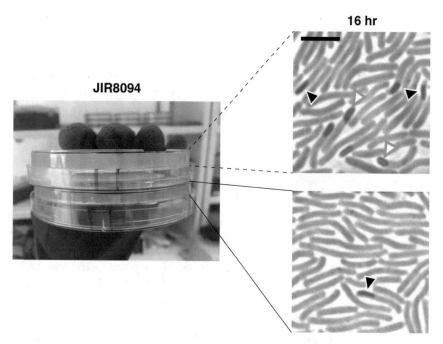

Fig. 3 Effect of 70:30 plate thickness on the sporulation of JIR8094. Inoculums taken from the same overnight BHIS(TA) plate were used to inoculate the plates shown on the *left* and incubated for 16 h. *Black arrows* indicate immature phase-dark forespores; *blue arrows* demarcate phase-dark forespores that appear to have completed engulfment as indicated by the phase-dark outline surrounding the forespore. Scale bars represent 5 μm

6. The age of the inoculum can affect the efficiency of sporulation, although it probably varies depending on anaerobic chamber conditions and thus may vary between labs. In our experience, overnight growth between 20 and 26 h leads to maximal spore formation.

7. The plates need to pre-dried because excess water on the plates reduces sporulation. In addition, high humidity in the chamber can also reduce sporulation.

8. The 70:30 media was optimized for maximizing sporulation of JIR8094 [5]. In our experience, the 70:30 media works for a wider range of *C. difficile* strains, but it should be noted that SM(C) media [8, 9, 13, 26] may give maximum sporulation yields for certain strains. It may be beneficial to empirically determine the optimal sporulation media for your strain of interest (Fig. 1).

9. Large colonies should be visible at this time. The inoculum size can affect the efficiency of spore formation—too light of an inoculum will lead to reduced sporulation, as will too much. If the colonies obtained from re-streaking from frozen stock are small, scrape up more of the plate to acquire enough cells to inoculate the 70:30 plate.

10. Continuously rotate the plate slightly to ensure that the inoculum is spread across the entire plate. The goal is to create an even lawn of *C. difficile* over the entire plate.

11. In our hands, we have observed that frequently refreshing the gas mix in the chamber enhances sporulation.

12. Sporulation is asynchronously induced from the initial inoculum. In our hands and in other reports, it does not appear to significantly increase over the course of 2 days [8, 13], although others have reported an increase in sporulation levels [26, 27]. Sporulation can be partially synchronized during growth in broth culture [13].

13. For RNA analyses, we typically harvest sporulating cells at 18 h to maximize sporulation-related transcript levels. For Western blot analyses, we typically harvest sporulating cells at 24 h, although the harvesting time points used can be empirically determined to maximize detection of the protein of interest. For heat resistance assays, we typically harvest samples 22–24 h after sporulation induction.

14. Do not include antibiotics in these plates even if the strains used are carrying a plasmid encoding thiamphenicol resistance, since thiamphenicol will cause significantly slower growth.

15. Prior to performing a heat resistance assay, we always check the level of sporulation by phase-contrast microscopy to ensure that the samples are sporulating. In our experience primarily working with the JIR8094 strain, sporulation levels can be quite variable from day-to-day, and there are periods of times where sporulation does not work very well due to variation in humidity, plates, etc. in the chamber.

16. If harvesting samples for RNA, we resuspend the pellet directly into RNA*pro*™ solution and isolate RNA as per the manufacturer's directions (MP Biomedicals, [6])

17. We typically save Western blot samples in duplicate.

18. Ideally, the sample will form a continuous line across the slide to facilitate the sample being spread across the entire slide when the coverslip is added.

19. The goal is to flatten the sample sufficiently so that the cells are present in a single layer, i.e., the cells are densely arranged, the cells are immobilized, and the overlapping cells should be minimized (Fig. 2).

20. Developing forespores will appear phase-dark typically after engulfment has been completed (or at least initiated in some mutants with engulfment defects, Fig. 2, black arrows). Sporulating cells that have completed engulfment and produce cortex but fail to localize coat around the forespore will frequently have a phase-dark forespore that appears to be out-

lined in black ([5, 25], Fig. 2, blue arrows). Mature forespores appear phase-bright, typically when the coat surrounds the forespore ([5, 25], Fig. 2, white arrows). Mature spores will be phase-bright in their center and outlined in a black (Fig. 2, red arrows). It should be noted that phase-contrast microscopy will not detect cells that have initiated sporulation and/or completed asymmetric division [6].

21. These can be analyzed using the Cell Counter in ImageJ to determine percent sporulation.

22. We normally mark the bottom of the round bottom wells with a Sharpie marker (different colors for each column) to help visualize the column being plated when the dilutions are in the chamber. It can be difficult to keep track of which column you are plating, and the colored bottom of the plate can be beneficial.

23. Depending on the reliability of your heat block, it may be helpful to add water to the heat block to ensure uniform and rapid heating of the sample.

24. Since the heat resistance assay is quite time sensitive, particularly with respect to oxygen exposure (see note below), ensure that you have enough 0.1–10 μL filter tips in the chamber for plating the samples onto BHIS(TA) plates as well as the filter tips for performing the sample dilutions on your bench. Heat treatments vary from 60 to 70 °C for between 25 and 40 min [6, 8, 9, 13, 23].

25. It is important to work quickly to minimize exposure of the "Untreated" sample to oxygen. A decrease in the number of viable vegetative cells will artificially inflate the measurement of the efficiency of heat-resistant spore formation. We typically measure $\sim 1 \times 10^7$ cells in 10 μL of sample using the described protocol. If you anticipate it will take more than 5 min to prepare your dilutions, perform the dilutions in the chamber.

26. Each time a 10 μL sample dilution is added to 90 μL PBS on the plate, mark that you have added the sample to the indicated row using a Sharpie marker to ensure that you do not skip a dilution.

27. We use the lid of the 96-well plate to cover up samples that have not been plated yet. After you plate the dilutions for a given sample, move the plate to uncover the next set of samples. Along with the colored marker on the bottom of the round bottom plate, this strategy helps to ensure that the correct sample is plated onto the correct plate.

28. Depending on the strain background, it may not be necessary to plate all the dilutions indicated, since strains can vary widely in their sporulation efficiency (Fig. 1, [23]). For JIR8094, we plate the undiluted sample through to the 10^{-5} dilution, but

for the R20291 and 630 strain backgrounds, we plate up to the 10^{-6} dilution. The dynamic range of the experiment thus depends on the level of sporulation of the wild type strain being studied (e.g., $<10^{-6}$ for JIR8094, $<10^{-7}$ for R20291 and 630 strain backgrounds).

29. The dilution should contain at least 3 CFUs and generally less than 30 CFUs for accurate counting. It may be necessary to count the second lowest dilution as well, if the CFUs are close to the upper or lower limits of this range cells per condition). The 20–22 h time point for measuring CFUs is chosen to minimize the chance that the colonies overgrow into each other, reducing the CFU count. However, it may be necessary to optimize this time point based on the culturing conditions in the chamber and strain background used.

30. In order to determine the sporulation efficiency of a given strain relative to a reference strain or growth condition, the heat resistance assay must be performed in triplicate. Some strains exhibit greater variability in their sporulation efficiency between replicates, since many factors can affect the efficiency of sporulation as described in the notes.

Acknowledgments

K.F. is supported by T32 AI055402 from the National Institute of Allergy and Infectious Disease. A.S. is a Pew Scholar in the Biomedical Sciences, supported by The Pew Charitable Trusts; work in this manuscript was supported by start-up funds from Award Number P20 GM103496 and R01GM108684 from the National Institute of General Medical Sciences. The content is solely the responsibility of the authors and does not necessarily reflect the views of the Pew Charitable Trusts, the National Institute of Allergy and Infectious Disease, the National Institute of General Medical Sciences, or the National Institute of Health.

References

1. Rupnik M, Wilcox M, Gerding D (2009) Clostridium difficile infection: new developments in epidemiology and pathogenesis. Nat Rev Microbiol 7(7):526–536. doi:10.1038/nrmicro2164

2. Paredes-Sabja D, Shen A, Sorg JA (2014) Clostridium difficile spore biology: sporulation, germination, and spore structural proteins. Trends Microbiol. doi:10.1016/j.tim.2014.04.003

3. Jump RL, Pultz MJ, Donskey CJ (2007) Vegetative Clostridium difficile survives in room air on moist surfaces and in gastric contents with reduced acidity: a potential mechanism to explain the association between proton pump inhibitors and C. difficile-associated diarrhea? Antimicrob Agents Chemother 51(8):2883–2887. doi:10.1128/AAC.01443-06

4. Deakin LJ, Clare S, Fagan RP, Dawson LF, Pickard DJ, West MR, Wren BW, Fairweather NF, Dougan G, Lawley TD (2012) The Clostridium difficile spo0A gene is a persistence and transmission factor. Infect Immun 80(8):2704–2711. doi:10.1128/IAI.00147-12, IAI.00147-12 [pii]

5. Putnam EE, Nock AM, Lawley TD, Shen A (2013) SpoIVA and SipL are *Clostridium difficile* spore morphogenetic proteins. J Bacteriol 195(6):1214–1225. doi:10.1128/JB.02181-12

6. Fimlaid KA, Bond JP, Schutz KC, Putnam EE, Leung JM, Lawley TD, Shen A (2013) Global analysis of the sporulation pathway of *Clostridium difficile*. PLoS Genet 9(8):e1003660. doi:10.1371/journal.pgen.1003660

7. Sorg JA, Sonenshein AL (2008) Bile salts and glycine as cogerminants for *Clostridium difficile* spores. J Bacteriol 190(7):2505–2512. doi:10.1128/JB.01765-07, JB.01765-07 [pii]

8. Pereira FC, Saujet L, Tome AR, Serrano M, Monot M, Couture-Tosi E, Martin-Verstraete I, Dupuy B, Henriques AO (2013) The spore differentiation pathway in the enteric pathogen *Clostridium difficile*. PLoS Genet 9(10):e1003782. doi:10.1371/journal.pgen.1003782

9. Saujet L, Pereira FC, Serrano M, Soutourina O, Monot M, Shelyakin PV, Gelfand MS, Dupuy B, Henriques AO, Martin-Verstraete I (2013) Genome-wide analysis of cell type-specific gene transcription during spore formation in *Clostridium difficile*. PLoS Genet 9(10):e1003756. doi:10.1371/journal.pgen.1003756

10. Adams C, Eckenroth B, Putnam E, Doublie S, Shen A (2013) Structural and functional analysis of the CspB protease required for Clostridium spore germination. PLoS Pathog 9(2):e1003165

11. Francis MB, Allen CA, Shrestha R, Sorg JA (2013) Bile acid recognition by the *Clostridium difficile* germinant receptor, CspC, is important for establishing infection. PLoS Pathog 9(5):e1003356. doi:10.1371/journal.ppat.1003356

12. Edwards AN, Nawrocki KL, McBride SM (2014) Conserved oligopeptide permeases modulate sporulation initiation in *Clostridium difficile*. Infect Immun 82(10):4276–4291. doi:10.1128/IAI.02323-14

13. Dembek M, Barquist L, Boinett CJ, Cain AK, Mayho M, Lawley TD, Fairweather NF, Fagan RP (2015) High-throughput analysis of gene essentiality and sporulation in *Clostridium difficile*. mBio 6(2):e02383. doi:10.1128/mBio.02383-14

14. Dineen SS, Villapakkam AC, Nordman JT, Sonenshein AL (2007) Repression of *Clostridium difficile* toxin gene expression by CodY. Mol Microbiol 66(1):206–219. doi:10.1111/j.1365-2958.2007.05906.x, MMI5906 [pii]

15. Sebaihia M, Wren B, Mullany P, Fairweather N, Minton N, Stabler R, Thomson N, Roberts A, Cerdeño-Tárraga A, Wang H, Holden M, Wright A, Churcher C, Quail M, Baker S, Bason N, Brooks K, Chillingworth T, Cronin A, Davis P, Dowd L, Fraser A, Feltwell T, Hance Z, Holroyd S, Jagels K, Moule S, Mungall K, Price C, Rabbinowitsch E, Sharp S, Simmonds M, Stevens K, Unwin L, Whitehead S, Dupuy B, Dougan G, Barrell B, Parkhill J (2006) The multidrug-resistant human pathogen *Clostridium difficile* has a highly mobile, mosaic genome. Nat Genet 38(7):779–786. doi:10.1038/ng1830

16. Wang S, Shen A, Setlow P, Li YQ (2015) Characterization of the dynamic germination of individual *Clostridium difficile* spores using Raman spectroscopy and differential interference contrast microscopy. J Bacteriol 197(14):2361–2373. doi:10.1128/JB.00200-15

17. He M, Sebaihia M, Lawley T, Stabler R, Dawson L, Martin M, Holt K, Seth-Smith H, Quail M, Rance R, Brooks K, Churcher C, Harris D, Bentley S, Burrows C, Clark L, Corton C, Murray V, Rose G, Thurston S, van Tonder A, Walker D, Wren B, Dougan G, Parkhill J (2010) Evolutionary dynamics of *Clostridium difficile* over short and long time scales. Proc Natl Acad Sci U S A 107(16):7527–7532. doi:10.1073/pnas.0914322107

18. Lawley T, Clare S, Walker A, Goulding D, Stabler R, Croucher N, Mastroeni P, Scott P, Raisen C, Mottram L, Fairweather N, Wren B, Parkhill J, Dougan G (2009) Antibiotic treatment of *Clostridium difficile* carrier mice triggers a supershedder state, spore-mediated transmission, and severe disease in immunocompromised hosts. Infect Immun 77(9):3661–3669. doi:10.1128/iai.00558-09

19. Heap J, Kuehne S, Ehsaan M, Cartman S, Cooksley C, Scott J, Minton N (2010) The ClosTron: mutagenesis in Clostridium refined and streamlined. J Microbiol Methods 80(1):49–55. doi:10.1016/j.mimet.2009.10.018

20. van Eijk E, Anvar SY, Browne HP, Leung WY, Frank J, Schmitz AM, Roberts AP, Smits WK (2015) Complete genome sequence of the *Clostridium difficile* laboratory strain 630Deltaerm reveals differences from strain 630, including translocation of the mobile element CTn5. BMC Genomics 16:31. doi:10.1186/s12864-015-1252-7

21. Stabler R, He M, Dawson L, Martin M, Valiente E, Corton C, Lawley T, Sebaihia M, Quail M, Rose G, Gerding D, Gibert M, Popoff M, Parkhill J, Dougan G, Wren B (2009) Comparative genome and phenotypic analysis of *Clostridium difficile* 027 strains provides insight into the evolution of a hypervirulent bacterium. Genome Biol 10(9):R102. doi:10.1186/gb-2009-10-9-r102

22. Sorg JA, Dineen SS (2009) Laboratory maintenance of *Clostridium difficile*. Curr Protoc Microbiol Chapter 9:Unit 9A 1. doi:10.1002/9780471729259.mc09a01s12

23. Burns DA, Minton NP (2011) Sporulation studies in *Clostridium difficile*. J Microbiol Methods 87(2):133–138.doi:10.1016/j.mimet.2011.07.017

24. Kevorkian Y, Shirley DJ, Shen A (2015) Regulation of *Clostridium difficile* spore germination by the CspA pseudoprotease domain. Biochimie. doi:10.1016/j.biochi.2015.07.023

25. Pishdadian K, Fimlaid KA, Shen A (2015) SpoIIID-mediated regulation of sigma(K) function during *Clostridium difficile* sporulation. Mol Microbiol 95(2):189–208. doi:10.1111/mmi.12856

26. Permpoonpattana P, Tolls E, Nadem R, Tan S, Brisson A, Cutting S (2011) Surface layers of *Clostridium difficile* endospores. J Bacteriol 193(23):6461–6470. doi:10.1128/jb.05182-11

27. Phetcharaburanin J, Hong HA, Colenutt C, Bianconi I, Sempere L, Permpoonpattana P, Smith K, Dembek M, Tan S, Brisson MC, Brisson AR, Fairweather NF, Cutting SM (2014) The spore-associated protein BclA1 affects the susceptibility of animals to colonization and infection by *Clostridium difficile*. Mol Microbiol 92(5):1025–1038. doi:10.1111/mmi.12611

28. Ng YK, Ehsaan M, Philip S, Collery MM, Janoir C, Collignon A, Cartman ST, Minton NP (2013) Expanding the repertoire of gene tools for precise manipulation of the *Clostridium difficile* genome: allelic exchange using *pyrE* alleles. PLoS One 8(2):e56051. doi:10.1371/journal.pone.0056051

Chapter 11

Characterization of Functional Prophages in *Clostridium difficile*

Ognjen Sekulović and Louis-Charles Fortier

Abstract

Bacteriophages (phages) are present in almost, if not all ecosystems. Some of these bacterial viruses are present as latent "prophages," either integrated within the chromosome of their host, or as episomal DNAs. Since prophages are ubiquitous throughout the bacterial world, there has been a sustained interest in trying to understand their contribution to the biology of their host. *Clostridium difficile* is no exception to that rule and with the recent release of hundreds of bacterial genome sequences, there has been a growing interest in trying to identify and classify these prophages. Besides their identification in bacterial genomes, there is also growing interest in determining the functionality of *C. difficile* prophages, i.e., their capacity to escape their host and reinfect a different strain, thereby promoting genomic evolution and horizontal transfer of genes through transduction, for example of antibiotic resistance genes. There is also some interest in using therapeutic phages to fight *C. difficile* infections.

The objective of this chapter is to share with the broader *C. difficile* research community the expertise we developed in the study of *C. difficile* temperate phages. In this chapter, we describe a general "pipeline" comprising a series of experiments that we use in our lab to identify, induce, isolate, propagate, and characterize prophages. Our aim is to provide readers with the necessary basic tools to start studying *C. difficile* phages.

Key words *Clostridium difficile*, Prophage, Temperate phage, Lysogen, Electron microscopy, Mitomycin C

1 Introduction

Bacteriophages (or phages) are viruses that infect bacteria. Their role in genome evolution and virulence of many bacterial species has been largely described in the literature (for reviews *see* refs. 1, 2). Contrary to virulent (or strictly lytic) phages that kill their host at the end of the infection cycle, "temperate" phages are capable of integrating into the chromosome of their host, or to remain as latent episomal DNAs, thereby establishing a stable prophage–host relationship. The genome of these prophages is replicated along with the bacterial genomic DNA during cell division, and can persist almost "unnoticed" within the bacterial population for

Adam P. Roberts and Peter Mullany (eds.), *Clostridium difficile: Methods and Protocols*, Methods in Molecular Biology, vol. 1476, DOI 10.1007/978-1-4939-6361-4_11, © Springer Science+Business Media New York 2016

prolonged periods of time. However, in certain cases, prophages can lead to profound modifications of the biology of their host [1, 2]. Indeed, although the expression of most prophage genes is silenced during lysogeny (i.e., latency), a number of genes are expressed to maintain lysogeny and prevent the prophage from engaging into a lytic cycle [3]. Many prophages also carry additional genes that have been acquired through horizontal transfer, like toxins and other virulence factors, and these genes can also be expressed during latency [4]. One of the most notorious consequences of this is lysogenic conversion of non-toxigenic bacterial strains into deadly toxigenic pathogens through the expression of phage-encoded toxins, like the Shiga toxins in *Escherichia coli* O157:H7 [5] and the botulinum toxin in *Clostridium botulinum* [6]. Prophages can modify the lifestyle and fitness of their host in multiple other ways, for example by encoding various virulence factors, by inactivating the gene into which they integrate, by interfering with bacterial gene transcription, by causing genome rearrangements, and by providing immunity to infection by similar phages [1, 2]. As such, there has been a sustained interest in understanding the impact of prophages on the biology of their host. The enteric pathogen *Clostridium difficile* is no exception to the rule and several temperate phages have been isolated and characterized over the last decade [7–19]. The whole genome sequencing of hundreds of *C. difficile* isolates in the past few years [20–22] now provides a fertile ground for genome mining in search of integrated prophages [23]. Yet one fundamental question arising is how prophages impact their host's lifestyle and virulence. One way of addressing this is to isolate the prophage after inducing it from a lysogenic strain, to amplify the phage to high titers and then to characterize it, which often implies transferring the phage into different strains. The following paragraphs give an overview of a general pipeline that can be used to identify, induce, isolate, propagate, and characterize prophages.

1.1 Identification of Prophages in Bacterial Genomes

Identifying prophages is not always an easy task, and with the increasing amount of genomic sequences available in databases, fast and reliable methods of identifying prophages are necessary. Different bioinformatics tools and web servers have been developed and described in the literature to identify prophage sequences within bacterial genomes, including Phage_Finder [24], Prophage finder [25], Prophinder [26], PHAST [27], PhiSpy [28], and PhAnToMe (http://www.phantome.org). These tools use different approaches and algorithms to identify potential prophage sequences. Some require pre-annotated genomes while others like PHAST can perform annotation of raw fasta DNA sequences followed by prophage identification [27]. Comparison of these various tools revealed that none of them predict prophages with 100% accuracy [27, 28]. This is partly due to the fact that novel phages sometimes encode multiple genes with no homologs in public databases and functional assignment is impossible based on simple Blast comparisons. Therefore, when using bioinformatics approaches to find prophages in bacterial genomes, it is a good idea to compare the results generated by more than one tool to get reliable results. It is not the objective of this chapter to describe all the prophage identification tools available and we do not go into more details here.

Based on our experience, we suggest running automated prophage identification tools and then manually scrutinizing the corresponding bacterial sequences as a confirmation. Most of the time, prophages share genome synteny, i.e., genes associated with a particular function (e.g., capsid or tail morphogenesis) are grouped in clusters or functional modules that are themselves often organized in a similar order in different phages. This is true for a majority of tailed phages characterized from various bacterial species including *C. difficile* [29–31].

1.2 Prophage Induction

Prophages are generally stable once integrated into the chromosome of their host, but spontaneous excision and replication through the lytic cycle can be observed under standard culture conditions. Depending on the phage-host partner and on environmental conditions, this frequency can vary greatly [32]. When searching for potential prophages in the absence of a sequenced bacterial genome, or if the functionality of a prophage identified using bioinformatics tools needs to be verified, it is of common practice to perform prophage induction, i.e., forcing prophages to switch to a lytic mode of replication. DNA-damaging treatments are well known to promote prophage induction via a RecA-dependent SOS response. This leads to inactivation of the phage CI (pronounce C "one") repressor and causes reactivation of the lytic cycle [3]. Among the DNA-damaging treatments, mitomycin C and ultra-violet (UV) light are the most frequently used, but other antimicrobial agents that induce an SOS response or that interfere with DNA replication, such as norfloxacin, levofloxacin and moxifloxacin have also been used successfully [11, 17, 33]. The aim of prophage induction is to generate infectious phage particles to facilitate further isolation and analysis. In the absence of a suitable replicating host (see next section), it is still possible to get enough phage particles using this approach to perform a number of characterization experiments such as transmission electron microscopy (TEM), phage DNA extraction and restriction enzyme analysis (REA), or pulsed-field gel electrophoresis (PFGE). It is important to note that not all prophages are induced equally in a given condition. For example, one prophage might be induced with mitomycin C, while a different prophage will be induced after treatment with another antibiotic or with UV [10, 15, 17]. It is thus highly recommended to test different inducing agents and conditions to maximize prophage induction. In our lab, UV and mitomycin C have proven to be very effective [14, 15]. The induction can be performed in liquid broth or on agar surfaces depending on the needs (see below).

1.3 Identification of a Propagating Host

In order to characterize a newly identified phage, it is essential to isolate and purify that phage from other potential contaminating particles released during prophage induction. Bacterial isolates often carry more than one prophage (complete and/or partial) and as such, induction lysates sometimes contain more than one type of phage particle, including phage tail-like particles (PTLPs) and defective phages [11, 14]. Therefore, the phage needs to be propagated (through a lytic cycle) on an appropriate sensitive host. A bacterial lysogen carrying a given prophage in its chromosome is intrinsically immune to lytic reinfection by the same phage or related phages. This generally results from a CI repressor-mediated phenomenon [3], but other mechanisms are also possible, like superinfection exclusion [34]. Hence, a temperate phage that has been induced from a specific bacterial strain cannot reinfect that same strain, and another host lacking that phage is required for further isolation and propagation. To do this, different approaches can be used depending on the inducing strategy. For low through-put applications, lysogenic bacterial cultures can be treated with UV, mitomycin C, or other antibiotics and cleared supernatants containing phage particles can be spotted directly on top of soft agar overlays containing a test strain forming a bacterial lawn. Alternatively, a phage dilution can be incorporated directly into the soft agar layer [35]. If the test strain in the soft agar is sensitive to the phage, the latter will replicate and propagate and zones of lysis, or plaques, will form. Another approach is to combine prophage induction with the identification of a sensitive host in a single step using UV induction on agar plates. In this case, diluted bacterial spots deposited on bottom agar are irradiated with UV light and then a soft agar overlay containing a test strain is poured on top. If a prophage is induced from the bacterial spots and the bacterial strain in the soft agar is sensitive to it, zones of lysis will be observed. Phages present in the agar can be further propagated, isolated as single plaques and purified to get pure phage lysates.

1.4 Observation of Phage Particles by Transmission Electron Microscope (TEM)

Most phages described in the literature and that have been observed under the electron microscope fall within the group of tailed phages of the order *Caudovirales* [36]. These phages are characterized by an isometric or prolate capsid (elongated head), with a long contractile tail (*Myoviridae* family) or a long flexible non-contractile tail (*Siphoviridae* family). A third family, the *Podoviridae*, comprises phages with very short tails. All phages of *C. difficile* that have been described so far are tailed phages of the *Myoviridae* and *Siphoviridae* families. PTLPs and defective phage particles have been observed in many lysogens as well [10, 11, 13, 14]. Thus, observing crude lysates resulting from prophage induction and purified phage particles is an important step in the general characterization of phages associated with a lysogenic strain. In addition to providing morphological information on the phages under study, TEM can also reveal the presence of different phages within an induction lysate (based on size and morphotype) as well defective particles and PTLPs.

High-quality phage preparations for TEM analysis are not always easy to obtain, especially when analyzing crude phage lysates following prophage induction. Therefore, a purification step is highly recommended. Multistep processes involving concentration of phage particles with polyethylene glycol (PEG) followed by cesium chloride density gradient centrifugations and dialysis can be performed. However, this can become time consuming if several preparations need to be analyzed. A rapid and reliable method that we use routinely in our lab with *C. difficile* phages consists in washing phage particles or crude induction lysates in ammonium acetate buffer [14, 15]. Various staining procedures can then be used to increase contrast of viral particles before observation by electron microscopy, uranyl acetate (UA) and phosphotungstic acid (PTA) being the most commonly used [37]. Note that titers of at least 10^8 phages (or plaque forming units, pfu)/mL are necessary to obtain good results in TEM without having to screen the grids for hours to find particles.

1.5 Whole Phage Genome Analyses

Phages with similar morphologies (shape and size) can be completely unrelated genetically, so classification based on morphology should be complemented with whole genome analyses. Before proceeding to whole genome sequencing, it is recommended to perform a simple genome characterization using restriction enzyme analysis (REA). Optionally, PFGE can also be performed if the appropriate system is available. To do this, a mini-preparation of genomic DNA from 1 to 5 mL of phage lysate is generally sufficient to obtain enough DNA for REA and/or PFGE analysis. Ideally, two or three restriction enzymes should be used to generate different profiles to facilitate differentiation of closely related phages. In the case of PFGE, undigested DNA should also be run on gel to estimate the total genome size. Phage DNA can be extracted from crude prophage induction lysates if a suitable propagating host is not available, keeping in mind that a mixture of more than one phage particle might be obtained. Ideally DNA extraction should be performed on purified phage lysates whenever possible. Purification columns and kits are commercially available (e.g., Qiagen Lambda kits), but low-cost in-house protocols can also be used, especially for small-scale phage DNA preparations. High-titer phage lysates (>10^8 phages/mL) are necessary for most downstream applications.

1.6 Isolation of Bacterial Lysogens Carrying a Newly Identified Phage

An interesting question about temperate phages, in particular those infecting pathogenic bacteria such as *C. difficile*, is their potential contribution to the virulence and fitness of their host [2, 12, 16, 38–41]. Curing a bacterial lysogen from its natural prophage(s) is not an easy task. It implies extensive screening of hundreds of colonies in order to find one that lost the prophage. Phages isolated after prophage induction are certainly capable of reintegrating the chromosome of another susceptible host to create a new lysogen. Thus, it is generally easier to transfer a newly isolated phage into a different strain to study phage-host interactions. In addition, the procedure for generating lysogens can be very useful to determine whether a phage isolated from the environment (e.g., sewage, feces) is strictly lytic (i.e., virulent) or temperate, without the need to sequence the whole phage genome to search for lysogeny-associated genes such as integrases and phage repressors.

A classic approach is to search for phage plaques with turbid centers on soft agar overlays, indicating that lysogens formed and started to regrow after lysis of the susceptible cells. An agar "plug" containing the mixture of phages and lysogens is crushed and eluted in a suitable growth medium, and then plated on agar to get isolated colonies, which should be lysogens. In our lab we routinely use a rapid method of generating new lysogens which takes advantage of the fact that high MOI favor lysogeny [3]. To do this, we simply use a reversed version of the standard soft agar overlay [16]. Briefly, instead of incorporating bacteria into the soft agar to get a bacterial lawn into which phage dilutions are added to get isolated phage plaques, we incorporate high phage titers into the soft agar and then plate bacterial dilutions on top of it. The fact that isolated bacteria lie on top of a phage lawn creates high MOI conditions, which increase the chances of obtaining lysogens following multiple simultaneous phage infections of the same cell. These colonies are then purified by successive streaking on plates without phages and then checked for the presence of the incorporated prophage. This can be done by inducing the prophage using DNA-damaging treatments such as mitomycin C or UV irradiation, followed by reisolation of the phage and restriction enzyme analysis to confirm that it is the same as the one used initially for infection. If the phage sequence is known, a more rapid approach is to use phage-specific PCR primers in order to detect the presence of the prophage in bacterial genomic DNA preparations from isolated colonies.

2 Materials

For all bacterial cultures in broth and agar, we recommend using tryptose yeast extract (TY) broth (3% tryptose (Oxoid Canada, Cat. No. LP0047), 2% yeast extract (BioShop Canada, Cat. No. YEX401.500), pH 7.4) because less precipitate is formed when cationic ions are added for phage infection. However, brain heart infusion (BHI) broth (BD, Cat. No. 237500) can also be used.

When required, agar (BioShop Canada, Cat. No. FB0010) is incorporated at 10 g/L before autoclaving for standard plates, or 5 g/L for soft agar overlays.

All liquid and solid media are degassed overnight in the anaerobic chamber before use to avoid toxic effects of oxygen on *C. difficile* viability, especially when preparing bacterial lawns in soft agar (*see* **Note 1**). Likewise, we recommend working in the anaerobic chamber as much as possible to avoid compromising viability of *C. difficile*.

All materials (glass tubes, polypropylene tubes, syringes, filters, etc.) must be sterile.

Electronic equipment like the spectrophotometer used inside the anaerobic chamber should be taken out of the chamber after use because we have noticed that on the long term, the anaerobic gas damages some electronic devices that are not specifically designed to operate under such conditions.

2.1 Mitomycin C Prophage Induction in Broth

1. Degassed TY broth.

2. Mitomycin C (BioShop Canada, Cat. No. MIT232.10). Prepare a 10 mg/mL stock solution in sterile distilled water and store aliquots at −20 °C. Avoid repeated freeze-thaw cycles. Old solutions generally tend to loose activity and are less efficient in inducing prophages.

3. Borosilicate glass tubes with caps suitable for optical density measurements (16×150 mm, Fisher Scientific, Cat. No. 14-961-31).

4. Spectrophotometer adjusted to a 600 nm wavelength (OD_{600}) with adapter for glass tubes.

5. Conical 15 and 50 mL polypropylene centrifuge tubes (Sarstedt, Cat. No. 62.554.205 and 62.547.205 or equivalent).

6. Disposable 10 mL syringes (BD, Cat. No. 309604, or equivalent).

7. Disposable syringe filters, 0.45 μm (Sarstedt, Cat. No. 83.1826, or equivalent).

8. Refrigerated centrifuge equipped with a rotor capable of spinning 15 mL tubes at $\geq 3000 \times g$.

2.2 UV Prophage Induction in Broth and on Agar Plates

1. Degassed TY broth.

2. Degassed 1 % TY bottom agar plates (TY with 10 g/L agar).

3. UV transilluminator (302–365 nm wavelengths). The transilluminator of a conventional gel documentation system is perfect.

4. Conical 15 and 50 mL polypropylene centrifuge tubes (Sarstedt, Cat. No. 62.554.205 and 62.547.205 or equivalent).

5. Borosilicate glass tubes with caps suitable for optical density measurements (16×150 mm, Fisher Scientific, Cat. No. 14-961-31).

6. Inoculation spreader (Sarstedt, Cat. No. 86.1569.001, or equivalent) or glass beads (3 mm diameter, Fisher Scientific, Cat. No. S80024).

7. Sterile, 1.5 mL microcentrifuge tubes (BioBasic, Cat. No. BT620-NS, or equivalent).

8. $MgCl_2$, 5 M stock solution, filter-sterilized (dry powder, BioShop Canada, Cat. No. MAG520).

9. $CaCl_2$, 2 M stock solution, filter-sterilized (dry powder, BioShop Canada, Cat. No. CCL444).

10. Dry block heater adjusted at 55 °C and capable of holding 13×100 mm glass tubes.

11. Disposable 10 mL serological pipettes (Sarstedt, Cat. No. 86.1254.025, or equivalent).

12. Refrigerated centrifuge equipped with a rotor capable of spinning 15 mL tubes at $3000 \times g$.

13. Disposable 10 mL syringes (BD, Cat. No. 309604, or equivalent).

14. Disposable syringe filters, 0.45 μm (Sarstedt, Cat. No. 83.1826, or equivalent).

2.3 Phage Propagation in Broth and Soft Agar

1. Degassed TY broth.

2. Degassed 1% TY bottom agar plates (TY with 10 g/L agar).

3. Degassed 0.5% TY soft agar (TY with 5 g/L agar) melted and kept at 55 °C in a block heater.

4. Borosilicate glass tubes with caps suitable for optical density measurements (16×150 mm, Fisher Scientific, Cat. No. 14-961-31).

5. Borosilicate glass tubes with caps (13×100 mm, Fisher Scientific, Cat. No. 14-961-27).

6. UV transilluminator (302–365 nm wavelengths).

7. Sterile, 1.5 mL microcentrifuge tubes (BioBasic, Cat. No. BT620-NS, or equivalent).

8. $MgCl_2$, 5 M stock solution, filter-sterilized (BioShop Canada, Cat. No. MAG520).

9. $CaCl_2$, 2 M stock solution, filter-sterilized (BioShop Canada, Cat. No. CCL444).

10. Dry block heater adjusted at 55 °C and capable of holding 13×100 mm glass tubes.

11. Sterile truncated 200 μL pipet tips, or sterile Pasteur pipets.

12. Disposable 10 mL syringes (BD, Cat. No. 309604, or equivalent).

13. Syringe filters, 0.45 μm (Sarstedt, Cat. No. 83.1826, or equivalent).

2.4 Observation of Phages and Lysates by Transmission Electron Microscopy

1. Microcentrifuge tubes (1.5 mL, BioBasic, Cat. No. BT620-NS, or equivalent).

2. Ammonium acetate, 0.1 M filter-sterilized, pH 7.5 (BioShop Canada, Cat. No. ACE601).

3. Formvar/carbon-coated copper grids 400-mesh (Electron Microscopy Sciences, Cat. No. FF400-CU-UL).

4. Refrigerated centrifuge, equipped with a fixed-angled rotor capable of spinning 1.5 mL microcentrifuge tubes at $24,000 \times g$.

5. Uranyl acetate, 2% solution pH 4–4.5 (Electron Microscopy Sciences, Cat. No. 22400-2). Dissolve the powder in distilled water and adjust the pH with 1 M KOH or NaOH and then filter-sterilize. Stable for several months at 4 °C.

6. Phosphotungstic acid, 2%, pH 7.2 (Electron Microscopy Sciences, Cat. No. 12501-23-4) Dissolve in distilled water and adjust the pH with 1 M KOH or NaOH. Stable for several months at 4 °C.

7. Pointed tweezers.

8. Whatman paper.

9. Transmission electron microscope.

2.5 Extraction of Phage DNA (In-House Mini-Prep Protocol)

1. $MgCl_2$, 5 M stock solution, filter-sterilized (BioShop Canada, Cat. No. MAG520).

2. DNaseI, 10 mg/mL (dry powder, Roche Life Science, Cat. No. 10104159001).

3. RNase, 10 mg/mL (dry powder, Roche Life Science, Cat. No. 10109134001).

4. SDS-Mix solution (0.25 M EDTA, 0.5 M Tris–HCl pH 9, 2.5% SDS).

5. Potassium acetate, 8 M solution (BioShop Canada, Cat. No. POA303).

6. Phenol–chloroform–isoamyl alcohol (25:24:1) solution, pH 8 (Amresco, Cat. No. 0883-100ML).

7. Isopropanol (BioShop Canada, Cat. No. PRP001.1).

8. Ethanol 70% solution, high grade (Amresco, Cat. No. E505-500ML).

9. Tris–HCl buffer solution, 10 mM, pH 8.

10. Microcentrifuge tubes (1.5 mL, BioBasic, Cat. No. BT620-NS, or equivalent).

11. Refrigerated centrifuge, equipped with a rotor capable of spinning 1.5 mL plastic tubes at $\geq 10,000 \times g$.

3 Methods

3.1 Mitomycin C Prophage Induction in Liquid Broth

1. In a 16×150 mm glass tube, inoculate 5 mL of TY broth using a fresh isolated colony or a frozen glycerol stock (-80 °C). Incubate overnight under anaerobic atmosphere at 37 °C.

2. The next day, use 0.4 mL of the overnight culture to inoculate 40 mL of fresh TY broth in a 50 mL tube. Mix well by inversion and divide this freshly inoculated broth into four 10 mL aliquots in disposable 16×150 glass tubes (*see* **Note 1**).

3. Monitor the optical density at 600 nm (OD_{600}) using a spectrophotometer installed inside the anaerobic chamber.

4. When cells reach an $OD_{600} = 0.1$ (early exponential growth phase), add three different concentrations of mitomycin C in three of the four tubes. One tube is left untreated and serves as a positive control for bacterial growth (*see* **Note 2**).

5. Continue monitoring the OD_{600} at regular intervals (e.g., 30–60 min). Typically, the OD_{600} will continue rising for 2–3 h and then will start dropping rapidly, which is indicative of cell lysis (*see* **Note 3**). When the OD_{600} does not decrease anymore, proceed to the next step.

6. Transfer the culture into a 15 mL conical tube and centrifuge at $\geq 3000 \times g$ for 10 min at 4 °C to pellet unlysed cells and bacterial debris.

7. Filter the supernatant through 0.45 μm syringe filters to obtain an induction lysate containing phage particles. Store at 4 °C until use (*see* **Note 4**) or proceed to the identification of a propagating host (Subheading 3.3).

3.2 UV Prophage Induction in Liquid Broth

Some phages will not induce with mitomycin C or DNA-damaging antibiotics like fluoroquinolones, but will induce with UV [15]. The following method allows inducing cultures with UV and monitoring bacterial lysis in broth using optical density measurement.

1. Follow **steps 1–3** from Subheading 3.1 to prepare four tubes of bacterial culture to be used for induction.

2. When the OD_{600} reaches 0.2, transfer each 10 mL bacterial culture into a 15 mL polypropylene conical tube, screw cap tightly within the anaerobic chamber before taking out for centrifugation at $\geq 3000 \times g$ for 10 min at 4 °C.

3. Transfer tubes back inside the anaerobic chamber. Discard the supernatant and suspend bacteria from each 10 mL culture in 0.1 mL of pre-reduced TY broth.

4. Spread each 0.1 mL fraction of bacterial suspension on top of a pre-reduced TY bottom agar plate using a sterile inoculation spreader or glass beads (remove them after spreading). Make

sure to spread uniformly, and that all the liquid has been absorbed into the agar.

5. Take the plates outside the anaerobic chamber and place a first plate upside-down, without the lid, directly on the surface of a UV transilluminator. Irradiate for 5 s at 302 nm. Close the dish and quickly repeat the same procedure with two other plates, while increasing the irradiation time to 10 s and 15 s, respectively. The last plate is left non-irradiated and serves as a positive control of bacterial growth.

6. Rapidly bring back the plates inside the anaerobic chamber, and collect bacterial cells by flooding the surface of the plates with 10 mL of pre-reduced TY broth. Collect with a serological pipet and transfer the suspended cells into 16×150 mm glass tubes and monitor the OD_{600} at regular intervals (30–60 min).

7. Follow **steps 5** through **7** as in Subheading 3.1.

3.3 Identification of a Susceptible Host for Phage Propagation

1. In a 16×150 mm glass tube, inoculate 5 mL of TY broth using fresh isolated colonies or frozen glycerol stocks (−80 °C) of the strains to be tested. Incubate overnight under anaerobic atmosphere at 37 °C (*see* **Note 1**).

2. The next day, inoculate 5 mL of fresh TY broth with 0.05 mL of the overnight culture and incubate until the OD_{600} reaches the mid-log phase (OD_{600} 0.3–0.6) (*see* **Note 5**).

3. TY soft agar (0.5 %) can be prepared in advance and sterilized by autoclaving. Just before use, melt the agar using a microwave oven (make sure to open the recipient to avoid pressure build-up). Dispense 3 mL aliquots into sterile 13×100 mm glass tubes. There is no need to further degas the agar, since melting it will remove most of the oxygen. Once melted, keep at 55 °C in a dry block heater inside the anaerobic chamber until use, but do not prepare too much in advance to avoid dehydration.

4. To a tube containing 3 mL of melted soft agar at 55 °C, add 0.3 mL of a 5 M $MgCl_2$ solution and 0.020 mL of a 2 M $CaCl_2$ solution (final concentrations of ~0.4 M and 0.01 M, respectively) and mix gently, avoiding introducing bubbles (*see* **Note 6**). Then add 0.5 mL of a log-phase (OD_{600} = 0.3–0.6) culture from a propagating host strain, swirl gently and rapidly poor on top of a TY bottom agar plate. Rock the plates gently to ensure uniform distribution of the soft agar overlay and let stand on a leveled surface for a few minutes until the agar has solidified.

5. In microcentrifuge tubes containing 0.5 mL TY broth, prepare tenfold serial dilutions of the phage lysate. For the spot test assay follow **step 6**. For the conventional plaque assay, follow **step 7**.

6. Spot test assay. Deposit 5 μL of each dilution side by side on the soft agar prepared in **step 4** leaving enough space to avoid merging of the spots (*see* **Note 7**). Carefully transfer the plates

on a leveled surface in the incubator and incubate in an upright position overnight at 37 °C under anaerobic condition.

7. Plaque assay. The spot test assay gives a rough estimation of the sensitivity of a strain towards a phage. The plaque assay allows determining the efficiency of plaquing (EOP), i.e., the proportion of each infecting phage that gives rise to an isolated plaque [42]. It also informs us about the size of the phage plaques, which is often indicative of the fitness of the phage on that strain (larger plaques suggest faster replication and larger phage progeny, or burst size). To do a plaque assay, simply follow **steps 3–5** above and after adding bacteria to the soft agar, add 0.1 mL of a phage dilution directly into the soft agar. Try different dilutions on different plates in order to get at least one plate with isolated phage plaques.

8. If the bacterial strain in the soft agar is susceptible to infection by the phage lysate tested, zones of lysis will form at the point where phages were deposited in the spot test assay (*see* **Note 7**), or isolated phage plaques will form in the soft agar if the lysate was incorporated directly into the agar. For pinpoint size phage plaques, use a colony counter to help visualization and counting.

3.4 UV Prophage Induction with Simultaneous Identification of a Propagating Host

It can be advantageous to combine prophage induction with the identification of a sensitive host into one single step using UV induction on agar plates. This also allows screening multiple lysogenic hosts at once.

1. In a 16×150 mm glass tube, inoculate 5 mL of TY broth using a fresh isolated colony or a frozen glycerol stock (-80 °C). Inoculate as many different strains you want to test for prophage induction and susceptibility to phage infection. Incubate overnight under anaerobic atmosphere at 37 °C (*see* **Note 1**).

2. The next day, prepare in microcentrifuge tubes containing 1 mL of degassed TY broth tenfold serial dilutions of the strain(s) to be induced. Dilute down to 1/1000 and prepare all dilutions inside the anaerobic chamber.

3. Spot 5 μL of the 1/10, 1/100, and 1/1000 dilutions on top of a pre-reduced 1 % TY bottom agar plate. Replicate this plate for every potential host strain to be tested. For example, if you want to screen four *C. difficile* strains potentially carrying prophages against ten potential susceptible strains, spot the four lysogenic strains (three dilutions each) and replicate on ten different plates. Incubate for 4 h at 37 °C to allow bacteria to reach the exponential growth phase.

4. Meanwhile, inoculate 5 mL of pre-reduced TY broth with 0.05 mL of an overnight culture from one of the bacterial strains to be tested as a susceptible propagating host. Incubate at 37 °C under anaerobic conditions. After 4 h of incubation,

all strains should be in exponential phase of growth with OD_{600} values around 0.3–0.6 (*see* **Note 5**).

5. Prepare melted soft agar as in **step 3** of Subheading 3.3.

6. After incubating the bacterial spots for 4 h, take the plates out of the anaerobic chamber and place them directly on the surface of a UV transilluminator, face down without lids, and irradiate for 10 s at 302 nm. Rapidly bring back the plates inside the anaerobic chamber (shorter and longer irradiation times can be tested if desired).

7. Combine $MgCl_2$ and $CaCl_2$ salts and bacterial test strains in soft agar as in **step 4** of Subheading 3.3 and pour on top of the irradiated plates. Distribute uniformly the soft agar overlay but do not rock the plates too much as this will cause bacterial spots to mix and spread with the soft agar, which will lead to smearing of phage plaques. Let stand on a leveled surface for 10–20 min until the agar has solidified. Stack the plates upside down and incubate overnight at 37 °C under anaerobic condition.

8. If the spotted bacterial strains contained inducible prophages capable of infecting the test strain within the bacterial lawn, zones of lysis or isolated plaques will be visible in the soft agar on top of it. The agar containing the released phages can be scraped off using a sterile truncated pipet tip or a Pasteur pipet and used to further purify, and propagate the phage(s) (*see* Subheading 3.5).

3.5 Phage Purification by Plaque Assay

Once a susceptible host has been identified for phage propagation, successive rounds of plaque isolation are necessary to purify the phage from other contaminants (PTLPs, other complete and defective phages, etc.).

1. Using a sterile truncated pipet tip or a Pasteur pipet, pick up from the soft agar overlay an isolated phage plaque in the form an agar "plug." Alternatively, scrape off a sample of agar containing a zone of lysis resulting from UV induction.

2. Transfer and crush the agar plug into a microcentrifuge tube containing 0.5 mL of sterile TY broth supplemented with 10 mM each (final concentration) of $MgCl_2$ and $CaCl_2$ (some phages are stabilized in the presence of cations) and leave at room temperature at least 3 h to allow phage particles to diffuse into the medium.

3. Filter the supernatant containing the diffused phage through a 0.45 µm syringe filter. Pre-wet the filter with sterile water to fill the void volume and minimize loss of phage lysate. Alternatively, simply spin the microcentrifuge tubes at $13,000 \times g$ for 1 min to pellet debris and remaining cells and transfer the supernatant to a new tube. Store at 4 °C until use or proceed directly to the next step.

4. Prepare tenfold serial dilutions (down to 10^{-4}) of the filtrate in microcentrifuge tubes containing 0.5 mL TY broth.

5. Prepare 0.5 % soft agar overlays as in Subheading 3.3 with the appropriate susceptible host and add the phage dilutions (in different tubes). Poor on top of TY bottom agar plates and incubate overnight at 37 °C under anaerobic conditions until isolated phage plaques are obtained.

6. The next day, pick up a single isolated plaque and repeat **steps 1** through **5** for two additional rounds.

7. After the third round of plaque purification, pick up an agar plug containing a single isolated plaque using a truncated pipet tip or Pasteur pipet, and transfer to a 16×150 mm glass tube containing 5 mL of TY broth and proceed to a first amplification (Subheading 3.6).

3.6 Phage Propagation: First Amplification

1. To a tube containing 5 mL of TY broth and a phage plug, add 10 mM each (final concentration) of $MgCl_2$ and $CaCl_2$ and 0.05 mL of an overnight culture of the appropriate *C. difficile* host and incubate the culture overnight at 37 °C under anaerobic conditions (*see* **Note 8**).

2. The next day, centrifuge the culture at $\geq 3000 \times g$ for 10 min and then filter the supernatant containing the amplified phage through a 0.45 μm syringe filter. Store at 4 °C until use, or proceed to next step for titration of the phage.

3. Prepare tenfold serial dilutions of the first amplification lysate and poor soft agar overlays containing various dilutions as described in Subheading 3.3, **step** 7 and determine the titer of the phage lysate, i.e., the number of plaque forming units (pfu) per mL (pfu/mL).

3.7 Phage Propagation: Second Amplification

A first amplification does not always lead to high phage titers. Therefore, a second amplification using the first amplification as a "seed" should be performed. Note that the ratio of phage-to-bacteria, i.e., the multiplicity of infection (MOI), needs to be adjusted in order to get maximal phage amplification (*see* **Note 9**).

1. Inoculate 5 mL of TY broth using a fresh isolated colony or a frozen glycerol stock (−80 °C) of the sensitive host. Incubate overnight under anaerobic atmosphere at 37 °C (*see* **Note 1**).

2. The next day, use 0.4 mL of the overnight culture to inoculate 40 mL of fresh TY broth in a 50 mL tube. Mix well by inversion and divide this freshly inoculated broth into four 10 mL aliquots in disposable glass tubes.

3. Monitor the optical density at 600 nm (OD_{600}) using a spectrophotometer under anaerobic conditions.

4. When cells reach an $OD_{600} = 0.1$, add 10 mM each (final concentration) of $MgCl_2$ and $CaCl_2$ (*see* **Note 6**) and then 0.1 mL

of three different phage dilutions in three of the four tubes in order to obtain MOI values of 0.01, 0.1, and 1 (*see* **Note 9**). One tube is left uninfected and serves as a positive control of bacterial growth.

5. Continue monitoring the OD_{600} at regular intervals (e.g., 30–60 min). The OD_{600} should continue rising for 2–3 h (sometimes more) and then will start dropping rapidly, which is indicative of cell lysis (the larger the drop, the better the amplification). When the OD_{600} does not decrease anymore, proceed to the next step.

6. Transfer the culture into a 15 mL conical tube and centrifuge at $\geq 3000 \times g$ for 10 min at 4 °C to pellet unlysed cells and bacterial debris.

7. Filter the phage lysate through a 0.45 µm syringe filter and store at 4 °C until use (*see* **Note 4**), or proceed to phage titration as in Subheading 3.5, **step 3**.

3.8 Observation of Phage Particles Under the Electron Microscope

1. Transfer 1.5 mL of phage lysate containing at least 10^8 pfu/ mL into a 1.5 mL microcentrifuge tube and spin at $24,000 \times g$ for 60 min at 4 °C in a centrifuge equipped with a fixed angle rotor. Phages will concentrate near the bottom of the tube, but a pellet will not form.

2. Gently pipet and discard the upper fraction leaving ~0.1 mL at the bottom of the tube. Add 1.5 mL of filter-sterilized ammonium acetate 0.1 M, pH 7.5 and spin again at $24,000 \times g$ for 60 min at 4 °C.

3. Repeat **step 2** two more times.

4. After the last centrifugation, gently pipet the upper fraction and leave ~0.1 mL of the washed phage preparation at the bottom of the tube.

5. Pipette 5 µL of the washed phage preparation directly onto a 400-mesh Formvar/carbon-coated copper grid that you hold with pointed tweezers. After 60 s, pipette 5 µL of a 2% uranyl acetate staining solution and gently mix by pipetting up-and-down a few times. After 60 s, blot the liquid with a piece of Whatman paper by touching the side of the grid. Let the grid dry a few minutes and store until observation (*see* **Note 10**).

6. Observe grids under the electron microscope at 60–80 kV.

3.9 Extraction of Phage DNA for Whole Genome Analyses

Different protocols can be used to extract phage DNA, including commercial kits. Here, we will describe a simple in-house and low-cost method that gives reliable results for most downstream applications. For whole genome sequencing however, we recommend using a commercial kit such as the Lambda DNA Purification Kit. This will avoid contamination with phenol or other impurities that could interfere with sequencing.

1. Transfer 1 mL of a high-titer phage lysate (>10^8 pfu/mL) into a 1.5 mL microcentrifuge tube.

2. Add 1 µL each of DNase I and RNase A solutions (1 mg/mL each) and incubate at 37 °C for 30 min.

3. *Optional*: some protocols suggest adding 10 µL of proteinase K (20 mg/mL) and incubating at 37 °C for 10 min to remove the DNAse I and RNAse A before lysing the capsids and exposing the nucleic acid. We generally do no use proteinase K for our phage DNA preparations and the DNA is of good quality.

4. Add 0.1 mL of SDS-Mix, invert the tube a few times and incubate at 65 °C for 30 min.

5. Add 0.125 mL of 8 M potassium acetate, mix well and incubate on ice for 30 min. A white precipitate will form.

6. Centrifuge at 13,000×g for 10 min at 4 °C.

7. Transfer the supernatant in two 1.5 mL microcentrifuge tubes (~0.6 mL in each). Add an equivalent volume of phenol–chloroform–isoamyl alcohol solution and mix vigorously but do not vortex to avoid excessive DNA shearing.

8. Centrifuge at 13,000×g for 10 min at room temperature.

9. Carefully pipet the upper aqueous phase containing phage genomic DNA and transfer into another clean microcentrifuge tube. Perform another phenol–chloroform–isoamyl alcohol extraction as described in **steps 7** and **8**.

10. After the last extraction, collect the upper phases and transfer into a single microcentrifuge tube. Precipitate the phage DNA by adding 0.7 volumes of isopropanol and mix well.

11. Centrifuge at 13,000×g for 10 min at room temperature to precipitate the DNA.

12. Remove isopropanol and wash the pellet with a 70% ethanol solution taking care to avoid disrupting the pellet. Centrifuge at 13,000×g for 5 min at room temperature. Repeat the washing step two times.

13. After the last centrifugation, remove as much ethanol as possible and air-dry the pellet for a few minutes. Do not over dry.

14. Solubilize the pellet in 50 µL of 10 mM Tris–HCl, pH 8. Verify the quality and quantity of the DNA preparation by running an aliquot through a 0.8% agarose gel (*see* **Note 11**).

3.10 Analysis of Phage Genomes by REA

The purpose of REA is to determine whether the newly isolated phage corresponds to a known phage, or to the expected profile inferred from the prophage sequence identified in bacterial genomes (Subheading 1.1). It is also a good way to classify and compare different phages within a collection.

1. In a microcentrifuge tube, digest 1 µg of phage DNA with a suitable restriction enzyme following the manufacturer's recommendations. Prepare two to three reactions with different enzymes to get different profiles.

2. Following digestion, heat the restricted phage DNA at 75 °C for 10 min to dissociate cohesive termini (if present) and then rapidly chill on ice (*see* **Note 12**).

3. Add gel loading dye and run through a 0.8% agarose gel at constant voltage of 110 V in 1× TAE buffer. Use your favorite staining method and record the profiles using a gel documentation system.

3.11 Creation of New Lysogens

1. Inoculate 5 mL of TY broth using fresh isolated colonies or frozen glycerol stocks (−80 °C) of the strains to be tested. Incubate overnight under anaerobic atmosphere at 37 °C (*see* **Note 1**).

2. The next day, inoculate 5 mL of fresh TY with 0.05 mL of the overnight culture and incubate until the OD_{600} reaches the mid-log phase (OD_{600} 0.3–0.6) (*see* **Note 5**).

3. Prepare melted soft agar (0.5% TY agar) and dispense 3 mL aliquots in sterile 13 × 100 mm glass tubes. Keep at 55 °C in a dry block heater inside the anaerobic chamber until use.

4. To a tube containing 3 mL of melted soft agar at 55 °C, add 0.3 mL of a 5 M $MgCl_2$ solution and 0.020 mL of a 2 M $CaCl_2$ solution (final concentrations of ~0.4 M and 0.01 M, respectively) and mix gently, avoiding introducing bubbles (*see* **Note 6**). Then add 0.1 mL of a high-titer phage lysate (~10^8 to 10^9 pfu/mL) directly into the soft agar. Swirl gently and rapidly poor on top of a TY agar plate. Rock the plates gently to ensure uniform distribution of the soft agar overlay and let stand on a leveled surface for 10–20 min until the agar has solidified. Prepare two or three of these plates.

5. In microcentrifuge tubes containing 0.5 mL of sterile TY broth, prepare tenfold serial dilutions of the log phase culture prepared earlier (an overnight culture also works fine) and plate 0.1 mL of appropriate dilutions on top of different soft agar overlays containing phages. Select the dilutions that give a few dozens to a 100 colonies on a single plate. We recommend using sterile glass beads (3 mm diameter) to spread bacteria to avoid damaging the soft agar.

6. In parallel, plate the same bacterial dilutions on TY bottom agar plates in order to count the number of CFU in each dilution.

7. Incubate the plates upside down overnight at 37 °C under anaerobic conditions.

8. The next day, count colonies on each plate. You should get dozens of colonies that will be lysogens for the great majority.

9. Pick up two or three colonies and re-streak them on separate TY bottom agar plates without phages and incubate overnight at 37 °C. Repeat another round of colony purification by picking-up one isolated colony from each plate and repeating the same steps. The aim is to eliminate free phages that could contaminate the bacterial colonies.

10. After three successive rounds of colony purification, pick up one colony from each plate (two or three colonies in total) and analyze them for the presence of the prophage. This can be achieved by inducing the prophage with UV or mitomycin C following the procedures detailed in Subheadings 3.1–3.4.

11. If the phage genome sequence is known, PCR primers can be designed to detect the presence of the prophage in bacterial DNA preparations. In this case phage DNA can be extracted following the procedure described in Subheading 3.9.

12. An alternative method is to rapidly isolate genomic DNA from a colony using the cation exchange resin Chelex®. To do this, simply suspend an isolated colony in a microcentrifuge tube containing 0.1 mL of a 5 % (w/vol) suspension of Chelex® ion exchange resin (Bio-Rad Laboratories, Cat. No. 1421253). Mix well and boil in a water bath for 10 min (make sure to lock the caps securely). Alternatively, the suspension can be prepared in PCR tubes and heated in a PCR thermocycler (98 °C, 10 min). After heating, centrifuge at $13,000 \times g$ for 1 min to pellet debris and remaining cells. Use 1 or 2 μL of this crude DNA preparation in PCR reaction using phage-specific primers. Make sure to use a positive PCR control using primers specific for the bacterial strain (e.g., a toxin gene or the triose phosphate isomerase gene, *tpi* [43]).

4 Notes

1. *C. difficile* is very sensitive to oxygen and prolonged exposure to open air is often deleterious. It is therefore highly recommended to always use pre-reduced broth and agar media, by placing tubes and bottles (unscrew caps before) as well as petri dishes inside the anaerobic chamber at least 24 h prior to use, to ensure maximum growth. Some institutions might have restrictions regarding the maximum concentration of hydrogen that can be used in anaerobic chambers, but according to our experience, better anaerobic conditions are maintained using a gas mixture containing 10 % hydrogen (instead of 5 %), 5 % CO_2, and 85 % N_2.

2. Different DNA-damaging agents have been used successfully to induce *C. difficile* prophages, including mitocymin C, norfloxacin, ciprofloxacin, moxifloxacin, and levofloxacin [13, 17]. We routinely use mitomycin C at three different concentrations

in order to get optimal inducing conditions. Alternatively, a preliminary experiment aiming at determining the minimum inhibitory concentration (MIC) of the inducing agent on the strain can be performed to target the appropriate concentration range [44]. The objective is to reach a concentration of inducing agent which is high enough to induce the prophage, but not too much to cause significant growth inhibition. Final concentrations of mitomycin C and norfloxacin ranging between 0.5 and 3 µg/mL are generally adequate for good prophage induction but higher concentrations can be necessary if the *C. difficile* strain is less susceptible to the inducing agent [13, 17].

3. At sub-optimal concentrations of inducing agent, cultures will continue to grow to high densities, albeit sometimes with reduced growth rate and final biomass. On the other hand, if the concentration of inducing agent is too high, growth will be significantly impaired and it is likely that the induction will be unproductive. An increase in $OD_{600} > 0.2$–0.3 units followed by a similar drop is generally a good indication of productive prophage induction. The OD_{600} generally does not reach 0 at the end of the lysis, and a plateau is rather observed, after which regrowth sometimes occurs. It is therefore advisable to proceed to centrifugation and filtration when the OD_{600} has stabilized during two consecutive readings instead of leaving the tubes incubating overnight.

4. Phages are usually stable for several months at 4 °C when kept in the original filtered culture supernatant [35]. However, we have observed variation in stability from one phage to another. The presence of 10 mM each of $MgCl_2$ and $CaCl_2$ seems to stabilize some phages.

5. Although stationary phase cells from an overnight culture sometimes give good results, to get the most uniform and reproducible *C. difficile* bacterial lawns in soft agar overlays it is best to use exponentially growing cells ($OD_{600} = 0.3$–0.6). We also highly recommend to poor all soft agar overlays inside the anaerobic chamber to avoid prolonged exposure to open air and incorporation of oxygen into the soft agar. Otherwise, this might lead to nonuniform spotty bacterial lawns that will cause difficulty to detect phage plaques and zones of lysis.

6. Cationic ions such as Mg^{2+} and Ca^{2+} are often required to favor phage adsorption and phage infection [45]. With *C. difficile* phages, the addition of high $MgCl_2$ concentrations in soft agar overlays is critical for some phages [8], like φCD38-2 that forms plaques only in the presence of 0.4 M $MgCl_2$ [16]. Although not all phages require such high salt concentrations, we routinely use a combination of 0.4 M $MgCl_2$ and 10 mM $CaCl_2$ to propagate all of our *C. difficile* phages in soft agar.

Note that salts will generally form a precipitate after the addition to the melted agar, but it does not interfere with bacterial lawn formation and plaque formation. For phage amplification in broth, salts are also needed, but at lower concentrations (10 mM each of $CaCl_2$ and $MgCl_2$). The use of TY broth instead of BHI also reduces precipitation of $CaCl_2$. If using BHI, reduce the final $CaCl_2$ concentration to 1 mM.

7. Spotting concentrated phage lysates (i.e., $>10^8$ pfu) on bacterial lawns might induce early bacterial lysis called "lysis from without." This is due to the cell wall-degrading enzymatic activity (e.g., lysozyme) in some phage tail proteins [46]. At high multiplicity of infection, when several phages adsorb simultaneously to a cell, their cell wall-degrading activity can cause significant cell wall damage that leads to cell lysis, even if the phage is not able to replicate on that host. A consequence of that is the erroneous interpretation of the host sensitivity towards a given phage. Therefore, we recommend diluting the initial phage lysate and spotting 1/10 and 1/100 dilutions side by side. Lysis in the undiluted lysate but not in the 1/10 or 1/100 dilution would suggest a nonspecific lysis from without phenomenon. In case of doubt, we recommend testing the susceptibility of the host using the soft agar overlay technique in which phages are directly incorporated into the soft agar.

8. The same procedure can be used when starting from an old phage lysate, or reactivating a phage from a frozen stock [35]. In this case, simply replace the phage plug by a small volume (0.01–0.1 mL) of a phage lysate, or a sample of frozen lysate. After a first amplification, especially when starting from an isolated phage plaque, the final titer obtained (i.e., pfu/mL) is sometimes low (i.e., $<10^8$ pfu/mL). As such, clearing of the culture might not be visible and it might be difficult to conclude on the success of the infection. For this reason, we recommend proceeding to titration of the first amplification lysate (using the plaque assay, Subheading 3.3, **step 7**) in order to know how much phages have been generated and to decide whether a second amplification must be performed. Knowing the phage titer will allow optimizing the second amplification round with better-controlled infection parameters (e.g., multiplicity of infection).

9. With temperate phages, low MOI generally favor amplification of the phage via the lytic cycle while higher MOI generally favor lysogeny [3]. An MOI ranging between 0.01 and 0.1 is generally the best to get maximal amplification in broth. At lower MOI, the ratio of phages to bacteria is too low and the bacterial culture reaches the stationary phase before the phage has enough time to replicate to high titers. Inversely, at higher MOI bacteria are rapidly killed by the phage, thus limiting fur-

ther phage propagation. In addition, lysogens (which are immune to further reinfection) emerge early in the process, leading to growth of phage-resistant bacteria and poor phage production. It is therefore important to find the optimal phage-to-bacteria ratio (MOI) to favor maximal phage replication before bacteria enter the stationary phase. Typically, a culture of *C. difficile* at an OD_{600} of 0.1 contains roughly 10^7 CFU/mL. Therefore, in a phage amplification broth of 10 mL containing ~10^8 CFU, 10^6 or 10^7 phages need to be added to obtain an MOI of 0.01 and 0.1, respectively. Of course, these values are provided only as a reference based on our experience and the optimal MOI might be different with other phages and hosts.

10. Phosphotungstic acid, 2%, pH 7.2 (PTA) can also be used instead of, or ideally in parallel with uranyl acetate (UA) staining. Both staining solutions will give different results and PTA generally gives more negative staining than UA that tends to give positive staining under certain conditions. However, one advantage of UA is that both positive and negative staining can be obtained on a single grid. For further details and technical tips on the observation of phages by electron microscopy, we recommend reading the excellent book chapter written by Pr. Hans W. Ackermann, an expert in phage microscopy [37].

11. A phage lysate with a titer of 10^9 pfu/mL should yield enough DNA for a few restriction enzyme digestions, and for PFGE analysis. To increase the yield or if the titer of the lysate is a little lower, it is possible to simply scale up all the volumes according to the initial volume of phage lysate used.

12. Comparing a non-heated aliquot of the same restriction reaction side-by-side with a heated sample can be useful to determine whether cohesive termini are present in the phage genome analyzed. In the affirmative, a band in the non-heated sample will be split into two fragments in the heated reaction. Generating profiles with more than one enzyme can be helpful.

References

1. Brussow H, Canchaya C, Hardt W-D (2004) Phages and the evolution of bacterial pathogens: from genomic rearrangements to lysogenic conversion. Microbiol Mol Biol Rev 68:560–602. doi:10.1128/MMBR.68.3.560-602.2004

2. Fortier L-C, Sekulovic O (2013) Importance of prophages to evolution and virulence of bacterial pathogens. Virulence 4:354–365. doi:10.4161/viru.24498

3. Oppenheim AB, Kobiler O, Stavans J et al (2005) Switches in bacteriophage lambda development. Annu Rev Genet 39:409–429. doi:10.1146/annurev.genet.39.073003.113656

4. Juhala R, Ford M, Duda R et al (2000) Genomic sequences of bacteriophages HK97 and HK022: pervasive genetic mosaicism in the lambdoid bacteriophages. J Mol Biol 299:27–51

5. Hayashi T, Makino K, Ohnishi M et al (2001) Complete genome sequence of enterohemorrhagic Escherichia coli O157:H7 and genomic comparison with a laboratory strain K-12. DNA Res 8:11–22

6. Eklund MW, Poysky FT, Reed SM, Smith CA (1971) Bacteriophage and the toxigenicity of Clostridium botulinum Type C. Science (New York, NY) 172:480–482. doi:10.1126/science.172.3982.480

7. Hargreaves KR, Clokie MRJ (2014) Clostridium difficile phages: still difficult? Front Microbiol 5:184. doi:10.3389/fmicb.2014.00184

8. Goh S, Riley TV, Chang BJ (2005) Isolation and characterization of temperate bacteriophages of Clostridium difficile. Appl Environ Microbiol 71:1079–1083

9. Govind R, Fralick J, Rolfe R (2006) Genomic organization and molecular characterization of *Clostridium difficile* bacteriophage {Phi} CD119. J Bacteriol 188:2568–2577

10. Hargreaves KR, Colvin HV, Patel KV et al (2013) Genetically diverse Clostridium difficile strains harboring abundant prophages in an estuarine environment. Appl Environ Microbiol 79:6236–6243. doi:10.1128/AEM.01849-13

11. Shan J, Patel KV, Hickenbotham PT et al (2012) Prophage carriage and diversity within clinically relevant strains of Clostridium difficile. Appl Environ Microbiol 78:6027–6034. doi:10.1128/AEM.01311-12

12. Hargreaves KR, Kropinski AM, Clokie MRJ (2014) What does the talking?: quorum sensing signalling genes discovered in a bacteriophage genome. PLoS One 9:e85131. doi:10.1371/journal.pone.0085131

13. Nale JY, Shan J, Hickenbotham PT et al (2012) Diverse temperate bacteriophage carriage in *Clostridium difficile* 027 strains. PLoS One 7:e37263. doi:10.1371/journal.pone.0037263

14. Fortier L-C, Moineau S (2007) Morphological and genetic diversity of temperate phages in Clostridium difficile. Appl Environ Microbiol 73:7358–7366. doi:10.1128/AEM.00582-07

15. Sekulovic O, Garneau JR, Néron A, Fortier L-C (2014) Characterization of temperate phages infecting Clostridium difficile isolates of human and animal origins. Appl Environ Microbiol 80:2555–2563. doi:10.1128/AEM.00237-14

16. Sekulovic O, Meessen-Pinard M, Fortier L-C (2011) Prophage-stimulated toxin production in Clostridium difficile NAP1/027 lysogens. J Bacteriol 193:2726–2734. doi:10.1128/JB.00787-10

17. Meessen-Pinard M, Sekulovic O, Fortier L-C (2012) Evidence of in vivo prophage induction during Clostridium difficile infection. Appl Environ Microbiol 78:7662–7670. doi:10.1128/AEM.02275-12

18. Horgan M, O'Sullivan O, Coffey A et al (2010) Genome analysis of the Clostridium difficile phage PhiCD6356, a temperate phage of the Siphoviridae family. Gene 462:34–43. doi:10.1016/j.gene.2010.04.010

19. Mayer MJ, Narbad A, Gasson MJ (2008) Molecular characterization of a Clostridium difficile bacteriophage and its cloned biologically active endolysin. J Bacteriol 190:6734–6740

20. Didelot X, Eyre D, Cule M et al (2012) Microevolutionary analysis of Clostridium difficile genomes to investigate transmission. Genome Biol 13:R118. doi:10.1186/gb-2012-13-12-r118

21. Eyre DW, Fawley WN, Best EL et al (2013) Comparison of multilocus variable-number tandem-repeat analysis and whole-genome sequencing for investigation of Clostridium difficile transmission. J Clin Microbiol 51:4141–4149. doi:10.1128/JCM.01095-13

22. Eyre DW, Cule ML, Wilson DJ et al (2013) Diverse sources of C. difficile infection identified on whole-genome sequencing. N Engl J Med 369:1195–1205. doi:10.1056/NEJMoa1216064

23. Hargreaves KR, Otieno JR, Thanki A et al (2015) As clear as mud? Determining the diversity and prevalence of prophages in the draft genomes of estuarine isolates of Clostridium difficile. Genome Biol Evol 7(7):1842–1855. doi:10.1093/gbe/evv094

24. Fouts DE (2006) Phage_Finder: automated identification and classification of prophage regions in complete bacterial genome sequences. Nucleic Acids Res 34:5839–5851. doi:10.1093/nar/gkl732

25. Bose M, Barber RD (2006) Prophage Finder: a prophage loci prediction tool for prokaryotic genome sequences. In Silico Biol (Gedrukt) 6:223–227

26. Lima-Mendez G, Van Helden J, Toussaint A, Leplae R (2008) Prophinder: a computational tool for prophage prediction in prokaryotic genomes. Bioinformatics 24:863–865. doi:10.1093/bioinformatics/btn043

27. Zhou Y, Liang Y, Lynch KH et al (2011) PHAST: a fast phage search tool. Nucleic Acids Res 39:W347–W352. doi:10.1093/nar/gkr485

28. Akhter S, Aziz RK, Edwards RA (2012) PhiSpy: a novel algorithm for finding prophages in bacterial genomes that combines similarity- and composition-based strategies. Nucleic Acids Res 40:e126. doi:10.1093/nar/gks406

29. Grose JH, Casjens SR (2014) Understanding the enormous diversity of bacteriophages: the tailed phages that infect the bacterial family

Enterobacteriaceae. Virology 468–470C:421–443. doi:10.1016/j.virol.2014.08.024

30. Brussow H, Desiere F (2001) Comparative phage genomics and the evolution of Siphoviridae: insights from dairy phages. Mol Microbiol 39:213–222

31. Hargreaves KR, Flores CO, Lawley TD, Clokie MRJ (2014) Abundant and diverse clustered regularly interspaced short palindromic repeat spacers in Clostridium difficile strains and prophages target multiple phage types within this pathogen. mBio 5:e01045–13. doi:10.1128/mBio.01045-13

32. Rokney A, Kobiler O, Amir A et al (2008) Host responses influence on the induction of lambda prophage. Mol Microbiol 68:29–36. doi:10.1111/j.1365-2958.2008.06119.x

33. Ubeda C, Maiques E, Knecht E et al (2005) Antibiotic-induced SOS response promotes horizontal dissemination of pathogenicity island-encoded virulence factors in staphylococci. Mol Microbiol 56:836–844. doi:10.1111/j.1365-2958.2005.04584.x

34. Labrie SJ, Samson JE, Moineau S (2010) Bacteriophage resistance mechanisms. Nat Rev Microbiol 8:317–327. doi:10.1038/nrmicro2315

35. Fortier L-C, Moineau S (2009) Phage production and maintenance of stocks, including expected stock lifetimes. Methods Mol Biol 501:203–219. doi:10.1007/978-1-60327-164-6_19

36. Ackermann H-W, Prangishvili D (2012) Prokaryote viruses studied by electron microscopy. Arch Virol 157:1843–1849. doi:10.1007/s00705-012-1383-y

37. Ackermann H-W (2009) Basic phage electron microscopy. In: Kropinski AM, Clokie MRJ (eds) Bacteriophages: methods and protocols. Volume 1. Isolation, characterization, and interactions. Methods in molecular biology (Clifton, NJ). Humana Press, New York, pp 113–126

38. Hargreaves KR, Kropinski AM, Clokie MR (2014) Bacteriophage behavioral ecology: how phages alter their bacterial host's habits. Bacteriophage 4:e29866. doi:10.4161/bact.29866

39. Sekulovic O, Fortier L-C (2015) Global transcriptional response of *Clostridium difficile* carrying the φCD38 prophage. Appl Environ Microbiol 81:1364–1374. doi:10.1128/AEM.03656-14

40. Goh S, Chang BJ, Riley TV (2005) Effect of phage infection on toxin production by Clostridium difficile. J Med Microbiol 54:129–135

41. Govind R, Vediyappan G, Rolfe RD et al (2009) Bacteriophage-mediated toxin gene regulation in Clostridium difficile. J Virol 83:12037–12045. doi:10.1128/JVI.01256-09

42. Kutter E (2009) Phage host range and efficiency of plating. In: Clokie MRJ, Kropinski AM (eds) Bacteriophages: methods and protocols, vol 1. Humana Press, New York, pp 141–149

43. Dhalluin A, Lemee L, Pestel-Caron M et al (2003) Genotypic differentiation of twelve Clostridium species by polymorphism analysis of the triosephosphate isomerase (tpi) gene. Syst Appl Microbiol 26:90–96

44. Wiegand I, Hilpert K, Hancock REW (2008) Agar and broth dilution methods to determine the minimal inhibitory concentration (MIC) of antimicrobial substances. Nat Protoc 3:163–175. doi:10.1038/nprot.2007.521

45. Spinelli S, Veesler D, Bebeacua C, Cambillau C (2014) Structures and host-adhesion mechanisms of lactococcal siphophages. Front Microbiol 5:3. doi:10.3389/fmicb.2014.00003

46. Abedon ST (2011) Lysis from without. Bacteriophage 1:46–49. doi:10.4161/bact.1.1.13980

Chapter 12

Induction and Purification of *C. difficile* Phage Tail-Like Particles

John P. Hegarty, William Sangster, Robert E. Ashley, Roland Myers, Susan Hafenstein, and David B. Stewart Sr.

Abstract

Due to the inherent limitations of conventional antibiotics for the treatment of *C. difficile* infection (CDI), there is a growing interest in the development of alternative treatment strategies. Both bacteriophages and R-type bacteriocins, also known as phage tail-like particles (PTLPs), show promise as potential antibacterial alternatives for treating CDI. Similar to bacteriophages, but lacking a viral capsid and genome, PTLPs remain capable of killing target bacteria. Here we describe our experience in the induction and purification of *C. difficile* PTLPs. These methods have been optimized to allow production of concentrated, non-contractile, and non-aggregated samples for both sensitivity testing and structural electron microscopy studies.

Key words *Clostridium difficile*, Phage tail-like particles, Induction, Purification, Microscopy

1 Introduction

The most important risk determinant for the development of CDI beyond exposure to the organism itself is the use of antibiotics, due to their widespread effects which result in both the intended killing of their target organism and the unintended killing of a significant number of other host bacteria. The resultant perturbation to the bacterial component of the gut microbial community not only produces an environment conducive to the development of CDI, but it also promotes recurrences of CDI after initial treatment, which affects as many as 20–50 % of patients following their first episode of this infection [1, 2].

Bacteriophages and phage endolysins both show promise as potential antibacterial alternatives for treating CDI [3, 4]. In addition, many bacteria produce non-propagating PTLPs, often referred to as "defective prophages." Characterized by phage structural components with an absence of a phage capsid and phage genome, PTLPs can retain selective phage-like lytic activity by creating a channel in the wall of their target cell that leads to a rapid dissipation of

Adam P. Roberts and Peter Mullany (eds.), *Clostridium difficile: Methods and Protocols*, Methods in Molecular Biology, vol. 1476, DOI 10.1007/978-1-4939-6361-4_12, © Springer Science+Business Media New York 2016

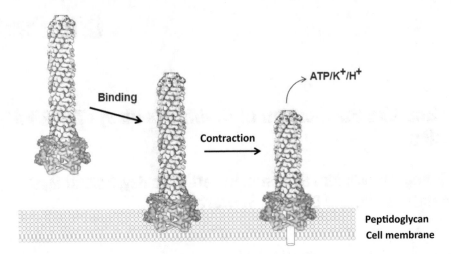

Fig. 1 PTLP bactericidal mechanism. Attachment is mediated by specific binding of the receptor-binding protein to a bacterial surface receptor. Subsequent sheath contraction and penetration of the PTLP core through the bacterial cell wall produce an open channel that results in cell death

membrane proton potential and cell death (Fig. 1). Since PTLPs are a form of bacteriocins, they can be broadly categorized into one of the two categories, either as contractile (R-type) or as non-contractile (F-type) forms. The former family is structurally similar to tails of T-even phages (*Myoviridae*), while the morphology of the latter family resembles the flexible tails of lambda phage (*Siphoviridae*) [5].

Studies have shown that PTLPs can, with a narrow specificity, effectively reduce target bacterial numbers both in vitro and in vivo. This may offer a means for construction of new therapeutic agents with directed action against specific bacteria. *C. difficile* is known to produce PTLPs ,[6, 7] and recently seminal data have demonstrated the efficacy of both natural and modified PTLPs to efficiently kill specific strains of *C. difficile* both in vitro [8, 9] and in vivo [10].

The structure of the contractile mechanisms of PTLPs produced by *P. aeruginosa* has recently been described [11]. Our group aimed to extend similar transmission and cryo-electron microscopy (cryo-EM) structural studies to *C. difficile* PTLPs, and in particular its tail-subunit which has a large, novel, receptor-binding protein. Cryo-EM studies necessitate high-quality samples at a high concentration. The initial PTLP purification work in our laboratory using ultracentrifugation pelleting ($90,000 \times g$, 2 h) and fast ($14,000 \times g$, 100 k MWCO) ultrafiltration concentration approaches resulted in non-ideal samples for cryo-EM study (Fig. 2). These samples typically contained (1) excessive cellular debris, (2) significant numbers of contracted and tail-sheared particles, and/or (3) extensive clumping of PTLPs due to aggregation of their "flower-like" receptor-binding proteins, especially at higher concentrations. Here we detail an alternative method for preparation of *C. difficile* PTLP samples that largely removes these contaminants and artifacts.

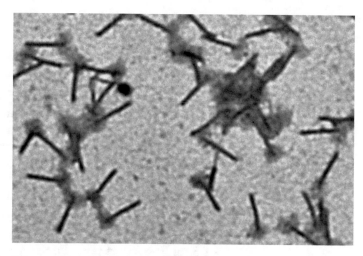

Fig. 2 Aggregation of PTLP receptor-binding proteins following concentration

2   Materials

2.1 C. difficile Growth and PTLP Induction

1. Sheep blood (5%) agar plates (TSA II—BBL 221261, BD Diagnostics, USA).

2. Pre-reduced brain–heart infusion supplemented with l-cysteine (BHIS) broth (AS-872, Anaerobe Systems, USA).

3. 50× Norfloxacin (150 μg/ml solution): Add 10 ml Milli-Q water to 6 mg norfloxacin (N9890 Sigma Aldrich, USA). Acidify with two drops 1 N HCL and vortex vigorously to dissolve. Add 30 ml DPBS and then 0.2 μm filter. Store at 4 °C.

4. Sterile cotton swab applicators.

2.2 PTLP Precipitation

1. SM buffer (100 mM NaCl, 8 mM $MgSO_4$, 50 mM Tris–HCL, pH 7.5), 0.2 μm filter.

2. 5 M NaCl (146 g NaCl in 500 ml water).

3. 0.2 μm Surfactant-free cellulose acetate syringe filters (190-9920, Nalgene).

4. Magnetic stirrer and stir bar.

5. 250 ml GSA centrifuge tubes.

6. Balance/scale.

7. PEG-8000/$MgSO_4$ solution: To 500 ml H_2O in a 1 L bottle add 1.8 g $MgSO_4 \cdot 7H_2O$.
   Slowly add 120 g polyethylene glycol 8000 (PEG8000; P5413 Sigma-Aldrich) with stirring. Cap and shake bottle until largely dissolved. Heat bottle in 50 °C water bath for 20 min to completely dissolve. 0.45 μm filter. Store at 4 °C.

8. DNase I (2000 U/ml, M0303L, New England Biolabs, USA).

9. RNase A (20 μg/ml, Life Technologies).

2.3 Electron Microscopy	1. 400-Mesh continuous-carbon copper grids (Electron Microscopy Sciences, PA, USA).

1. 400-Mesh continuous-carbon copper grids (Electron Microscopy Sciences, PA, USA).

2. Dumont Tweezer L5 (72882-D); Dumont self-closing N4-style forceps (72870-D, Electron Microscopy Sciences, USA).

3. 1.0% Uranyl acetate: Weigh 4 g of uranyl acetate (UA) under the fume hood (wear protection) and add to the 100 ml volumetric flask. Pipette 96 ml of near-boiling CO_2-free double-distilled water into the flask. Stir until uranyl acetate dihydrate crystals are dissolved (several hours). Allow solution cool down to room temperature (pH 4.5). Filter through a Whatman #1 filter into a lightproof bottle and cap tightly. Store at 4 °C.

4. 0.75% Uranyl formate: Weigh 0.0044 g of uranyl formate (UF) powder and mix into 0.587 ml of 12.5 mM NaOH in a 1.5 ml Eppendorf tube. Place capped Eppendorf tube in boiling water bath to solubilize UF. Vortex and repeat boiling until UF is dissolved. Pass through 0.22 μm syringe filter and adjust to pH to 4.5–5.5. Storage at room temperature away from light for up to 1 week.

5. Ultra-pure Milli-Q water.

6. Petri dishes.

7. Whatman #1 filter paper cut into wedges.

8. Timer.

2.4 CsCl Purification

1. 62.5% CsCl solution: 25 g CsCl + 15 ml deionized water, 0.2 μm filtered.

2. TE buffer: 10 mM Tris–HCl at a pH of 8.0, and 1 mM EDTA.

3. Thin-wall ultraclear centrifuge tubes (#344059, Beckman Coulter).

4. 9″ Glass borosilicate Pasteur pipettes.

5. Balance/scale.

6. 21-G disposable needle/syringes.

7. Slide-A-Lyzer Dialysis Cassettes 10,000 MWCO 3 ml capacity (#66380 Thermo Scientific, USA).

2.5 Concentration

1. 300 kDa MWCO spin filters (OD300C33; NanoSep Omega, Pall Corp., USA).

2. SM buffer.

3. 1.7 ml Sterile microfuge tubes with locking caps.

3 Methods

3.1 C. difficile Growth

1. Swab-culture *C. difficile* isolate HMC114 (*see* **Note 1**) under anaerobic conditions using an Anoxomat, or similar anaerobic system, at 37 °C for 48 h onto pre-reduced blood agar plates.

3.2 PTLP Induction

Although PTLPs are spontaneously produced by *C. difficile* in lower numbers, they cannot be propagated in the manner of bacteriophage. Production can raised by 2 orders of magnitude through induction of an SOS response using sub-inhibitory amounts of antibiotics or UV irradiation [12, 13] (*see* **Note 2**).

1. Resuspend bacteria from one half of plate into 3 ml BHIS broth and use to swab (*see* **Note 3**) 12–15 plates pre-swabbed (*see* **Note 4**) with 50× norfloxacin solution.

2. Incubate plates under anaerobic incubation for 16 h.

3.3 PTLP Precipitation

1. Collect induced cells from plate surfaces by flooding each with 5 ml SM buffer, pooling into a single tube, and thoroughly suspend by pipetting and vortexing.

2. Add 1/5 volume of 5 M NaCl.

3. Incubate at room temperature for 30 min with shaking to promote disaggregation of PTLPs from the cells.

4. Pellet cells and large debris at $12,000 \times g$ for 15 min at 4 °C.

5. Gently pass supernatant through 0.2 μm surfactant-free cellulose acetate filter.

6. Precipitate PTLPs by adding a half volume of PEG-8000/MgSO$_4$ solution for final concentrations of 8%/5 mM, respectively.

7. Slowly stir on ice for 30 min.

8. Precipitate PTLPs at 4 °C, overnight.

9. Split PTLP sample into 250 ml GSA tubes and balance.

10. Pellet the PTLPs by centrifugation at $3400 \times g$ for 40 min at 4 °C (*see* **Note 5**).

11. Decant supernatant, draining excess PEG onto paper towels.

12. Suspended pellet (*see* **Note 6**) in 3 ml SM buffer.

13. Allow PTLPs to solubilize in buffer for 1 h with gentle shaking at room temperature.

14. Digest with DNase I (8 μl; plus 300 μl 10× reaction buffer) and RNase A (10 μl) for 1 h at 37 °C.

15. Extract PEG with repeat equal volumes of CHCl$_3$ (*see* **Note 7**) carefully collecting the upper aqueous phase each time, until the interface is clear.

16. Store samples at 4 °C.

3.4 Cesium Chloride Gradient Purification

1. Prepare CsCl step-gradients in ultracentrifuge tubes using 62.5% CsCl diluted with TE buffer.

2. Use the following ratios (volumes) of CsCl to TE per tube: 1:2 (3 ml), 1:1 (3 ml), 2:1 (3 ml), 1:0 (1.5 ml). Layer sequentially denser CsCl solutions to the bottom of each tube using a Pasteur pipette.

3. Layer the PTLP sample (approximately 3 ml each) on top of step gradients.

4. Adjust and balance final tube volumes to 1 mm below rim using TE buffer.

5. Ultracentrifuge tubes in a Beckman SW41 rotor at $35,000 \times g$ at 4 °C for 2 h.

6. Two opaque bands are typically visible near the middle of the tube. Carefully collect the second band from the top (Fig. 3) in a minimal volume by gentle side puncture of tube with a 21-G needle/syringe.

7. Transfer collected PLTP sample to cassette and dialyze against $500 \times$ volume SM buffer at 4 °C, with two buffer changes.

3.5 Concentration of PTLP Samples

1. Pre-rinse 300 kDa MWCO filters with three washes of SM buffer (*see* **Note 8**).

2. Gently concentrate PTLPs by centrifuging 1 ml samples at $4000 \times g$ at 4 °C through 300 kDa MWCO filters until approximately 100 μl volume remains (*see* **Note 9**).

3. Wash PTLPs with two sequential 1 ml volumes of sterile-filtered SM buffer, again reducing the volume to 100 μl with each $1000 \times g$ spin.

4. Transfer concentrated PTLP samples to microfuge tubes. Seal lids with parafilm and store at 4 °C. Samples are ready for sensitivity testing (Fig. 4) and microscopy studies (Fig. 5).

3.6 Electron Microscopy

1. Hold the glow-discharged grid in forceps above filter paper-lined Petri dish and apply a 3 μl sample onto a copper grid (*see* **Note 10**). Allow PTLPs to absorb onto grid surface for

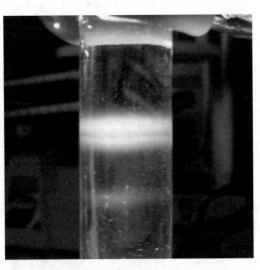

Fig. 3 CsCl gradient bands. The opaque, second band from the top of the gradient (bluish tint) is collected by syringe for dialysis

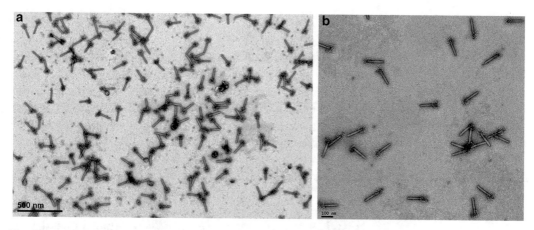

Fig. 4 Transmission electron microscopy of negatively stained phage tail-like particles

Fig. 5 Plate spot sensitivity testing. Clear zone of cell death is visible following spotting 10 µl PTLP for strain HMC114 onto ribotype 027 *C. difficile* bacterial lawn and anaerobic incubation for 16 h

1–5 min. Draw off excess sample from the edge of the grid with filter paper.

2. For UA stain:

    (a) Wash grid briefly by quickly placing grid surface atop two successive droplets of ultra-pure water.

    (b) Stain grid with 5 µl of 1.0 % uranyl acetate for 15 s. Draw off excess stain from the grid edge using filter paper.

3. For UF stain:

    (a) Wash with three drops of ultra-pure water, blotting grid from the side between each drop.

    (b) Stain with 6 µl 0.75 % uranyl formate for 10 s. Blot off excess stain from the grid edge using filter paper.

4. Air-dry stained covered grids, and then place in grid storage box.

5. Visualize grids using a JEOL JEM1400 transmission electron microscope at 120 kV.

6. In brief for cryo-EM: Glow discharge holey carbon Quantifoil electron microscopy grids for approximately 1 min. Place 3.5 μl aliquot of sample onto the carbon side of the glow-discharged grid. Blot and vitrify by plunging into a mixture of liquid ethane cooled by liquid nitrogen using a Gatan CP3 plunge-freezing robot operating at 90 % humidity.

4   Notes

1. HMC114 is a ribotype 078 *C. difficile* strain isolated from human stool by our laboratory and identified as consistently producing PTLPs in significant quantities following norfloxacin or mitomycin C induction.

2. Our *C. difficile* induction protocols use broth dosages of 6 μg/ ml norfloxacin, 3 μg/ml mitomycin C, or 100 J/m^2 UV light (G30T8, 30 W germicidal tube; with an incident dose rate of 20 ergs/mm^2/s for 22 s from 53 cm distance in open Petri dishes filled to depth of 3 mm with log-phage *C. difficile*). Our experience aligns with observations [14] that the induction efficacy for any given agent varies among individual isolates, likely due to sequence differences in regulatory regions flanking the PTLP clusters.

3. In our hands, induction of broth cultures produced disappointing PTLP yields with excessive cellular debris. We found that induction of cells grown on solid-media blood plates swabbed with 50× norfloxacin solution often yielded much better preparations.

4. For PTLP induction, swab each plate *immediately* before swabbing with bacterial culture.

5. When placed into the rotor, mark the outer side of each tube to assist in location of the pellet target area.

6. Suspend the precipitated PTLP pellet by repeat pipetting of buffer gently over the marked side wall of the tube. Using a plate-based induction, we observed very clean, barely visible, U-shaped pellets.

7. Use a glass pipette to transfer chloroform.

8. Rinsing removes trace manufacturing amounts of glycerin from the Omega membranes.

9. Low-speed centrifugation through the filters in a refrigerated centrifuge avoided PTLP receptor aggregation.

10. Glow-discharge carbon-coated and Quantifoil grids for 15 s and 1 min, respectively, using room oxygen at 20 mA in a plasma cleaner.

References

1. McFarland LV, Elmer GW, Surawicz CM (2002) Breaking the cycle: treatment strategies for 163 cases of recurrent *Clostridium difficile* disease. Am J Gastroenterol 97:1769–1775

2. Surawicz CM (2013) Infection: treating recurrent *C. difficile* infection-the challenge continues. Nat Rev Gastroenterol Hepatol 10(1):10–11

3. Hargreaves KR, Clokie MR (2014) *Clostridium difficile* phages: still difficult? Front Microbiol 28(5):184

4. Nakonieczna A, Cooper CJ, Gryko R. (2015) Bacteriophages and bacteriophage derived endolysins as potential therapeutics to combat gram positive spore forming bacteria. J Appl Microbiol. June 24 [Epub]

5. Michel-Briand Y, Baysse C (2002) The pyocins of *Pseudomonas aeruginosa*. Biochimie 84:449–510

6. Fortier LC, Moineau S (2007) Morphological and genetic diversity of temperate phages in *Clostridium difficile*. Appl Environ Microbiol 73:7358–7366

7. Nale JY, Shan J, Hickenbotham PT, Fawley WN, Wilcox MH, Clokie MR (2012) Diverse temperate bacteriophage carriage in *Clostridium difficile* 027 strains. PLoS One 7:e37263

8. Gebhart D, Williams SR, Bishop-Lilly KA, Govoni GR, Willner KM, Butani A et al (2012) Novel high-molecular-weight, R-type bacteriocins of *Clostridium difficile*. J Bacteriol 194:6240–6247

9. Sangster W, Hegarty JP, Stewart DB Sr (2015) Phage tail-like particles kill *Clostridium difficile* and represent an alternative to conventional antibiotics. Surgery 157(1):96–103

10. Gebhart D, Lok S, Clare S, Tomas M, Stares M, Scholl D, Donskey CJ, Lawley TD, Govoni GR (2015) A modified R-type bacteriocin specifically targeting *Clostridium difficile* prevents colonization of mice without affecting gut microbiota diversity. MBio 6(2):e02368-14

11. Ge P, Scholl D, Leiman PG, Yu X, Miller JF, Zhou ZH (2015) Atomic structures of a bactericidal contractile nanotube in its pre- and post-contraction states. Nat Struct Mol Biol 22(5):377–382

12. Goh S, Riley TV, Chang BJ (2005) Isolation and characterization of temperate bacteriophages of *Clostridium difficile*. Appl Environ Microbiol 71(2):1079–1083

13. Sekulovic O, Garneau JR, Néron A, Fortier LC (2014) Characterization of temperate phages infecting *Clostridium difficile* isolates of human and animal origins. Appl Environ Microbiol 80(8):2555–2556

14. Meessen-Pinard M, Sekulovic O, Fortier LC (2012) Evidence of in vivo prophage induction during *Clostridium difficile* infection. Appl Environ Microbiol 78(21):7662–7670

Chapter 13

Phage Transduction

Shan Goh

Abstract

Bacteriophages mediate horizontal gene transfer through a mechanism known as transduction. Phage transduction carried out in the laboratory involves a bacterial donor and a recipient, both of which are susceptible to infection by the phage of interest. Phage is propagated in the donor, concentrated, and exposed transiently to recipient at different multiplicity of infection ratios. Transductants are selected for the desired phenotype by culture on selective medium. Here we describe transduction of *ermB* conferring resistance to erythromycin by the *C. difficile* phage φC2.

Key words Phage, Transduction, Antibiotic resistance genes

1 Introduction

Transduction refers to phage-mediated transfer of DNA from a donor bacterial cell to a recipient bacterial cell. Since the discovery of transduction in the Salmonella phage, P22 [1], other phages were also shown capable of either generalized or specialized transduction. Generalized transduction occurs when phage transfers random bacterial DNA, usually not associated with phage DNA [2]. Specialized transduction occurs when phage transfers specific pieces of bacterial DNA together with phage DNA [2].

Transduction was used in early molecular investigations to map genes in *Escherichia coli* and *Salmonella* spp. These experiments used very high titers of phage ($\geq 10^9$ PFU/mL) propagated in a donor strain, and phage suspensions were mixed directly with recipient cells on selective agar plates [3]. Modifications of this protocol included mixing of cells in liquid media/buffers before plating, and the inclusion of controls for sterility of phage suspensions and for spontaneous mutations of the recipients [4]. Transduction of antibiotic resistance genes was measured using similar protocols. Otherwise, phages were induced at high titers of $\geq 10^8$ PFU/mL from a donor lysogen, either with mitomycin C or UV irradiation, and used directly for transduction with recipient

Adam P. Roberts and Peter Mullany (eds.), *Clostridium difficile: Methods and Protocols*, Methods in Molecular Biology, vol. 1476, DOI 10.1007/978-1-4939-6361-4_13, © Springer Science+Business Media New York 2016

strains [5]. Phage that was not induced at high titers has been assayed for transduction using larger volumes of induced phage [6]. Although this has not been attempted in *C. difficile*, it appears feasible provided only one phage type is induced from the donor strain, and presence of the phage can be validated in some way (i.e., plaque assay or transmission electron microscopy). This may be challenging as many *C. difficile* lysogens contain more than one phage type [7, 8], it is difficult to find *C. difficile* hosts for *C. difficile* phage to plaque on [9], and access to/availability of a transmission electron microscopy is not always easy.

The methods presented here are based on *C. difficile* phage φC2 transduction of *ermB* between *C. difficile* isolates [10]. They are similar to early methods used in terms of propagating the phage in donor cells, then mixed with recipient cells in liquid media, and plated onto selective plates. The main changes pertain to concentration of the phage so as to obtain a high titer of $\geq 10^8$ PFU/mL, and maintaining viability of *C. difficile* cells under anaerobic conditions.

2   Materials

2.1 Bacterial Growth and Phage Propagation Media

Anaerobe basal agar (ABA): dehydrated powder (Oxoid Thermo Scientific).

Brain heart infusion agar (BHIA): dehydrated powder (Oxoid Thermo Scientific).

Brain heart infusion broth (BHIB): dehydrated powder (Oxoid Thermo Scientific).

Blood agar: 5% defibrinated horse blood, dehydrated BHIA.

Soft agar (SA): anaerobe basal broth dehydrated powder (Oxoid Thermo Scientific), 0.74% Bacteriological agar no. 1 (Oxoid Thermo Scientific), 0.01 M $CaCl_2$, 0.4 M $MgCl_2 \cdot 6H_2O$.

Petri dishes 90 and 150 mm.

2.2 Broth Microdilution MIC Susceptibility Assays

0.22 μm syringe filters.

Schandlers broth (SB): dehydrated powder (Oxoid Thermo Scientific).

Clindamycin: dissolve clindamycin powder in 70% ethanol to obtain 50 mg/mL concentration, filter sterilize stock through 0.22 μm syringe filter.

Chloramphenicol: dissolve chloramphenicol powder in 95% ethanol to obtain 50 mg/mL concentration.

Erythromycin: dissolve erythromycin powder in 95% ethanol to obtain 50 mg/mL concentration.

Tetracycline: dissolve tetracycline powder in 70% ethanol to obtain 10 mg/mL concentration, filter sterilize stock through 0.22 μm syringe filter.

96-well plates.

Multichannel pipette.

Multichannel reagent reservoirs.

2.3 Phage Purification

Phage buffer: dissolve the following in water to indicated concentrations 0.15 M NaCl, 10 mM Tris–HCl, 10 mM $MgSO_4$, 1 mM $CaCl_2$, adjust pH to 7 with HCl and make up to a final volume of 1 L, autoclave.

0.22 µm syringe filters.

5–10 mL syringes.

1 M NaCl: dissolve NaCl in water to 1 M, autoclave.

PEG 8000.

Chloroform.

1 M KCl: dissolve KCl in water to 1 M, autoclave.

2.4 PCR

PCR grade water.

Phusion High-Fidelity PCR Master mix (Thermo Scientific).

Forward primer E5 (specific for *ermB*): CTCAAAACT TTTTAACGAGTG.

Reverse primer E6 (specific for *ermB*): CCTCCCGTTA AATAATAGATA.

Genomic DNA extracted with Qiagen Puregene yeast kit.

2.5 Transduction

BHIA.

BHIS-T (taurocholate) agar: dehydrated BHIA, 5 mg/mL yeast extract, 0.1% taurocholate, 0.1% l-cysteine, dissolve all in water and autoclave.

BHIA + Tet (10 µg/mL): dehydrated BHIA, 1/1000 tetracycline stock solution.

BHIA + Erm (50 µg/mL): dehydrated BHIA, 1/1000 erythromycin stock solution.

Disposable spreaders.

Phage buffer.

BHIB.

3 Methods

3.1 Finding Donors and Recipients of Antibiotic Resistant Genes (ARG) for Phage Transduction

C. difficile isolates that are hosts for plaque formation by phage must be tested for antibiotic susceptibility in order to determine appropriate donors and recipients for transduction of ARGs. Antibiotic susceptibility may be tested in a number of ways using standard guidelines provided by a number of organizations such as CLSI [11], BSAC [12], and EUCAST [13]. Here, a broth microdilution method following CLSI guidelines [11] is used.

1. Prepare a fresh 48 h culture of *C. difficile* on BA.

2. Pre-reduce SB for overnight (10 mL per *C. difficile* isolate to be tested).

3. For each *C. difficile* isolate, anaerobically subculture five colonies of similar sizes into 10 mL pre-reduced SB and incubate for 18–20 h.

4. Prepare 2× stock solutions of antibiotics in SB (2–256 mg/L). Dispense 50 µl of each antibiotic concentration per well in a 96-well plate, and include a no antibiotic control (i.e., 50 µl of SB) per antibiotic for each *C. difficile* isolate.

5. Dilute 18–20 h *C. difficile* culture in SB to obtain approximately 2×10^6 CFU/mL (*see* **Note 1**).

6. Within 15 min of preparing the standardized bacterial culture, inoculate 50 µl to wells containing antibiotics. For each antibiotic, leave a series of dilutions uninoculated with bacteria and add SB instead.

7. Incubate anaerobically for 46–48 h.

8. Score growth visually and record the minimum antibiotic concentration that prevents growth (MIC).

9. Compare MIC values with known MIC breakpoints from CLSI M11-A7 [11] to determine whether *C. difficile* test isolate is antibiotic resistant (a donor) or sensitive (a recipient).

3.2 PCR of Antibiotic Resistant Donor Isolates

Many mobilizable antibiotic resistant genes in *C. difficile* are sequenced. Presence of a resistance gene conferring an antibiotic resistant phenotype identified above should be confirmed by carrying out a PCR on the donor isolates, and the amplicon should be sequenced. For best results, the PCR template should be genomic DNA (gDNA) extracted from an overnight culture grown in BHIB. We use the Gentra Puregene Yeast/Bacteria kit (Qiagen) for gDNA extraction, and the Phusion High-Fidelity PCR Master Mix with HF Buffer (Life Technologies).

1. Prepare Phusion Master Mix on ice as follows: 1× Phusion Master Mix, 0.5 µM E5 primer, 0.5 µM E6 primer, and 10–50 ng gDNA in a final volume of 25 µl.

2. Mix by vortexing and spin down briefly. Run PCR using the following conditions (*see* **Note 2**): 98 °C for 30 s, 35 cycles of 98 °C for 10 s, 56 °C for 15 s, and 72 °C for 30 s, and a final extension at 72 °C for 5 min.

3. Analyze PCR products in a 1% agarose gel and an appropriate DNA ladder (e.g., 2-log ladder, New England Biolabs). The expected amplicon is 750 bp.

3.3 Propagate Phage in Donor (Agar Overlay Method)

Phage may be propagated either in liquid medium or on agar plates, and with overnight or log phase host cultures. This depends on phage preferences, which can be determined by methods described elsewhere. For example, φC2 propagates equally well in overnight and log phase cultures of CD062 (a recipient strain for transduction) but prefers log phase cultures of CD80 (a donor strain for transduction). φC2 does not propagate well in liquid medium, hence the method outlined is for propagation on agar plates in log phase cultures of CD80. Large agar plates (150 mm diameter) are preferable, otherwise standard agar plates (90 mm diameter) will work but yield lower volumes of harvested phage.

1. Inoculate 1–2 *C. difficile* colonies into 10 mL of pre-reduced BHIB and incubate for 18–20 h.

2. If phage prefers log phase cultures for propagation, prepare a log phase culture of the donor by inoculating 500 µl of an overnight culture into 5 mL pre-reduced BHIB. Incubate for 3–4 h, with occasional shaking by hand (*see* **Note 3**).

3. Prewarm labeled ABA plates to 37 °C. Melt SA thoroughly, ensuring there are no lumps and keep molten in a 50 °C water bath (*see* **Note 4**).

4. Inoculate a sterile universal bottle with 1 mL of phage suspension (~10^5 PFU/mL).

5. Remove log phase donor culture (tightly sealed in tube) from the anaerobic workstation.

6. Add 4 mL of donor, followed by 9 mL of SA into the universal bottle containing phage, and immediately overlay onto ABA plate by swirling gently but quickly to cover the entire surface.

7. Immediately transfer the plate into the anaerobic workstation. Lift off the lid slightly to let out trapped oxygen, then replace the lid and incubate overnight (*see* **Note 5**).

8. Include a no-phage control plate, which is a positive control for donor growth.

9. Semi-confluent lysis of bacteria should be obvious when compared to the no-phage control (*see* **Note 6**).

10. Harvest the phage by scrapping the layer of SA containing phage into a tube containing the same volume of phage buffer (i.e., 14 mL per plate).

11. Vortex vigorously to obtain a homogenous suspension.

12. Centrifuge at 11,000 × g for 15 min at 4 °C.

13. Filter the supernatant using a syringe and a 0.45 or 0.22 µm syringe filter to obtain a crude phage suspension. Store at 4 °C.

3.4 Semi-purify Crude Phage Suspension

Phage should be concentrated by PEG precipitation if the titer is less than 10^8 PFU/mL. Dialyzed phage suspensions are ideal for use in transduction, but require particle separation through a pre-formed density gradient using an ultracentrifuge, followed by several rounds of dialysis. The use of semi-purified phage suspensions for transduction gives satisfactory results, provided some controls are included.

1. To remove bacterial nucleic acid present in the phage suspension, treat with DNase I (10 μg/mL) and RNase A (10 μg/mL) for 30 min at 37 °C.

2. Add 1 M NaCl and dissolve by swirling.

3. Add 10 % w/v PEG 8000 and dissolve by stirring.

4. Place suspension on ice and inside a fridge for overnight.

5. Centrifuge suspension at $5,000 \times g$ for 20 min at 4 °C.

6. Remove the supernatant and resuspend the pellet in 1/50–1/100 the original volume with phage buffer and a transfer pipette. Pipette up and down to break up the PEG pellet.

7. Add the same volume of chloroform and vortex to mix well (*see* **Note 7**).

8. Centrifuge at $5,000 \times g$ for 20 min at room temperature.

9. Recover the aqueous phase (or supernatant if using KCl, *see* **Note 7**) and determine phage titer by plaque assays.

3.5 Determine Phage Titer

1. Prepare overnight or log phase cultures of an appropriate host strain as described in "Propagate phage in donor (agar overlay method)".

2. Make tenfold serial dilutions of the phage suspension in 1 mL phage buffer.

3. Dispense 100 μl of appropriate serial dilutions into sterile bijou bottles, and include a no phage control bottle. Routine dilutions used are 10^{-3}, 10^{-4}, 10^{-5}, 10^{-6}.

4. Pre-warm five labeled ABA plates (standard 90 mm size) to 37 °C. Melt SA thoroughly, ensuring there are no lumps and keep molten in a 50 °C water bath.

5. Remove *C. difficile* culture from the anaerobic workstation and add 600 μl to each bijou bottle.

6. Add 1.5 mL of SA and immediately overlay onto ABA plate by swirling gently but quickly to cover the entire surface (*see* **Note 5**).

7. Incubate plates overnight.

8. Select the plate with 30–300 plaques for counting and calculation of phage titer.

3.6 Transduction

Unless otherwise stated, the procedure is carried out in an anaerobic workstation. This protocol is based on ϕC2 transduction between donor CD80 and recipient CD062.

1. Prepare log phase culture of CD062 (3–4 h).

2. Bring materials needed for transduction into anaerobic cabinet. These are: semi-purified ϕC2/80 of a known titer, 1.5 mL microfuge tubes, P1000 pipette, tips, waste bin, four plates of each antibiotic type, two BHIA plates, phage buffer, disposable spreaders, tube rack.

3. Dilute log phase CD062 culture 1/10 (to achieve approx. 10^7 CFU/mL) with pre-reduced BHIB (see **Note 8**).

4. Add volumes of phage and bacteria in microfuge tubes to obtain expected MOI of 0.125, 0.25, and 0.5. i.e., 125 μl phage + 1000 μl bacteria for 0.125 MOI, 250 μl phage + 1000 μl bacteria for 0.25 MOI, 250 μl phage + 500 μl bacteria for 0.5 MOI. The actual multiplicity of infection (MOI) should be calculated the following day after viable counts of the recipient are carried out (see **Note 9**). Include a negative control tube with 250 μl phage buffer and 1000 μl bacteria.

5. Mix tubes by inverting several times and incubate for 1 h

6. Meanwhile, serially dilute log CD062 used for transduction tenfold, 5×.

7. Spread plate 100 μl of 10^{-4}, 10^{-5} dilutions onto BHIA plates for viable count.

8. Spread plate 100 μl of 10^{-4}, 10^{-5} dilutions onto BHIA + Tet (10 μg/mL) and BHIA + Erm (50 μg/mL) plates to detect spontaneous mutants.

9. Carrying on from **step 6**. Move tubes out of the anaerobic workstation and spin in a microfuge for 1 min, $10,000 \times g$ to pellet cells.

10. Transfer tubes back into cabinet, remove S/N and resuspend cells in 1 mL BHIB.

11. Repeat wash (**steps 9** and **10**).

12. Resuspend cells in 200 μl BHIB.

13. Plate 100 μl of each tube containing phage and bacteria onto BHIA + Tet (10 μg/mL) and BHIA + Erm (50 μg/mL) (see **Note 10**).

14. Plate 100 μl of phage suspension used for transduction onto BHIS-T plate for sterility (free of contaminating donor spores).

15. Check control plates from **steps 8** and **14**, which should be free of growth.

16. Count number of transductant colonies on antibiotic plates after 48 and 72 h.

17. Calculate actual CFU/mL of CD062 (using viable count plates from **step 7**) used for transduction and calculate actual MOI for each tube (see **Note 11**)

18. Transduction frequency was calculated as transductants per input PFU.

3.7 Validation of Transductants

Transductants should be validated by PCR detection of the antibiotic resistance gene, followed by sequencing of the PCR product. Colonies of transductants can be boiled and used for PCR following standard protocols.

1. Lightly touch a colony of erythromycin resistant transductant with a sterile toothpick.

2. Resuspend cells in 10 µl of PCR grade water.

3. Boil cells at 95 °C for 15 min.

4. Meanwhile prepare Phusion Master Mix on ice as follows: 1× Phusion Master Mix, 0.5 µM E5 primer, and 0.5 µM E6 primer in a final volume of 15 µl per reaction.

5. Mix by vortexing and spin down briefly.

6. Add 15 µl of the Phusion Master Mix to each tube of boiled cells to obtain a final volume of 25 µl.

7. Run PCR with conditions shown above for the donor.

4 Notes

1. We usually find a 1/50 dilution to be sufficient, but one should carry out viable counts on BHIA plates to be sure. This can be done by removing 10 µl of the diluted culture into 20 mL SB and then plating 100 µl onto a BHIA plate. After an overnight incubation, 100 colonies are expected from a 2×10^6 CFU/mL culture.

2. The melting temperatures of PCR primers used with Phusion Master Mix should be calculated using a Tm calculator specific for the enzyme: https://www.lifetechnologies.com/uk/en/home/brands/thermo-scientific/molecular-biology/molecular-biology-learning-center/molecular-biology-resource-library/thermo-scientific-web-tools/tm-calculator.html.

3. It may be necessary to determine the growth curve of your *C. difficile* isolate under your experimental conditions if cultures are not turbid after 3–4 h of incubation.

4. Repeated melting of solidified SA will lead to caramelizing (darkening) of the agar, reducing performance. It is advisable to prepare SA in small aliquots of 10–50 mL, which can be discarded after it has been melted several times or has darkened.

5. Log phase cultures are extremely sensitive to oxygen and will not produce good lawns if exposed to oxygen for more than 10 min. **Steps 5** and **6** must be carried out within 10 min.

6. Titrations of the phage suspension may be included to aid in visualizing single plaques, which will be difficult to see in a semi-confluent lysis plate.

7. If phage is sensitive to chloroform, add 1 M KCl to PEG suspension instead and dissolve by inverting, then leave on ice for 30 min for phage particles to dissociate from PEG.

8. CD062 4 h culture is approx. 10^8 CFU/mL. This should be tested for each isolate prior to transduction.

9. These MOI ratios are a good starting point but they can be increased or decreased according to needs. MOI > 0.5 tended to lead to low or no recovery of transductants, likely due to lysis of CD062 by ϕC2, as a bacterial cell pellet was not visible after **step 9** of transdcution. This observation was noted in early transduction studies involving *E. coli* transducing phages [4].

10. Volumes of recipient, phage, PB, and BHIB should be scaled up if screening for more than two antibiotic genes.

11. MOI = Plaque forming units (PFU) of phage used for infection / number of cells. For example, if 2×10^7 cells is infected by 0.5 mL of phage with a titer of 107 PFU/mL. The MOI will be $0.5 \times 10^7 / 2 \times 10^7 = 0.25$.

References

1. Zinder ND, Lederberg J (1952) Genetic exchange in Salmonella. J Bacteriol 64:679–699

2. Birge EA (2000) Bacterial and bacteriophage genetics, 4th edn. Springer, New York

3. Eisenstark A (1965) Transduction of *Escherichia coli* genetic material by Phage P22 in *Salmonella typhimurium* × *E. coli* hybrids. Proc Natl Acad Sci U S A 54:1557–1560

4. Mise K (1971) Isolation and characterization of a new generalized transducing bacteriophage different from P1 in *Escherichia coli*. J Virol 7:168–175

5. Minshew BH, Rosenblum ED (1972) Transduction of tetracycline resistance in *Staphylococcus epidermidis*. Antimicrob Agents Chemother 1:508–511

6. Stanton TB, Humphrey SB, Sharma VK, Zuerner RL (2008) Collateral effects of antibiotics: carbadox and metronidazole induce VSH-1 and facilitate gene transfer among *Brachyspira hyodysenteriae* strains. Appl Environ Microbiol 74:2950–2956

7. Nale JY, Shan J, Hickenbotham PT, Fawley WN, Wilcox MH, Clokie MR (2012) Diverse temperate bacteriophage carriage in *Clostridium difficile* 027 strains. PLoS One 7:e37263

8. Hargreaves KR, Colvin HV, Patel KV, Clokie J, Clokie MR (2013) Genetically diverse *Clostridium difficile* strains harbouring abundant prophages in an estuarine environment. Appl Environ Microbiol 80:2644

9. Goh S, Riley TV, Chang BJ (2005) Isolation and characterization of temperate bacteriophages of *Clostridium difficile*. Appl Environ Microbiol 71:1079–1083

10. Goh S, Hussain H, Chang BJ, Emmett W, Riley TV, Mullany P (2013) Phage phiC2 mediates transduction of Tn6215, encoding erythromycin resistance, between *Clostridium difficile* strains. mBio 4:e00840-00813

11. CLSI (2009) Methods for antimicrobial susceptibility testing of anaerobic bacteria; approved standard, 7th edn. CLSI, Wayne, PA

12. BSAC (2015) BSAC methods for antimicrobial susceptibility testing, version 14, January 2015. BSAC, UK

13. European Committee for Antimicrobial Susceptibility Testing of the European Society of Clinical M, Infectious D (2003) Determination of minimum inhibitory concentrations (MICs) of antibacterial agents by broth dilution. Clin Microbiol Infect 9:ix–xv

Chapter 14

Transfer of *Clostridium difficile* Genetic Elements Conferring Resistance to Macrolide–Lincosamide–Streptogramin B (MLS_B) Antibiotics

Fabrizio Barbanti, François Wasels, and Patrizia Spigaglia

Abstract

Molecular analysis is an important tool to investigate *Clostridium difficile* resistance to macrolide–lincosamide–streptogramin B (MLS_B). In particular, the protocols described in this chapter have been designed to investigate the genetic organization of *erm*(B)-containing elements and to evaluate the capability of these elements to transfer in *C. difficile* recipient strains using filter mating assay.

Key words Antimicrobial susceptibility, *erm*(B) detection, PCR-mapping, Filter mating, PCR-ribotyping

1 Introduction

Clostridium difficile infection (CDI) occurs when the endogenous flora of the intestinal tract is disturbed or altered by antibiotic treatment [1, 2].

Resistance to a wide range of antibiotics allows *C. difficile* to colonize and infect the host in the presence of antimicrobials. Resistance to macrolide–lincosamide–streptogramin B (MLS_B) is the most common phenotype in *C. difficile* clinical isolates [3–5]. In particular, resistance to clindamycin has been significantly associated to CDI [4].

In *C. difficile*, MLS_B resistance is commonly due to the methylation of the 23S rRNA, the target of MLS_B antibiotics, mediated by an *erm*(B) gene [6]. These genes are located on mobile elements [7–9]. Mobile elements are defined as any region of nucleic acid that can move within a genome or between genomes. In *C. difficile*, *erm*(B) genes are carried by both conjugative elements (CTns) and mobilisable elements (MTns) [10]. Both the first and the second group of elements transfer from a donor to a recipient cell using a conjugative-like mechanism but the mobilisable

Adam P. Roberts and Peter Mullany (eds.), *Clostridium difficile: Methods and Protocols*, Methods in Molecular Biology, vol. 1476, DOI 10.1007/978-1-4939-6361-4_14, © Springer Science+Business Media New York 2016

elements lack the genes for conjugation and, therefore, they use those of CTns or conjugative plasmids present in the donor cell.

Tn*5398* is the most extensively studied mobilisable element, however several other *erm*(B)-containing elements showing genetic diversity have been detected in *C. difficile* clinical isolates. In total, 17 different genetic organizations have been identified by PCR-mapping and named from E1 to E17 [9, 11]. In particular, the conjugative transposon Tn*6194* (genetic organization E4) has been recently detected in the majority of epidemic strains, including strains 027 resistant to MLS_B antibiotics [12–15]. The protocols described in this chapter have been designed to investigate the ability of *erm*(B)-containing elements to transfer in *C. difficile* recipient strains.

2   Materials

2.1   Culture and Isolation

1. Anaerobic cabinet under an atmosphere consisting of 85 % N_2, 10 % H_2, 5 % CO_2, at 35 °C.

2. BHI (Brain Heart Infusion) broth (Oxoid Ltd., Wade Road, Basingstoke, Hants, UK). Store at 4 °C.

3. BHI (Brain Heart Infusion) agar (Oxoid Ltd.,Wade Road, Basingstoke, Hants, UK). Store at 4 °C.

4. BHIS (broth and agar): BHI supplemented with 0.5 % Yeast Extract (Oxoid Ltd.) and 0.1 % l-cysteine (Sigma-Aldrich Co. LLC, Saint Louis, MO, USA). Store at 4 °C.

5. Erythromycin solution (20 mg/ml): powder (Sigma-Aldrich Co. LLC) dissolved in 1/10 final volume of 95 % ethanol, then brought to the proper volume with distilled water. Store at –20 °C.

6. Rifampin solution (20 mg/ml): powder (Sigma-Aldrich Co. LLC) dissolved in 1/10 final volume of methanol, then brought to the proper volume with distilled water. Store at –20 °C.

7. Plates supplemented with filter-sterilized solution of erythromycin and/or rifampin at a final concentration of 20 mg/L. Store at 4 °C.

2.2   Minimal Inhibitory Concentrations (MICs) Determination

1. Brucella broth (Oxoid Ltd.). Store at 4 °C.

2. Brucella agar plates: Brucella agar (Oxoid Ltd.) containing 5 % sheep blood, 0.5 mg/L vitamin K1 (Sigma-Aldrich Co. LLC), 5 mg/L hemin (Sigma-Aldrich Co. LLC) (*see* **Note 1**). Store at 4 °C.

3. Etest strips (bioMérieux S.A., Marcy l'Étoile, France) of erythromycin, clindamycin, and rifampin. Store at –20 °C.

4. McFarland standard 1.

5. Sterile inoculating loops.

6. Sterile swabs.

2.3 Filter Mating Assay

1. 0.45 μm pore-size nitrocellulose filters (Merck Millipore, Darmstadt, Germany).

2.4 Standard Molecular Biology Procedures

2.4.1 PCR Amplification of the erm(B) Gene

1. E5   (5′-CTCAAAACTTTTTAACGAGTG-3′)   and   E6 (5′-CCTCCCGTTAAATAATAGATA-3′) primers pair were designed for the amplification of *erm*(B) gene. Store at –20 °C.

2. Make up to a final concentration of 100 μM in sterile distilled water of gene-specific oligonucleotide primers.

3. Taq DNA polymerase and 10× PCR buffer with magnesium (Takara Bio Inc., Otsu, Shiga, Japan). Store at –20 °C.

4. dNTPs (Takara Bio Inc.): make up to a final concentration of 2 mM with distilled water and dispense in 50 μl aliquots. Store at –20 °C.

5. Genomic DNA template. Store at –20 °C.

6. Distilled autoclaved water.

2.4.2 Molecular Characterization of erm(B)-Containing Elements by PCR-Mapping

1. Genomic DNA extraction: Nucleobond AXG Columns and Nucleobond Buffer Set III (Macherey Nagel GmbH & Co. KG, Düren, Germany).

2. A set of primers (2980: 5′-AATAAGTAAACAGGTAA CGTCT-3′; 3106: 5′-CGGGAGGAAATAATTCTATGAG-3′; 3140: 5′-ATTTTATACCTCTGTTTGTTAG-3′; 4192: 5′-CA AGTCGGCACGAACACGAACC-3′; 4349: 5′-CATGAGC GAGTTAATTTTGGCA-3′; 4350: 5′-TGCCAAAATTA ACTCGCTCATG-3′; 6604: 5′-TAAGAGTGTGTTGA TAGTGC-3′; 9069: 5′-TACTGGCTTTTAGACGCA CCTG-3′; 10237: 5′-CATAACGGACATAACAACAGCC-3′; 11617: 5′-CCAAACAGGAAAGATAGCCATA-3′) designed for the *erm*(B)-containing element genetic organization analysis. Store at –20 °C.

3. Make up to a final concentration of 100 μM in sterile distilled water of each specific oligonucleotide primer.

4. Taq DNA polymerase, 10× PCR buffer with magnesium, dNTPs (Takara Bio Inc.), genomic DNA template, and distilled autoclaved water as required for the PCR amplification of the *erm*(B) gene.

2.4.3 PCR-Ribotyping

1. Primer pairs 16S (5′-GTGCGGCTGGATCACCTCCT-3′) and 23S (5′-CCCTGCACCCTTAATAACTTGACC-3′) were used in classic agarose gel-based PCR ribotyping. Store at –20 °C.

2. Make up to a final concentration of 100 μM in sterile distilled water the gene-specific oligonucleotide primers.

3. HotStar Taq Master Mix (Qiagen Inc., Valencia, CA, USA). Store at –20 °C.

4. Genomic DNA template. Store at –20 °C.

2.4.4   Gel Electrophoresis

1. TAE buffer: Prepare 50× stock with 2 M Tris, 2 M acetic acid, and 50 mM EDTA. Adjust pH to 7.5–8.0. Working solution (1×) is prepared by diluting 20 ml of 50× TAE with 980 ml of distilled water. Store at 4 °C.

2. Agarose (Lonza, Rockland, ME, USA): dissolve in TAE buffer to a concentration of 1 % (w/v) by heating to greater than 55 °C.

3. MetaPhor™ Agarose (Lonza, Rockland, ME, USA) for PCR-ribotyping: dissolve in TAE buffer to a concentration of 3 % (w/v) (*see* **Note 2**).

4. DNA molecular weight marker: 50 bp (New England BioLabs Inc., Ipswich, MA, USA). Store at −20 °C.

5. 6× DNA-loading dye: 30 % (v/v) glycerol, 0.3 % (w/v) bromophenol blue. Store at 4 °C.

6. DNA staining solution: 0.2 μg/ml of ethidium bromide in distilled water. Store at 4 °C (*see* **Note 3**).

2.5   Southern Blotting

1. ECL Direct Nucleic Acid Labeling and Detection Systems kit (GE Healthcare Europe GmbH, Freiburg, Germany).

2. Purified *C. difficile* genomic DNA extracted from putative *C. difficile* transconjugants.

3. *Hind*III or other appropriate restriction enzymes.

4. E5/E6 primers pair as described above.

5. Gel electrophoresis materials as detailed above.

6. Depurination solution: 250 mM HCl. Store at room temperature.

7. Denaturation solution: 0.5 M NaOH, 1.5 M NaCl. Store at room temperature.

8. Neutralizing solution: 1.5 M NaCl, 0.5 M Tris–HCl (pH 7.5). Store at room temperature.

9. Hybond-N+ membrane (GE Healthcare Europe GmbH). Store dry at room temperature.

10. Whatman 3 MM paper.

11. 20× SSC: 3 M NaCl, 300 mM tri-sodium citrate, pH 7.0. Dilute to desired concentration with distilled water immediately prior to use.

12. Primary wash buffer: Urea 6 M, SDS 0.4 % (w/v), 0.5 % SSC (V/V).

13. Secondary wash buffer: 2× SSC.

14. X-ray film-cassettes.

15. Hyperfilm ECL (GE Healthcare Europe GmbH).

16. Film developing reagents (developer and fixer liquids) (Sigma-Aldrich Co. LLC). Store at 4 °C.

3 Methods

3.1 MICs Determination of Erythromycin, Clindamycin, and Rifampin Using Etest Strip

1. Allow the Etest package to reach room temperature before opening (approx. 30 min from –20 °C freezer).

2. Perform following **steps 3–7** under anaerobic conditions as much as possible.

3. Homogenize viable colonies from 24 h plate in Brucella broth to achieve turbidity equivalent to 1 McFarland (*see* **Note 4**).

4. Ensure that the surface of the pre-reduced Brucella agar plate is dry before streaking. Gently press to remove excess fluid and use the saturated swab to streak the entire agar surface evenly in three directions, rotating the plate approx. 60° each time (*see* **Note 5**).

5. Allow the agar surface to dry for approx. 15–20 min and check that the surface is completely dry before applying the Etest strips.

6. Apply the Etest strips to the agar surface with forceps (*see* **Note 6**).

7. Incubate the plates anaerobically at 35 °C for 24 h (*see* **Note 7**).

8. Read the MIC at the point of complete inhibition of all growth (*see* **Note 8**).

9. The breakpoint used for both erythromycin and clindamycin was 8 mg/L, in accordance with the guidelines established by the Clinical and Laboratory Standards Institute [16]. The breakpoint for rifampin was 4 mg/L, in accordance with the CLSI interpretive categories approved for *Staphylococcus aureus*, since no values are provided for anaerobes [17].

3.2 erm(B) Detection

1. Resuspend a single bacterial colony of each strain from an overnight culture in 50 µl of sterile distilled water.

2. Boil for 10 min.

3. Centrifuge at $8000 \times g$ for 10 min.

4. Use the supernatant containing bacterial DNA as template for PCR.

5. Perform amplification in a final volume of 50 µl with a reaction mixture containing buffer, 200 mM each deoxynucleoside triphosphate, 100 pmol each primer, 2.5 U Taq, and 5 µl of DNA extracted by boiling method.

6. Set up PCR as follow: denaturation for 5 min at 94 °C and amplification for 30 cycles consisting of 1 min at 94 °C, 1 min at 50 °C, and 1 min at 72 °C. At the end of cycling held samples at 72 °C for 5 min.

7. Run 10 µl of the PCR products on a 1 % agarose gel.

8. The expected size for PCR fragments is approximately 711 bp.

3.3 Determination of the erm(B)-Containing Element Genetic Organization

1. Use the genomic DNA as template for PCR.

2. Prepare a set of seven PCR reactions with the following couples of primers:

   (a) 6604×3140.
   (b) 2980×4349.
   (c) 4350×3140.
   (d) 2980×4192.
   (e) 3139×4210.
   (f) 9069×10237.
   (g) 3106×11617.

   Perform amplifications in a final volume of 50 μl with a reaction mixture containing buffer, 200 mM each deoxynucleoside triphosphate, 100 pmol each primer, and 2.5 U Taq.

3. Set up PCR as follow: denaturation for 5 min at 94 °C and amplification for 30 cycles consisting of 1 min at 94 °C, 2 min at 50 °C, and 1 min at 72 °C. At the end of cycling held samples at 72 °C for 5 min.

4. Run 10 μl of the PCR products on a 1 % agarose gel.

5. Compare the pattern obtained to those already detected to determine the genetic organization of the erm(B)-containing element (Table 1).

3.4 Selection of Rifampin—Resistant Colonies

1. If recipient strain is susceptible to rifampin, select resistant derivative colonies by streaking out exponentially grown cells (10^{10} cfu) on agar plates supplemented with 20 mg/L of rifampin.

2. Streak a single colony on plates without antibiotic.

3. Evaluate resistant phenotype using rifampin Etest strip.

4. Re-streak the selected colony on plates without antibiotic at least for two passages and verify the stability of the MIC value by Etest.

3.5 Filer Mating Assay

1. Separately grow C. *difficile* culture of both donor and recipient strains for 18 h on BHIS agar at 35 °C in anaerobic conditions.

2. Separately inoculate single well-isolated colonies of the donor and recipient strains in 20 ml BHIS pre-reduced broth.

3. Grow cultures until mid-exponential phase ($OD_{600} \cong 0.5$–0.6).

4. Harvest cells by centrifugation at $1500 \times g$ for 10 min at room temperature.

5. Discard the supernatants and resuspend cell pellets of both donor and recipient cultures in 1 ml of pre-reduced BHIS broth.

6. Spread 100 μl aliquots of both donor and recipient cultures onto pre-reduced BHIS agar supplemented with both erythromycin 20 mg/L and rifampin 20 mg/L to evaluate and measure the possibility of spontaneous mutations.

Table 1

Genetic organization of *erm*(B)-containing elements

ErmB determinant arrangements	Length in bp of the PCR fragments obtained						
	1	2	3	4	6	7	8
E1	610	1506	1044	1247/2219	–	1166	2759
E2	610	–	–	1247	–	–	–
E3	388	1527	–	2219	–	–	–
E4	388	1527	–	–	–	–	–
E5	–	–	–	1247	–	–	–
E6	388	–	–	–	–	–	–
E7	2500	–	–	–	–	–	–
E8	610	–	2000	1247/1500	–	–	–
E9	610	–	–	1247	–	1166	2759
E10	610	–	–	2500	–	–	–
E11	610	–	–	1247	–	1166	–
E12	388/610	1506	–	1247	–	1166	–
E13	2000	–	–	–	–	1166	–
E14	388	1506	1044	1247/2219	–	1166	2759
E15	388	1506	–	1247/2219	–	–	–
E16	388	–	–	1247/2219	–	–	–
E17	388	–	–	1247	–	–	–

7. Mixed together aliquots (*see* **Note 9**) of the donor and recipient suspensions on 0.45 μm pore-size nitrocellulose filters (*see* **Note 10**) on pre-reduced BHIS agar.

8. Incubate for 24 h at 35 °C in anaerobic conditions.

9. Aseptically remove the filters from the plates and place in 50 ml sterile tube containing 1 ml BHIS pre-reduced broth.

10. Vigorously wash the filter.

11. Spread 100 μl aliquots of cell mixture onto BHIS agar supplemented with both erythromycin 20 mg/L and rifampin 20 mg/L (*see* **Note 11**).

12. Plate tenfold dilution series of cell mixture onto BHIS agar supplemented with erythromycin 20 mg/L and BHIS agar supplemented with rifampin 20 mg/L to count donor and recipients cells separately.

13. Incubate for 48 h.

14. Count transconjugant colonies from plates supplemented with both erythromycin 20 mg/L and rifampin 20 mg/L.

15. Count donor cells from plates supplemented with erythromycin 20 mg/L.

16. Calculate the conjugation frequency per donor as the number of transconjugants divided by the number of bacteria isolated from plates supplemented with erythromycin 20 mg/L (*see* **Note 12**).

17. Subculture putative transconjugants on fresh selective plates and incubate for a further 48 h.

18. Verify and characterize putative transconjugants by PCR-ribotyping (*see* **Note 13**), presence of the *erm*(B) gene, MICs determination and Southern blotting.

3.6 PCR-Ribotyping

1. Use DNA extracted by boiling method as template for PCR.

2. Perform amplification in a final volume of 50 μl with a reaction mixture containing buffer, 200 mM each deoxynucleoside triphosphate, 100 pmol each primer, 2.5 U Taq and 5 μl of template.

3. Set up PCR as follows: denaturation for 6 min at 95 °C and amplification for 35 cycles consisting of 1 min at 95 °C, 1 min at 57 °C, and 1 min at 72 °C. At the end of cycling held samples at 74 °C for 7 min.

4. Run 10 μl of the PCR products on a 3 % agarose gel at 130 V for 5 h.

3.7 Southern Blotting

3.7.1 DNA Hybridization

Probe Synthesis

1. In this protocol, ECL Direct Nucleic Acid Labeling and Detection Systems kit, genomic DNA containing a *erm*(B) and oligonucleotide primers E5 and E6 are used for *erm*(B) probe synthesis, following the manufacturer's instruction.

2. After the PCR reaction is complete, a 5 μl aliquot is analyzed by gel electrophoresis as described previously.

3. Labeled probes can be stored at 4 °C until use.

Transfer of DNA

1. Purify transconjugant's genomic DNA.

2. Digest 5 μg of genomic DNA with appropriate restriction enzymes overnight, according to the manufacturer's instructions.

3. Mix digested DNA with DNA-loading dye and loaded into the wells of a 0.8 % agarose gel prepared using TAE buffer.

4. Run the gel overnight in TAE buffer at 30 V.

5. Depurinate the larger gDNA fragments submerging the gel in 250 mM HCl with gentle shaking at room temperature for 10–12 min. Depurination improves the transfer of DNA fragments greater than 10 kb in size.

6. Briefly rinse the gel in distilled water and then submerge it in denaturation solution for 25 min at room temperature with gentle shaking.

7. Briefly rinse in distilled water and submerge it in neutralizing solution for 30 min at room temperature with gentle shaking.

8. Transfer the DNA from the gel onto a nylon membrane overnight as described below:

    (a) Soak a piece of Whatman 3 MM with 10× SSC and placed on top of a bridge resting in a reservoir of 20× SSC.

    (b) Invert the gel and place it on the soaked Whatman 3 MM paper. Roll out air bubbles between the gel and the paper.

    (c) Cut the Hybond-N+ membrane equal the gel size, soak in 20× SSC and place on the gel. Roll out air bubbles.

    (d) Cut three pieces of Whatman 3 MM equal to the gel size, soak in 10× SSC and place on membrane.

    (e) Cut three pieces of dry Whatman 3 MM paper equal to the gel size and place on the wet Whatman 3 MM paper.

    (f) Cut paper towels equal to the gel size and place on the dried Whatman 3 MM paper.

    (g) Place a glass plate and weight on stack. Make sure that the stack is vertical.

9. After overnight transfer at room temperature, briefly rinse the membrane in 6× SSC and dry at room temperature for approximately 10 min.

10. Cross-link the DNA to the membrane by expo-sure to UV light (254 nm) for 3 min.

3.7.2 Hybridization

1. Add 0.5 mM NaCl and 5 % (w/v) blocking agent to the hybridization buffer.

2. Preheat the hybridization buffer at 42 °C for 1 h.

3. Place the membrane in a suitable container containing the hybridization buffer (0.2 ml/cm² filter surface area) and incubate for at least 15 min at 42 °C.

4. Prepare the labeled *erm*(B) DNA probe as described below:

    (a) Boil 100 ng of the probe in 10 μl of water for 5 min.

    (b) Place on ice for 5 min.

    (c) Add 10 μl of labeling reagent to the cooled DNA.

    (d) Add 10 μl glutaraldehyde solution.

    (e) Incubate for 10 min at 37 °C.

5. Add the labeled probe to the hybridization buffer containing the membrane; incubate overnight at 42 °C with gentle shaking.

6. Remove the membrane from the hybridization buffer and wash twice in primary wash buffer for 20 min at 42 °C with gentle shaking.

7. Wash the membrane twice in secondary wash buffer for 5 min at room temperature with gentle shaking.

3.7.3 Detection

1. Using buffers and reagents of the ECL Direct Nucleic Acid Labeling and Detection Systems kit, submerge the membrane in washing buffer for 5 min at room temperature with gentle shaking.

2. Mix an equal volume of detection reagent 1 and detection reagent 2 ($0.125 \ ml/cm^2$ of the membrane).

3. Remove the membrane from the secondary wash buffer and place in a fresh container. Drain off the excess of secondary wash buffer.

4. Add the detection reagent directly to the blot and incubate for 1 min at room temperature.

5. Drain off the detection reagent in excess and place the blot in the film cassette.

6. Take to darkroom, place a sheet of autoradiography film on the top of the blot, and close the film cassette.

7. Expose from 30 s to 10 min at room temperature.

8. Develop the film using standard procedures.

4   Notes

1. Pre-reduce media (both broth and plates) into the anaerobic cabinet to maximize rapid anaerobiosis for at least 2 h.

2. Dissolve the agarose by heating in a microwave oven at 500 W. Gently mix the agarose with a magnetic stirrer avoiding bubbles (use only stirrers that are coated in plastic. Do not put metal stirrers in microwave oven). Be careful not to overboil the agarose.

3. It is possible to use alternative new generation of fluorescent DNA stains instead of the highly toxic ethidium bromide.

4. Homogenize carefully to minimize aeration, do not vortex. Do not allow inoculum suspension to stand for more than 10 min prior to use.

5. Ensure that swab is soft and absorbent to ensure enough inoculum is drawn up into the swab. Dip the swab in the inoculum suspension and allow swab to soak up the inoculum.

6. Apply the Etest strip with the MIC scale facing upwards (towards the opening of the plate) and with the handle towards the rim of the plate. Once applied, do not remove the strip.

7. Always confirm clindamycin results at 48 h, due to inducible resistance.

8. For clindamycin read the MIC at the first point of significant inhibition of growth as detected by eye (the so-called 80% inhibition).

9. Use different ratios of donor and recipient strains to optimize the conjugation event (e.g., 2:1, 4:1, 1:2, 1:4 donor–recipient cell pellets volume ratio).

10. The use of 0.45 μm pore-size nitrocellulose filters bring the bacteria into close proximity and hold them in intimate contact. It is recommended that filter mating be carried out on the front side of a filter.

11. Plate also a 1:10 dilution to be sure to have a correct cell count.

12. If the conjugation frequency per recipient is required, count recipient cells from plates supplemented with rifampin 20 mg/L and divide the number of transconjugants by the number of recipient cells.

13. Verify that colonies growing on plates supplemented with both erythromycin 20 mg/L and rifampin 20 mg/L are not spontaneous rifampin mutants of donor strain by PCR-ribotyping. The PCR-ribotype of putative transconjugants must be the same of recipient strain.

References

1. Bartlett JG (2002) Antibiotic-associated diarrhea. N Engl J Med 346:334–339

2. Gerding DN, Johnson S, Peterson LR, Mulligan ME, Silva J Jr (1995) *Clostridium difficile* associated diarrhea and colitis. Infect Control Hosp Epidemiol 16:459–477

3. Freeman J, Vernon J, Morris K, Nicholson S, Todhunter S, Longshaw C, Wilcox MH, and the Pan-European Longitudinal Surveillance of Antibiotic Resistance among Prevalent *Clostridium difficile* Ribotypes' Study Group (2014) Pan-European longitudinal surveillance of antibiotic resistance among prevalent *Clostridium difficile* ribotypes. Clin Microbiol Infect. 21:248.e9–248.e16. doi:10.1016/j.cmi.2014.09.017

4. Johnson S, Samore MH, Farrow KA, Killgore GE, Tenover FC, Lyras D, Rood JI, De Girolami P, Baltch AL, Rafferty ME, Pear SM, Gerding DN (1999) Epidemics of diarrhea caused by a clindamycin-resistant strain of *Clostridium difficile* in four hospitals. N Engl J Med 341:1645–1651

5. Weisblum B (2002) Resistance to macrolide-lincosamide-streptogramin antibiotics. In: Fischetti VA, Novick RP, Ferretti JJ et al (eds) Gram-positive pathogens. ASM Press, Washington, DC, pp 694–710

6. Leclercq R, Courvalin P (1991) Bacterial resistance to macrolide, lincosamide, and streptogramin antibiotics by target modification. Antimicrob Agents Chemother 35:1267–1272

7. Farrow KA, Lyras D, Rood JI (2001) Genomic analysis of the erythromycin resistance element Tn*5398* from *Clostridium difficile*. Microbiology 147:2717–2728

8. Farrow KA, Lyras D, Rood JI (2000) The macrolide-lincosamide streptogramin B resistance determinant from *Clostridium difficile* 630 contains two *erm*(B) genes. Antimicrob Agents Chemother 44:411–413

9. Spigaglia P, Carucci V, Barbanti F, Mastrantonio P (2005) ErmB determinants and Tn*916*-like elements from clinical isolates of *Clostridium difficile*. Antimicrob Agents Chemother 49:2550–2553

10. Roberts, A.P., Allan, E., and Mullany, P. (2014) The Impact of Horizontal Gene Transfer on the Biology of Clostridium difficile. Adv Microb Physiol; 65: 63–82

11. Spigaglia P, Barbanti F, Mastrantonio P, on behalf of the European Study Group on *Clostridium difficile* (ESGCD) (2011) Multidrug resistance in European *Clostridium difficile* clinical isolates. J Antimicrob Chemother 66:2227–2234

12. Brouwer MSM, Roberts AP, Mullany P, Allan E (2012) In silico analysis of sequenced strains of *Clostridium difficile* reveals a related set of conjugative transposons carrying a variety of accessory genes. Mob Genet Elements 2:8–12

13. He M, Miyajima F, Roberts P, Ellison L, Pickard DJ, Martin MJ, Connor TR, Harris SR, Fairley D, Bamford KB, D'Arc S, Brazier J, Brown D, Coia JE, Douce G, Gerding D, Kim HJ, Koh TH, Kato H, Senoh M, Louie T, Michell S, Butt E, Peacock SJ, Brown NM, Riley T, Songer G, Wilcox M, Pirmohamed M, Kuijper E, Hawkey P, Wren BW, Dougan G, Parkhill J, Lawley TD (2012) Emergence and global spread of epidemic healthcare-associated *Clostridium difficile*. Nat Genet 45:109–113

14. He M, Sebaihia M, Lawley TD, Stabler RA, Dawson LF, Martin MJ, Holta KE, Seth-Smith HMB, Quail MA, Rance R, Brooks K, Churcher C, Harris D, Bentley SD, Burrows C, Clark L, Corton C, Murray V, Rose G, Thurston S, van Tonder A, Walker D, Wren BW, Dougan G, Parkhill J (2010) Evolutionary dynamics of *Clostridium difficile* over short and long time scales. Proc Natl Acad Sci U S A 107:7527–7532

15. Wasels F, Spigaglia P, Barbanti F, Mastrantonio P (2013) *Clostridium difficile erm*(B)-containing elements and the burden on the *in vitro* fitness. J Med Microbiol 62:1461–1467

16. Clinical and Laboratory Standards Institute (2007) Methods for antimicrobial susceptibility testing of anaerobic bacteria-seventh edition: approved standard M11-A7. CLSI, Wayne, PA

17. Clinical and Laboratory Standards Institute (2008) Performance standards for antimicrobial susceptibility testing: eighteenth informational supplement M100-S18. CLSI, Wayne, PA

Chapter 15

Methods for Determining Transfer of Mobile Genetic Elements in *Clostridium difficile*

Priscilla Johanesen and Dena Lyras

Abstract

Horizontal gene transfer by mobile genetic elements plays an important role in the evolution of bacteria, allowing them to rapidly acquire new traits, including antibiotic resistance. Mobile genetic elements such as conjugative and mobilizable transposons make up a considerable part of the *C. difficile* genome. While sequence analysis has identified a large number of these elements, experimental analysis is required to demonstrate mobility and function. This chapter describes the experimental methods utilized for determining function and transfer of mobile genetic elements in *C. difficile* including detection of the circular transfer intermediate and the analysis and confirmation of mobile genetic element transfer to recipient cells.

Key words *Clostridium difficile*, Horizontal transfer, Transposon, Mobilizable element, Mating, Antibiotic resistance, Mobilization, Conjugation

1 Introduction

Mobile genetic elements play a crucial role in the evolution and genome plasticity of *Clostridium difficile*. Evidence for this phenomenon is provided by genome sequence data, which indicates that over a tenth of the genome comprises mobile genetic elements, in particular conjugative transposons [1, 2]. The number and variety of mobile genetic elements present in *C. difficile* were recently reviewed in depth by Mullany et al. [3] and Amy et al. [4].

Two categories of transposons capable of horizontal gene transfer have been identified in *C. difficile* to date: conjugative transposons, epitomised by the well-characterized Tn*916*-like transposon, Tn*5397*[5], and mobilizable transposons, represented by the erythromycin resistance-encoding element Tn*5398* and the chloramphenicol resistance-encoding transposon Tn*4453*[6, 7].

The mechanism of both intra- and intercellular transfer of conjugative transposons is well understood [8]. In the process of intercellular transfer the conjugative transposon excises from the donor chromosome and forms a covalently closed circular intermediate.

Adam P. Roberts and Peter Mullany (eds.), *Clostridium difficile: Methods and Protocols*, Methods in Molecular Biology, vol. 1476, DOI 10.1007/978-1-4939-6361-4_15, © Springer Science+Business Media New York 2016

The circular intermediate is nicked at the origin of transfer (*oriT*), after which a single strand is transferred to the recipient cell in a process very similar to that described for conjugative plasmids [8]. In both the donor and recipient cell the single strand undergoes a process of replication to a double-stranded DNA molecule, which then integrates at the target site [8]. Conjugative transposons are capable of mobilizing other elements that are incapable of self-transfer, including mobilizable transposons. To facilitate the transfer process the mobilizable element must have an *oriT* site and, in some cases, the element must also encode cognate mobilization proteins [9]. The methods which have been developed to study transposition allow the transfer of both conjugative and mobilizable transposons from donor to recipient cell to be examined and for the steps required to achieve transfer to be dissected, including the formation of a circular intermediate.

Many genome sequences of *C. difficile* isolates are now available. Bioinformatic analysis of these sequences has allowed many mobile elements to be identified, including putative conjugative and mobilizable transposons [1, 2, 10, 11]. Detailed functional and phenotypic analysis of many of these elements has not been carried out.

This chapter discusses protocols used to determine whether genetic elements are capable of excision, transfer, and insertion in *C. difficile*. The well-characterized *C. difficile* mobilizable transposons Tn*4453*, a 6.3 kb element encoding chloramphenicol resistance [7], and Tn*5398*, a 9.6 kb element encoding erythromycin resistance [6], will be used as exemplars. Note that the protocols detailed here can also be applied to the analysis of other mobile genetic elements such as conjugative transposons or plasmids. This is especially important in the study of mobilizable elements since their transfer depends on the presence of a co-resident conjugative element. Detection of transfer of any of these elements is made easier and simpler by the presence of an antibiotic resistance marker within the element. While not discussed in this chapter, the most efficient way of studying elements that do not encode antibiotic resistance is to introduce such a marker, which can be achieved using standard homologous recombination-based methods or newer technologies such as TargeTron or Clostron, as outlined in Brouwer et al. [2].

2 Materials

2.1 Detection of Excision of Elements from the Genome

1. Genomic DNA template.

2. Oligonucleotide primers designed to read outward from the transposon Tn*4453* ends. *See* Fig. 1 and Table 1 for oligonucleotide primer sequences. Oligonucleotide primers are reconstituted to a concentration of 100 μM in sterile distilled water and then diluted to a working stock of 50 μM in sterile distilled water. Oligonucleotides are stored at –20 °C.

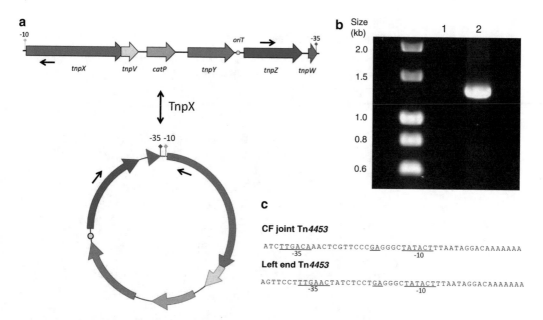

Fig. 1 Detection of the Tn*4453* circular intermediate. (**a**) Transposition of Tn*4453* involves a circular inter-mediate. Excision and insertion is mediated by TnpX. Oligonucleotide primers (indicated by the arrowheads) that read out from the ends of the transposon are used in PCR to detect the circular form. Figure adapted from Amy et al. [4]. (**b**) PCR results obtained after performing the circular intermediate PCR on strain W1 (Lane 2), which contains one copy each of Tn*4453a* and Tn*4453b*, and the negative control CD37 (Lane 1). (**c**) Nucleotide sequence analysis of the circular form joint and the left end of the element when integrated within the chromo-some. When integrated into the chromosome a promoter sequence is present (Left end). A strong promoter is also formed upon circularisation of the element (CF joint). These promoters control the expression of *tnpX*. Figure adapted from Lyras and Rood [14]

3. 10× PCR buffer with magnesium and Taq DNA polymerase (Roche Life Sciences). Stored at –20 °C.

4. Deoxynucleotides (dNTPs) are an equimolar solution of dATP, dCTP, dGTP, and dTTP, made up to a final concentration of 5 mM (1.25 mM of each dNTP) with 1× TE and dispensed in 50 μl aliquots. Stored at –20 °C.

5. Sterile distilled water. Distilled water is autoclaved and stored at room temperature.

6. TAE electrophoresis buffer: 40 mM Tris–acetate, 1 mM EDTA, pH 8.5. Stored at room temperature.

7. Seakem LE Agarose: Dissolve in TAE buffer to a concentration of 0.8 % (w/v) using a microwave, cool before pouring.

8. 6× DNA-loading dye: 30 % (v/v) glycerol, 0.3 % (w/v) bromo-phenol blue, 0.3 % (w/v) xylene cyanol. Stored at room temperature.

9. DNA molecular weight markers: Hyperladder I (Bioline) and λ-*Hin*dIII DNA size standards, with DNA-loading dye added.

10. QIAquick PCR Purification Kit (Qiagen).

Table 1
Synthetic oligonucleotide primers

PCR Target	Nucleotide Sequence
Tn4453 Circular Intermediate	5'-CCGATGTTCCGAGCTTCGTACAGC-3' 5'-GCAGATAGTTTCGTCCTAATCGGCTC-3'
tnpX	5'-GAGGGCTAAGCTTTAATAGGAC-3'
	5'-GGGAATTCTGCGGTTAAGC-3'
tnpV	5'-CATTGGAATTTTTCCACCATAAAAAAG-3'
	5'-AGCAATGCAGGATATAGTTTC-3'
catP	5'-TCGGCAAGCTTTCAAGAAGTTA-3'
	5'-TTAGTTCTAGACAAACCTGAAG-3'
tnpY	5'-AACCACAGGTTAGTGCAAAGAC-3'
	5'-AAAGATGTCGTGGGCAAGGGTG-3'
tnpZ	5'-CAAAAGGATCCCAAGGGGGAAC-3'
	5'-CGCTTCTAGAAAAGGTCTGCAC-3'
tnpW	5'-CGCTAAGCTTCTGCCTGTGGTG-3'
	5'-GGAACGAGTTTGTCTAGATGAT-3'
catP-probe	5'-ACTACCCCTGCTTAACCGCAGA-3' 5'-CCTTTGAGAGCAGGGCGGCGAT-3'

2.2   Determination of Transfer: Filter and Plate Matings

1. *C. difficile* strains include strain 630 (contains Tn5397 and Tn5398) and JIR8156 (strain 630::Tn4453) as donors, and *C. difficile* strain CD37 as a recipient.

2. BHIS medium (*see* **Note 1**): Brain–heart infusion 37 g/L, yeast extract 5 g/L (and agar 15 g/L for solid media). All media is autoclaved and solid media is cooled to 50–55 °C before pouring into petri dishes. Liquid media is allowed to cool and stored at room temperature. Before use, liquid media is pre-reduced by boiling for 10 min, or by incubation in an anaerobic environment for 4 h. Immediately prior to use of any media, sterile l-cysteine to a final concentration of 0.1 % (add 1 ml 10 % (w/v) filter-sterilized l-cysteine per 100 ml of media) and 1.5 ml per 100 ml sterile glucose (25 % (w/v) sterile glucose) are added.

3. Erythromycin: Dissolve 200 mg of erythromycin in 10 ml of absolute ethanol (final concentration 20 mg/ml) and store at −20 °C.

4. Rifampicin: Dissolve 500 mg of rifampicin in 10 ml of methanol (final concentration 50 mg/ml). Wrap tube in foil to protect from light and store at −20 °C.

5. Tetracycline: Dissolve 100 mg of tetracycline in 10 ml of absolute ethanol (final concentration 10 mg/ml). Wrap tube in foil to protect from light and store at –20 °C.

6. Thiamphenicol (*see* **Note 2**): Dissolve 100 mg of thiamphenicol in 10 ml of methanol (final concentration 10 mg/ml). Store at –20 °C.

7. Filters for matings: Nitrocellulose 0.45 μm (Whatman).

2.3 Analysis of C. difficile Transconjugants by PCR

1. PCR amplification materials as detailed in Subheading 2.1.

2. Oligonucleotide primers for the element, *see* Table 1.

3. Gel electrophoresis materials as detailed in Subheading 2.1.

2.4 Analysis of C. difficile Transconjugants by Southern Blot

1. PCR DIG Probe Synthesis Kit (Roche Life Sciences).

2. Purified pJIR1377 (pUC18 carrying Tn*4453*) plasmid DNA.

3. *catP*-specific oligonucleotides (*see* Table 1). Oligonucleotide primers are dissolved in sterile distilled water to a final concentration of 100 μM. Stored at –20 °C.

4. Gel electrophoresis materials, as in Subheading 2.1.

5. QIAquick PCR Purification Kit (Qiagen).

6. Genomic DNA extracted from *C. difficile* transconjugants and control strains (donor and recipient).

7. *Eco*RI restriction enzyme and buffer. Stored and used according to the manufacturer's instructions.

8. DIG-labeled λ*Hin*dIII DNA molecular weight markers (Roche Life Sciences).

9. Depurination solution: 250 mM HCl. Store at room temperature.

10. Denaturation solution: 0.2 M NaOH, 0.5 M NaCl. Store at room temperature.

11. Neutralization solution: 165 mM Trisodium citrate, 1.5 M NaCl, 0.25 M Tris–HCl (pH 7.5). Store at room temperature.

12. Hybond-N+ membrane (Amersham). Store dry at room temperature.

13. Whatman 3MM paper.

14. Stock solution of 20× SSC: 3 M NaCl, 300 mM trisodium citrate, pH 7.0. Dilute to desired concentration with distilled water immediately prior to use.

15. Pre-hybridization solution: 83 mM Trisodium citrate, 0.75 mM NaCl, 0.05 % (w/v) blocking reagent (Roche Life Sciences or skim milk powder), 1 % (w/v) *N*-lauroylsarcosine, 0.02 % (w/v) SDS. Make up fresh immediately prior to use.

16. Hybridization solution: 5 ml Pre-hybridization solution containing 50–75 ng of probe DNA.

17. Wash solution 1: 2× SSC, 0.1 % (v/v) SDS. Make fresh and use immediately.

18. Wash solution 2: 0.2× SSC, 0.1 % (v/v) SDS. Make fresh and use immediately.

19. Buffer 1 (maleic acid buffer): 0.1 M Maleic acid, 0.15 M NaCl, adjust to pH 7.5 with NaOH. Store at room temperature.

20. Buffer 2 (blocking buffer): Maleic acid buffer with 1 % (w/v) skim milk powder.

21. Wash buffer: Maleic acid, 0.3 % (v/v) Tween-20. Store at room temperature.

22. Anti-DIG-AP conjugate (Roche Life Sciences). Stored at 4 °C.

23. Buffer 3 (detection buffer): 0.1 M Tris–HCl, 0.1 M NaCl, 50 mM $MgCl_2$, pH 9.5. Store at room temperature.

24. CDP-Star Chemiluminescent substrate (Roche Life Sciences): Stored at 4 °C and protect from light.

25. X-ray film. Store at room temperature and protect from light.

3   Methods

3.1 Detection of Exciton of Elements from the Genome

1. Oligonucleotide primers are designed to read outward from the ends of the transposon and will amplify an approximately 1.3 kb product if the element forms a circular intermediate (see Fig. 1a). Genomic DNA (see **Note 3**) derived from a C. difficile isolate carrying Tn4453 is used as the template for the PCR reaction.

2. The components of the PCR are outlined in Table 2. Optimal PCR conditions should be determined for the combination of oligonucleotide primers (their melting temperatures) and template that is being utilized in the PCR. Note that there is no positive control available for this PCR but an appropriate negative control should be prepared.

3. Typical PCR conditions are outlined as follows: 94 °C for 3 min; 30 cycles of 94 °C for 30 s, 58 °C for 30 s, and 72 °C for 2 min (extension time of 1 min/kb); then a final extension of 72 °C for 10 min.

4. PCR products are analyzed via TAE agarose gel electrophoresis. Five microliters of the PCR product is mixed with DNA loading dye and electrophoresed alongside a DNA molecular weight marker at 100 V for 45 min. The gel is subsequently stained with ethidium bromide (see **Note 4**) and destained in water, and then visualized using a UV transilluminator. The

Table 2
Standard PCR Conditions

Component	Amount (volume)	Final Concentration
10x PCR Buffer with MgCl$_2$	5 µl	1 x
Taq DNA polymerase	0.5 µl	0.05 units/µl
DNA template (10-100 ng)	variable	200 pg/µl
Forward Primer (50 µM)	0.5 µl	0.5 µM
Reverse Primer (50 µM)	0.5 µl	0.5 µM
dNTPs (1.25 mM)	8 µl	200 µM
Water	variable	
	50 µl (Final volume)	

expected result for the Tn*4453* circular intermediate PCR is shown in Fig. 1b.

5. If the correct sized product is obtained, and to confirm that the product represents the joint of the circular form, the remainder of the PCR product is purified using the QIAquick PCR Purification Kit and sequence analysis is performed (*see* **Note 5**). Results obtained from sequencing the joint product from the Tn*4453* circular intermediate are shown in Fig. 1c.

3.2   Determination of Transfer

Transfer of mobile DNA from *C. difficile* to *C. difficile* can be performed *via* two different methodologies involving either plate or filter mating (first described in Mullany et al. [12]). Recent research in the Lyras laboratory has utilized plate matings rather than filter matings, because they yield higher transfer efficiencies and are more reproducible. Both protocols are described here, demonstrating transfer of the mobilizable transposons Tn*5398* and Tn*4453*, respectively. All *C. difficile* cultures and experiments are incubated at 37 °C and performed in an atmosphere of 10% (v/v) H$_2$ and 10% (v/v) CO$_2$ in N$_2$.

3.2.1   Filter Mating Transfer of Tn5398 from 630 to CD37

1. Streak donor and recipient strain on BHIS agar supplemented with erythromycin (50 µg/ml) for the donor and rifampicin (20 µg/ml) for the recipient strain. Incubate cultures overnight.

2. Take five colonies from the overnight culture, inoculate a pre-reduced 20 ml BHIS broth, and incubate until the optical density at 650 nm is approximately 0.45 (mid-exponential phase).

3. Harvest cells by centrifugation (1500×*g* for 10 min) at room temperature.

4. Discard the supernatant and resuspend the pellet in 1 ml BHIS broth.

5. Mix 100 µl of donor with 100 µl of recipient on a sterile 0.45 µm nitrocellulose filter (Whatman), which has been previously placed on a thick BHIS plate (40 ml of agar per plate).

6. For the controls, plate 100 µl of donor and 100 µl of recipient cells separately onto nitrocellulose filters.

7. Incubate plates for 24 h (with the lid facing up, agar down).

8. In addition to the mating mixture and controls, also plate a tenfold dilution series of donor on BHIS erythromycin medium (50 µg/ml) in triplicate and incubate for 48 h to obtain a viable count for the number of donors.

9. Following incubation, recover bacterial growth by placing each filter in a sterile bottle containing 1 ml of BHIS broth and resuspend by gentle vortexing or pipetting across the surface of the filter.

10. Plate 100 µl aliquots of the resuspended cultures as well as dilutions of 10^{-1} and 10^{-2} onto BHIS supplemented with erythromycin (50 µg/ml) and rifampicin (20 µg/ml). As negative controls plate 100 µl of donor or recipient cells separately onto the same selective medium. *See* **Note 6**.

11. Incubate plates for 48 h.

12. Following incubation, colonies will be visible on the double selection of erythromycin (50 µg/ml) and rifampicin (20 µg/ml) if transfer of Tn*5398* has occurred. Typically Tn*5398* transfer occurs at a very low frequency; when originally performed in the laboratory only four transconjugants were obtained. Assess the number of donors (derived at **step 8**) and the number of transconjugants (derived at **step 10**).

13. Calculations can then be performed to determine the frequency of transfer (number of transconjugants per donor cell input):

$$\text{Transconjugants per donor cell} = \frac{\text{number of transconjugants in 1 ml}}{\text{number of donors in 1 ml}}$$

Published results on the transfer frequency of MLS resistance mediated by Tn*5398*, from strain 630 to CD37, range from 1.2×10^{-9} to 3.6×10^{-8} transconjugants per donor cell [13].

3.2.2 Plate Matings: Transfer of Tn4453 from JIR8156 (630:: Tn4453) to CD37

1. Streak donor JIR8156 (630::Tn*4453*) and recipient (CD37) strains on BHIS agar supplemented with thiamphenicol (10 µg/ml) for the donor and rifampicin (20 µg/ml) for the recipient strain. Incubate cultures overnight.

2. Prepare overnight-grown cultures of donor (630::Tn*4453*) and recipient (CD37) strains in BHIS broth (20 ml).

3. Following incubation inoculate a pre-reduced 20 ml BHIS broth with 0.4 ml of the overnight culture and incubate for approximately 6 h.

4. Plate 100 μl aliquots of donor and recipient onto thick BHIS plates (with no selection). As controls, plate the donor and recipient strains separately on the same medium. Incubate plates for 24 h.

5. Scrape the growth from each plate into 3 ml of BHIS broth and plate 100 μl aliquots onto enrichment plates containing thiamphenicol (10 μg/ml). Incubate for 24 h.

6. Following enrichment, scrape the growth from the plates into 1 ml of BHIS broth and plate 100 μl aliquots and serial tenfold dilutions of 10^{-1} and 10^{-2} onto plates containing the double selection of thiamphenicol (10 μg/ml) and rifampicin (20 μg/ml). Incubate plates for 48 h. *See* **Note 6**.

7. Following incubation, colonies should be visible on the double selection of thiamphenicol (10 μg/ml) and rifampicin (20 μg/ml) if Tn*4453* has successfully been transferred to CD37. Perform plate counts. Transfer typically occurs at low frequency so data is expressed as total number of transconjugants per mating. Typical colony counts from this mating range from 50 to 100 colonies per plate. To calculate the frequency of transfer at **step 4** serially dilute in tenfold the donor culture and plate dilutions onto BHIS supplemented with thiamphenicol (10 μg/ml). Incubate for 48 h. Similar calculations to those described under **step 13** for filter matings can then be performed.

3.3 Confirmation of Transconjugants by PCR

To confirm transfer of the element to the recipient cell, PCR analysis can be performed on genomic DNA extracted from transconjugants, using oligonucleotide primers that bind to regions which are within the element of interest (*see* **Note 7**). Donor and recipient DNA act as positive and negative controls within the same PCR analysis.

1. For example, for the confirmation of the transfer of Tn*4453*, PCRs were performed with oligonucleotide primers specific for *tnpX*, *tnpY*, *tnpV*, *tnpZ*, and *catP* (*see* Table 1), using standard PCR components (*see* Table 2) and reaction conditions as follows: 94 °C for 3 min; 30 cycles of 94 °C for 30 s, 50 °C for 30 s, and 72 °C for 1 min/kb, and then a final extension of 72 °C for 10 min.

2. Upon completion of the cycling program, PCR products are analyzed via TAE agarose gel electrophoresis. Ten microliters of the reaction volume is mixed with DNA loading dye and electrophoresed alongside a DNA molecular weight marker at 100 V for 45 min. The gel is subsequently stained with ethidium bromide (*see* **Note 4**), destained in water, and then visualized using a UV transilluminator.

3.4 Confirmation of Transconjugants by Southern Hybridization

To determine the chromosomal location and also the copy number of the transferred element in the recipient cell Southern hybridization analysis can be performed. The protocol involved utilizes a non-radioactive labeling and detection methodology, the DIG system. Verification of Tn4453-carrying transconjugants from the plate mating methodology via Southern hybridization will be given as an example. Genomic DNA is probed with a specific DNA fragment, which will hybridize to *catP* present on Tn4453.

1. To synthesize the *catP*-specific gene probe, pJIR1377 (pUC18 carrying Tn4453) plasmid DNA is used as the PCR template together with oligonucleotide primers that are specific for the *catP* gene (*see* Table 1) [7]. Reaction components are identical to the standard components outlined in Table 2 apart from the addition of 1 μl of DIG-labeled dNTPs (PCR DIG Probe Synthesis Mix). A separate reaction without labeling mix should also be prepared as a control. Reaction conditions are as follows: 94 °C for 3 min; 30 cycles of 94 °C for 1 min, 50 °C for 2 min, and 72 °C for 3 min, and then a final extension time of 72 °C for 5 min.

2. The PCR reactions and products are then analyzed via TAE agarose gel electrophoresis. Ten microliters of the PCR product is mixed with DNA loading dye and electrophoresed alongside a DNA molecular weight marker at 100 V for 45 min. The gel is subsequently stained with ethidium bromide (*see* **Note 4**), destained in water, and then visualized using a UV transilluminator. The labeled and unlabeled PCR products should be compared to determine whether the product has been successfully labeled. The labeled product should appear slightly larger than the unlabeled product.

3. If the correct sized product is obtained, the remainder of the PCR product is purified using the QIAquick PCR Purification Kit and can be stored at 4 °C until use. The efficiency of the labeling reaction can be determined by the quantification protocol supplied by the manufacturer.

4. Genomic DNA (*see* **Note 3**) from the donor, recipient, and transconjugant (approximately 5 μg) is digested overnight with the appropriate enzyme, according to the manufacturer's instructions. For the analysis of Tn4453 the restriction enzyme *Eco*RI is utilized since Tn4453 does not contain any internal *Eco*RI restriction sites; therefore the entire element will be located on a single chromosomal fragment. If more than one copy of the transposon is located within the same cell, multiple bands are observed.

5. Following overnight incubation, a small aliquot of the reaction is assessed via TAE gel electrophoresis, to determine if digestion has proceeded to completion. If overnight digestion has been successful (*see* **Note 8**) the remainder of the digested

DNA is mixed with DNA-loading dye and loaded into the wells of an 18.2 cm × 15 cm 0.8 % (w/v) agarose gel prepared using TAE buffer. A well of DIG-labeled λHindIII DNA molecular weight marker is also loaded.

6. This gel is subjected to 100 V for 10 min to allow the DNA to migrate out of the wells and then electrophoresed overnight in TAE buffer at 35 V. To determine if the digested DNA has been well separated the gel is stained with ethidium bromide (*see* **Note 4**), destained in water, and then visualized with UV light by placing the gel onto a UV transilluminator.

7. Following visualization and confirmation of complete digestion, larger genomic DNA fragments are depurinated (to improve transfer of fragments greater than 10 kb) by submerging the gel in 0.25 M HCl with gentle shaking at room temperature for 15 min. As only larger fragments require depurination, the low-molecular-weight end of the gel needs to be elevated out of the solution.

8. The gel is then rinsed with distilled water and placed in denaturation solution for 30 min at room temperature with gentle shaking.

9. The gel is rinsed with distilled water again and placed in neutralization solution for 30 min at room temperature with gentle shaking. This step is then repeated.

10. The DNA is then transferred from the gel to the nylon membrane (Hybond-N+) overnight by capillary transfer. To achieve this transfer requires the assembly of a blotting apparatus (*see* **Note 9**). Typically the gel tank in which the agarose gel was electrophoresed is used as the holding vessel for the blotting step.

- To construct a wick, a piece of Whatman 3MM paper is soaked with 2×SSC and placed on top of a bridge resting in a reservoir of 10×SSC.

- The gel is placed upside down on top of the wick and any air bubbles formed must be removed.

- The nylon membrane is cut to exactly the same size as the gel and is pre-soaked in 2×SSC after which it is placed on top of the gel. Once again, any air bubbles that may have formed must be removed.

- Following this process, two pieces of Whatman 3MM paper cut to the size of the gel and pre-soaked in 2×SSC are placed on top of the nylon membrane. These are followed by a stack of paper towels, a glass plate, and a 500 g weight, which are added to the top of the stack.

- The DNA transfer is then left to proceed overnight at room temperature.

11. Following overnight transfer the apparatus is disassembled. The nylon membrane is removed and allowed to air-dry (approximately 10–15 min) on a piece of Whatman 3MM paper.

12. The DNA is then cross-linked to the membrane by exposure to UV light (254 nm) for 2–3 min. Following the cross-linking step the membrane can be stored between two sheets of Whatman 3MM paper and wrapped in foil or utilized in downstream steps immediately.

13. Hybridization requires pre-preparation of a probe prior to this step, as described above. Following cross-linking, the membrane is placed in a hybridization bottle or bag with pre-hybridization solution (20 ml per 100 cm^2 filter surface area), which is then placed in a hybridization oven and incubated for 3–4 h at 65 °C.

14. To prepare the hybridization solution, which should occur close to the completion of the pre-hybridization step, between 50 and 75 ng of probe DNA is added to 5 ml of pre-hybridization solution. This is boiled for 10 min to denature the DNA and then immediately quenched on ice for 5 min.

15. Following pre-hybridization, the pre-hybridization solution is removed and replaced with 6 ml of hybridization solution and returned to the hybridization oven for overnight incubation at 65 °C.

16. After hybridization the filter paper is removed from the solution and the membrane washed twice at room temperature in wash solution 1 (2×SSC, 0.1 % [w/v] SDS) for 5 min and twice at 65 °C in wash solution 2 (0.2×SSC, 0.1 % [w/v] SDS) for 15 min, before proceeding to the detection step.

17. There are a number of options available for the detection of DNA:DIG-labeled probe hybrids. The detection procedure outlined here assumes the use of the CDP-Star detection kit (Roche Life Sciences) for the chemiluminescent detection of probe-target hybrids.

18. Following the wash steps the membrane is washed briefly in buffer 1 for 5 min at room temperature with gentle shaking.

19. The membrane is then placed in 100 ml of buffer 2 (the blocking step) for 30 min at room temperature with gentle shaking.

20. Following blocking, the membrane is placed in 20 ml antibody solution (2 μl of the anti-DIG-AP conjugate in 20 ml of buffer 2) and incubated for 30 min at room temperature with gentle shaking.

21. Unbound anti-DIG-AP conjugate is then removed by washing the membrane twice in 100 ml of washing buffer (buffer 1 containing Tween 20 at 0.3 % [v/v]) for 15 min at room temperature with gentle shaking.

22. The membrane is then equilibrated by placing it in 20 ml of buffer 3 (detection buffer) for 3–5 min at room temperature with gentle shaking.

23. While the blot is equilibrating, a dilution of 20 μl CDP-Star reagent in 2 ml of buffer 3 (1:100) is prepared.

24. Following equilibration, the membrane is placed in a hybridization bag and the 2 ml diluted CDP-Star reagent (1 ml per 100 cm² filter surface area) is added, ensuring that the solution covers the entire blot and that air bubbles are not present. The bag is sealed and incubated for 5 min at room temperature.

25. Following incubation, excess solution is removed from the blot and the bag is resealed. The membrane is placed DNA side up in a film cassette.

26. The remainder of the steps are performed in a darkroom, and the membrane is exposed to X-ray film for 5–20 min at room temperature (*see* **Note 10**). The X-ray film is then developed according to standard protocols.

27. As a representative example, a blot in which a *catP* probe was used to examine Tn*4453* transconjugants is shown in Fig. 2.

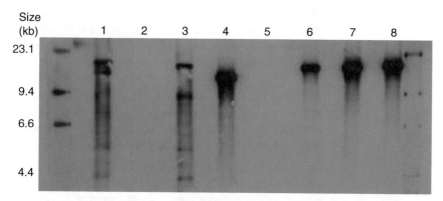

Fig. 2 Southern hybridisation analysis of Tn*4453* transconjugants. All lanes contain *Eco*RI digested genomic DNA. Digested DNA was subjected to electrophoresis using an 0.8% TAE agarose gel followed by DNA transfer to a nylon membrane as outlined in Methods. Southern hybridisation was then performed under stringent conditions using a *catP* gene probe. The size of λ*Hind*III DNA molecular weight markers is indicated and are contained in two lanes at the left and right ends of the blot. Lane (1): Strain W1, which contains 2 copies of Tn*4453* on *Eco*RI fragment sizes of 15.5 kb (Tn*4453a*) and 11 kb (Tn*4453b*). Lane (2): strain 630. Lane (3): Strain JIR8156, a transconjugant obtained from a mating between W1 and *C. difficile* strain 630, which contains two copies of Tn*4453* on *Eco*RI fragments of approximately 9 kb and 14 kb in size. Lane (4): Strain JIR8159, an independently derived transconjugant obtained from a mating between W1 and *C. difficile* strain 630, which contains one copy of Tn*4453* on an *Eco*RI fragment size of approximately 10 kb. Lane (5): the negative control strain CD37. Lanes (6) (7) and (8): transconjugants obtained from a mating between JIR8156 and CD37. These transconjugants all contain one copy of Tn*4453* on *Eco*RI fragment sizes of approximately 14 kb

4 Notes

1. For the experiments described in this chapter, strains were routinely grown in brain–heart infusion (BHIS) broth or agar. Some laboratories may have restricted access to BHIS and, since 2010, our laboratory has switched from BHIS to heart infusion (HIS), the formulation for the latter being identical but for the absence of brain reagents.

2. Thiamphenicol is a derivative of chloramphenicol, which is often used instead of chloramphenicol for selective purposes in clostridial matings.

3. There are a number of different protocols and commercial kits that can be utilized for the extraction of total genomic DNA.

4. Ethidium bromide is a carcinogen, so care should be taken in its use. In recent years ethidium bromide has been replaced with alternatives such as SYBR Safe and Gel Red.

5. For nucleotide sequencing, a number of different systems are available. For the work described here, sequencing reactions were performed using the ABI Prism BigDye Terminator Cycle Sequencing Ready Reaction kit.

6. The transfer of Tn5398 (filter mating method) or Tn4453 (plate mating method) from strain 630 to CD37 probably relies on the presence of one of the seven co-resident conjugative transposons. While examining transfer of the element of interest, such as Tn5398 or Tn4453, co-transfer of Tn5397 can be monitored by plating on selective medium containing tetracycline (10 μg/ml) for Tn5397 and either erythromycin (50 μg/ml) for Tn5398 or thiamphenicol (10 μg/ml) for Tn4453, and rifampicin (20 μg/ml) for the recipient cell. Alternatively, any transconjugants that are obtained on double selection can be patched onto media containing tetracycline to monitor co-transfer on Tn5397.

7. In addition to PCR screening for the element it is useful to utilize a set of oligonucleotide primers that distinguish the donor from recipient strain. In the case of the donor 630 and recipient CD37, PCR analysis for the presence of PaLoc can be performed, as described in [2].

8. If digestion of genomic DNA is not complete after overnight incubation, another 1 μl of restriction enzyme is added and the reaction continued for another 4–6 h.

9. A Southern blot assembly apparatus can be seen at http://www.sigmaaldrich.com/technical-documents/articles/biology/southern-and-northern-blotting.html.

10. Film exposure times may vary from 15 s to 20 min.

Acknowledgments

Research in the Lyras laboratory at Monash University is supported by Project Grants from the Australian National Health and Medical Research Council (NHMRC) and Discovery Grants from the Australian Research Council (ARC). Associate Professor Lyras is supported by an Australian Research Council Future Fellowship. We acknowledge laboratory work performed by Dr. Kylie Farrow, Mr. Jacob Amy, and Ms. Pauline Howarth.

References

1. Sebaihia M, Wren BW, Mullany P et al (2006) The multidrug-resistant human pathogen *Clostridium difficile* has a highly mobile, mosaic genome. Nat Genet 38(7):779–786. doi:10.1038/ng1830

2. Brouwer MS, Warburton PJ, Roberts AP, Mullany P, Allan E (2011) Genetic organisation, mobility and predicted functions of genes on integrated, mobile genetic elements in sequenced strains of *Clostridium difficile*. PLoS One 6(8):e23014. doi:10.1371/journal.pone.0023014

3. Mullany P, Allan E, Roberts AP (2015) Mobile genetic elements in *Clostridium difficile* and their role in genome function. Res Microbiol 166(4):361–367

4. Amy J, Johanesen PA, Lyras D (2015) Extrachromosomal and integrated genetic elements in *Clostridium difficile*. Plasmid 80:97–110. doi:10.1016/j.plasmid.2015.04.006

5. Roberts AP, Johanesen PA, Lyras D, Mullany P, Rood JI (2001) Comparison of Tn*5397* from *Clostridium difficile*, Tn*916* from *Enterococcus faecalis* and the CW459*tet*(M) element from *Clostridium perfringens* shows that they have similar conjugation regions but different insertion and excision modules. Microbiology 147(Pt 5):1243–1251

6. Farrow KA, Lyras D, Rood JI (2001) Genomic analysis of the erythromycin resistance element Tn*5398* from *Clostridium difficile*. Microbiology 147(Pt 10):2717–2728

7. Lyras D, Storie C, Huggins AS, Crellin PK, Bannam TL, Rood JI (1998) Chloramphenicol resistance in *Clostridium difficile* is encoded on Tn*4453* transposons that are closely related to Tn*4451* from *Clostridium perfringens*. Antimicrob Agents Chemother 42(7):1563–1567

8. Salyers AA, Shoemaker NB, Stevens AM, Li LY (1995) Conjugative transposons: an unusual and diverse set of integrated gene transfer elements. Microbiol Rev 59(4):579–590

9. Bellanger X, Payot S, Leblond-Bourget N, Guedon G (2014) Conjugative and mobilizable genomic islands in bacteria: evolution and diversity. FEMS Microbiol Rev 38(4):720–760. doi:10.1111/1574-6976.12058

10. Brouwer MS, Roberts AP, Mullany P, Allan E (2012) In silico analysis of sequenced strains of *Clostridium difficile* reveals a related set of conjugative transposons carrying a variety of accessory genes. Mob Genet Elements 2(1):8–12. doi:10.4161/mge.19297

11. He M, Sebaihia M, Lawley TD, Stabler RA, Dawson LF, Martin MJ, Holt KE, Seth-Smith HM, Quail MA, Rance R, Brooks K, Churcher C, Harris D, Bentley SD, Burrows C, Clark L, Corton C, Murray V, Rose G, Thurston S, van Tonder A, Walker D, Wren BW, Dougan G, Parkhill J (2010) Evolutionary dynamics of *Clostridium difficile* over short and long time scales. Proc Natl Acad Sci U S A 107(16):7527–7532

12. Mullany P, Wilks M, Lamb I, Clayton C, Wren B, Tabaqchali S (1990) Genetic analysis of a tetracycline resistance element from *Clostridium difficile* and its conjugal transfer to and from *Bacillus subtilis*. J Gen Microbiol 136(7):1343–1349

13. Mullany P, Wilks M, Tabaqchali S (1995) Transfer of macrolide-lincosamide-streptogramin B (MLS) resistance in *Clostridium difficile* is linked to a gene homologous with toxin A and is mediated by a conjugative transposon, Tn*5398*. J Antimicrob Chemother 35(2):305–315

14. Lyras D, Rood JI (2000) Transposition of Tn*4451* and Tn*4453* involves a circular intermediate that forms a promoter for the large resolvase, TnpX. Mol Microbiol 38:588–601

Chapter 16

Investigating Transfer of Large Chromosomal Regions Containing the Pathogenicity Locus Between *Clostridium difficile* Strains

Michael S.M. Brouwer, Peter Mullany, Elaine Allan, and Adam P. Roberts

Abstract

The genomes of all sequenced *Clostridium difficile* isolates contain multiple mobile genetic elements. The chromosomally located pathogenicity locus (PaLoc), encoding the cytotoxins TcdA and TcdB, was previously hypothesized to be a mobile genetic element; however, mobility was not demonstrated. Here we describe the methods used to facilitate and detect the transfer of the PaLoc from a toxigenic strain into non-toxigenic strains of *C. difficile*. Although the precise mechanism of transfer has not yet been elucidated, a number of controls are described which indicate transfer occurs via a cell-to-cell-mediated conjugation-like transfer mechanism. Importantly, transfer of the PaLoc was shown to occur on large chromosomal fragments of variable sizes, indicating that homologous recombination is likely to be responsible for the insertion events.

Key words Pathogenicity locus, Conjugation, Transfer, Chromosomal transfer, Recombination, Next-generation sequencing, SNP analysis

1 Introduction

Many studies have shown that *Clostridium difficile* engages in frequent gene transfer as mobile genetic elements and heterologous acquired DNA can comprise more than 10 % of its genome [1–4]. In addition, whole-genome analysis of recent and historic isolates has shown that *C. difficile* genomes have undergone chromosomal rearrangement and exchange between isolates of distinct evolutionary lineages [4–6].

The pathogenicity locus (PaLoc) of *Clostridium difficile* encodes both cytotoxins, TcdA and TcdB, along with regulatory genes and a conserved hypothetical gene of unknown function [7, 8]. Early genetic analysis of the region suggested that it was potentially a remnant of a mobile genetic element [7]. Whole-genome sequence comparisons of various *C. difficile* ribotypes supported the idea that the PaLoc had been mobile at some point [5]; however, the mobility of the region was proven only recently [9].

Adam P. Roberts and Peter Mullany (eds.), *Clostridium difficile: Methods and Protocols*, Methods in Molecular Biology, vol. 1476, DOI 10.1007/978-1-4939-6361-4_16, © Springer Science+Business Media New York 2016

Conjugation experiments selecting for the transfer of the genetically marked conjugative transposon CTn*1* from donor strain 630Δ*erm* into the non-toxigenic strain CD37 [10] resulted in the co-transfer of the PaLoc, converting the recipient into a toxin-producing strain [9]. Furthermore, PaLoc transfer could be directly selected for using a genetically marked PaLoc [11]. The most likely explanation for these events is that a chromosomally integrated mobile genetic element was responsible for the transfer of a chromosomal fragment containing the PaLoc. This type of transfer has been previously reported for other bacterial species [12, 13].

Next-generation sequencing of multiple transconjugants showed that the PaLoc had integrated into the recipient chromosome at identical locations; however, single-nucleotide polymorphism (SNP) and insertion deletion (indel) analysis of the region flanking the PaLoc showed that it had transferred as part of a larger, variable-sized fragment [9]. The donor-specific sequence which flanked the PaLoc in the transconjugants was never the same in different transconjugants, suggesting that the transferred region was inserted into the chromosome through homologous recombination as opposed to a site-specific recombination reaction associated with transposition. Although the precise method of chromosomal mobilization and transfer has not yet been defined, control experiments demonstrated that transformation and transduction were both unlikely to be responsible [9].

A recent study of the erythromycin resistance-conferring genetic elements Tn*5398*, Tn*6215*-like, and Tn*6194*-like also showed the integration of large chromosomal fragments into a naïve recipient strain, converting it from an erythromycin susceptible to a resistant phenotype [14]. One important difference between these experiments and the PaLoc transfer results we reported [12] is that, in contrast to our experiments, transfer of the erythromycin resistance-encoding elements was inhibited in the presence of DNase with some recipient strains. This suggests that there is likely to be some variability in the mechanisms of transfer of chromosomal fragments between *C. difficile*.

2 Materials

2.1 Bacterial Strains

1. Suitable donor strains contain a selectable resistance marker in the region that is to be tested for transfer. If no appropriate markers are present in the desired chromosomal region, these can be specifically inserted (*see* **Note 1**).

2. Suitable recipient strains should contain at least a single selectable resistance marker. If no appropriate markers are present, spontaneous rifampicin-resistant mutants can be selected from most *C. difficile* isolates (*see* **Note 2**). It is advisable that the resistance marker in the recipient strain is not located close to the chromosomal location of the fragment that is transferred as

it could be lost during homologous recombination and produce false-negative results.

2.2 Growth Media

1. Liquid medium: BHI broth (Oxoid Ltd, Basingstoke, UK), prereduced (*see* **Note 3**).

2. Solid medium: BHI agar (Oxoid Ltd, Basingstoke, UK) supplemented with 5% horse blood (E&O Laboratories, Bonnybridge, UK) and appropriate selective antibiotics.

3. The choice of antibiotics depends on the donor and recipient strains. In the example described here we use lincomycin 40 μg/ml and rifampicin 25 μg/ml (Sigma-Aldrich Company Ltd, Gillingham, UK).

2.3 Transfer via Conjugation

1. Nitrocellulose filters, 0.45 μm pore size (Sartorius, Epsom, UK).

2. DNase (Sigma-Aldrich Ltd) can be added to agar plates at 50 μg/ml.

2.4 Confirmation of Transconjugants

1. PCR reagents and equipment.

2. Oligonucleotides to perform PCR for identifying transconjugants (*see* **Note 4**).

2.5 Mitomycin C Induction and Phage Infection

1. Mitomycin C.

2. 1 M NaCl (Sigma-Aldrich Ltd).

3. PEG 6000.

4. PBS (Sigma-Aldrich Ltd).

2.6 Next-Generation Sequencing (See Note 5)

1. Next-generation sequencing (NGS) sequencing was carried out on the Illumina GAII-X platform.

2. For DNA extraction we have used the Gentra Puregene Yeast/Bact. Kit (Qiagen).

3. For library preparation we used the Encore NGS multiplex system (Nugen, Leek, The Netherlands).

4. Analysis software: Velvet software suite [15], xBase [16], ACT [17], eBioX [18].

3 Methods

3.1 Transfer via Conjugation

1. We have chosen for transfer via conjugation using a filter-mating protocol as previously described [19].

2. *C. difficile* is cultured at 37 °C under anaerobic conditions (80% N_2, 10% H_2, 10% CO_2). Liquid cultures can be incubated shaking at 200 rpm to promote gaseous exchange.

3. Overnight cultures of both donor and recipient were grown to logarithmic phase, i.e., $OD_{600} \sim 0.5$. 10 ml of donor culture and 50 ml of recipient culture were each centrifuged for 10 min

at $4500 \times g$ and the recovered bacteria were resuspended into 500 μl of fresh broth. The cell suspensions were mixed and 200 μl was spread onto a filter on an agar plate containing no antibiotics. DNase was added to some plates to test if transformation occurred (*see* **Note 6**). The agar plates containing the filters were incubated for 24 h at 37 °C anaerobically.

4. After the incubation period, the filters were placed into 20 ml tubes containing 1 ml broth using sterile forceps and vortexed for 30 s to wash the bacteria off the filters. Serial dilutions were spread onto plates selecting for either donors or recipients. Neat cell suspensions were spread onto plates selecting for transconjugants.

5. Cells were grown for approximately 72 h before the colonies were counted and putative transconjugants were restreaked onto fresh selective plates.

3.2 Confirmation of Transconjugants

1. To analyze putative transconjugants, whole-cell lysates are made by resuspending a colony in 100 μl H_2O and heating the sample for 10 min at 100 °C.

2. PCR on the lysate is carried out using standard protocols to confirm chromosomal transfer and identity of the putative transconjugant (*see* **Note 4**).

3.3 Mitomycin C Induction and Phage Infection

1. To check if the endogenous mitomycin C-inducible temperate phages have a role in the transfer of large chromosomal fragments they can be induced using mitomycin C at 3 μg/ml.

2. A 50 ml culture of donor cells is induced with mitomycin C for 4 h under anaerobic conditions.

3. The culture is centrifuged ($7800 \times g$, 10 min, 4 °C).

4. 1 M NaCl and 20 % PEG 6000 are added and the phages are left to precipitate overnight at 4 °C.

5. The phage suspension is centrifuged ($7800 \times g$, 10 min, 4 °C) and the pellet is resuspended in 2 ml PBS. The presence of phages is determined using a plaque assay (*see* **Note 7**).

6. Ten milliliters of an overnight culture of the recipient strain is incubated with 1 ml of phage suspension for 2 h. The cells are centrifuged for 10 min at $4500 \times g$ after which the pellet is resuspended in 1 ml BHI broth.

7. The cell suspension is plated out on single- and double-selective plates (*see* **Note 8**).

3.4 Next-Generation Sequencing

1. DNA is isolated using the Gentra Puregene Yeast/Bact. Kit (Qiagen), according to the manufacturers' instructions.

2. DNA libraries are prepared using the Encore NGS multiplex system (Nugen, Leek, The Netherlands), according to the manufacturers' instructions.

3. Seventy-two basepair, paired-end runs are performed on the Illumina GAII-X platform.

4. Quality control and read trimming are performed using custom Illumina software.

5. The Velvet software suite [15] is used to perform initial *de novo* assembly of the reads.

6. Mapping of the contigs against the reference genomes of both the donor and recipient genomes is performed using xBase [16].

7. Analysis to determine if the expected fragment was integrated in the transconjugant chromosome is done using ACT [17]. Using a whole-genome sequence comparison tool and comparing the transconjugant sequence with that of the donor and recipient can easily identify if the region of interest is present in the transconjugant and if it is integrated at the same chromosomal location as in the donor; *see* Fig. 1. It is likely/possible that some specific sequence of the recipient strain is lost at this location; in our study the 115 bp sequence present in nontoxigenic strains that replaces the PaLoc in non-toxigenic strains [7] was absent in all seven transconjugants we examined.

8. SNP analysis to determine the precise ends of these fragments is performed using eBioX [18]. Transconjugants will have the same SNPs as the donor for the entire transferred fragment and SNPs will be identical to the sequence of the recipient outside of the transferred fragment. However, between these SNPs there will be a number of nucleotides for which it is unknown if they originate from the donor or recipient chromosome as these are identical in both; *see* Fig. 1. Therefore for each transconjugant we can only determine the minimum and maximum possible size of the DNA fragment that has integrated in the recipient chromosome.

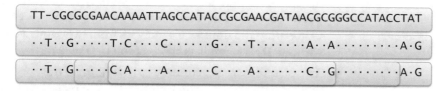

Fig. 1 Analysis for SNPs in the chromosomal sequence results in a minimum and maximum number of nucleotides that were derived from the donor sequence that has been transferred. The top strand in green represents the donor sequence; the middle strand in blue represents the recipient sequence. The bottom sequence represents the transconjugant sequence, SNPs provide evidence for the source of the sequence indicated by shading of the sequence. For the conserved bases shaded in orange the origin cannot be determined

4   Notes

1. The donor strain must contain an antibiotic resistance marker within the chromosomal region that is to be transferred. The recipient strain must be susceptible to this antibiotic. The ClosTron site-directed mutagenesis system [20–22] can be used to incorporate an erythromycin resistance gene into any region of interest if no resistance genes naturally occur in this region.

2. Mutations in the *rpoB* gene encoding RNA polymerase can result in spontaneous rifampicin-resistant mutants. Selection for these can be done by spreading a large number of cells (approximately 10^{10}) on agar plates supplemented with rifampicin. Any colonies should be subcultured on fresh selective plates to confirm their resistance [9, 23].

3. Liquid media are prereduced before inoculation by incubating for at least 4 h in an anaerobic environment.

4. Spontaneous mutants occur at low frequency, especially against rifampicin, and the identity of true transconjugants needs to be checked by PCR before performing downstream experiments or costly analysis such as whole-genome sequencing.

   Oligonucleotide sets need to be designed against distinct genes within both the fragment that is transferred from the donor and for a location in the recipient chromosome away from the expected insertion point.

   When either the donor or recipient genomes have not been sequenced, sequencing of genes used for the MLST typing scheme may suffice in characterizing putative transconjugants [24].

5. Many NGS platforms are available and the choice of kits for DNA isolation, library preparation, and downstream software packages is vast. We describe here which kits and software are used in our study.

6. To determine if chromosomal DNA was transferred to recipient cells via transformation, some filter-mating experiments were carried out using agar plates containing DNase. Any naked DNA that would be transferred via transformation is degraded while DNA transferred via conjugation is protected. Comparing the transfer frequencies from experiments with and without DNase predicts the method of transfer.

7. The plaque assay is necessary to determine if the concentrated phages have the capacity to infect the recipient cell; a positive control strain which is proven susceptible to the phage can be used to confirm the phage induction and isolation was successful [25].

8. The single-selective plates are used to determine the total number of recipient cells in the suspension. The double-selective plates are used to determine if any transductants are present which have received the specific chromosomal fragment.

Acknowledgements

The work described in this chapter was funded by the Medical Research Council (grant no. G0601176) and the European Community's Seventh Framework programme (FP7/207-2013) under grant agreement no. 223585.

References

1. Sebaihia M, Wren BW, Mullany P, Fairweather NF, Minton N, Stabler R, Thomson NR, Roberts AP, Cerdeno-Tarraga AM, Wang H, Holden MT, Wright A, Churcher C, Quail MA, Baker S, Bason N, Brooks K, Chillingworth T, Cronin A, Davis P, Dowd L, Fraser A, Feltwell T, Hance Z, Holroyd S, Jagels K, Moule S, Mungall K, Price C, Rabbinowitsch E, Sharp S, Simmonds M, Stevens K, Unwin L, Whitehead S, Dupuy B, Dougan G, Barrell B, Parkhill J (2006) The multidrug-resistant human pathogen Clostridium difficile has a highly mobile, mosaic genome. Nat Genet 38:779–786

2. Stabler RA, Gerding DN, Songer JG, Drudy D, Brazier JS, Trinh HT, Witney AA, Hinds J, Wren BW (2006) Comparative phylogenomics of Clostridium difficile reveals clade specificity and microevolution of hypervirulent strains. J Bacteriol 188:7297–7305

3. Scaria J, Ponnala L, Janvilisri T, Yan W, Mueller LA, Chang YF (2010) Analysis of ultra low genome conservation in Clostridium difficile. PLoS One 5:e15147

4. He M, Sebaihia M, Lawley TD, Stabler RA, Dawson LF, Martin MJ, Holt KE, Seth-Smith HM, Quail MA, Rance R, Brooks K, Churcher C, Harris D, Bentley SD, Burrows C, Clark L, Corton C, Murray V, Rose G, Thurston S, van Tonder A, Walker D, Wren BW, Dougan G, Parkhill J (2010) Evolutionary dynamics of Clostridium difficile over short and long time scales. Proc Natl Acad Sci U S A 107:7527–7532

5. Dingle KE, Griffiths D, Didelot X, Evans J, Vaughan A, Kachrimanidou M, Stoesser N, Jolley KA, Golubchik T, Harding RM, Peto TE, Fawley W, Walker AS, Wilcox M, Crook DW (2011) Clinical Clostridium difficile: clonality and pathogenicity locus diversity. PLoS One 6:e19993

6. Monot M, Eckert C, Lemire A, Hamiot A, Dubois T, Tessier C, Dumoulard B, Hamel B, Petit A, Lalande V, Ma L, Bouchier C, Barbut F, Dupuy B (2015) Clostridium difficile: new insights into the evolution of the pathogenicity locus. Sci Rep 5:15023

7. Braun V, Hundsberger T, Leukel P, Sauerborn M, von Eichel-Streiber C (1996) Definition of the single integration site of the pathogenicity locus in Clostridium difficile. Gene 181:29–38

8. Rupnik M, Dupuy B, Fairweather NF, Gerding DN, Johnson S, Just I, Lyerly DM, Popoff MR, Rood JI, Sonenshein AL, Thelestam M, Wren BW, Wilkins TD, von Eichel-Streiber C (2005) Revised nomenclature of Clostridium difficile toxins and associated genes. J Med Microbiol 54:113–117

9. Brouwer MS, Roberts AP, Hussain H, Williams RJ, Allan E, Mullany P (2013) Horizontal gene transfer converts non-toxigenic Clostridium difficile strains into toxin producers. Nat Commun 4:2601

10. Brouwer MS, Allan E, Mullany P, Roberts AP (2012) Draft genome sequence of the nontoxigenic Clostridium difficile strain CD37. J Bacteriol 194:2125–2126

11. Kuehne SA, Cartman ST, Heap JT, Kelly ML, Cockayne A, Minton NP (2010) The role of toxin A and toxin B in Clostridium difficile infection. Nature 467:711–713

12. Hochhut B, Marrero J, Waldor MK (2000) Mobilization of plasmids and chromosomal DNA mediated by the SXT element, a constin found in Vibrio cholerae O139. J Bacteriol 182:2043–2047

13. Whittle G, Hamburger N, Shoemaker NB, Salyers AA (2006) A bacteroides conjugative transposon, CTnERL, can transfer a portion of itself by conjugation without excising from the chromosome. J Bacteriol 188:1169–1174

14. Wasels F, Spigaglia P, Barbanti F, Monot M, Villa L, Dupuy B, Carattoli A, Mastrantonio P (2015) Integration of (B)-containing elements through large chromosome fragment exchange in. Mob Genet Elements 5:12–16

15. Zerbino DR, Birney E (2008) Velvet: algorithms for de novo short read assembly using de Bruijn graphs. Genome Res 18:821–829

16. Chaudhuri RR, Pallen MJ (2006) xBASE, a collection of online databases for bacterial comparative genomics. Nucleic Acids Res 34:D335–D337

17. Carver TJ, Rutherford KM, Berriman M, Rajandream MA, Barrell BG, Parkhill J (2005) ACT: the Artemis Comparison Tool. Bioinformatics 21:3422–3423

18. Barrio AM, Lagercrantz E, Sperber GO, Blomberg J, Bongcam-Rudloff E (2009) Annotation and visualization of endogenous retroviral sequences using the Distributed Annotation System (DAS) and eBioX. BMC Bioinformatics 10(Suppl 6):S18

19. Hussain H, Roberts AP, Whalan W, Mullany P (2010) In: Mullany P, Roberts AP (eds) Clostridium difficile, vol 1, 1st edn, Methods in molecular biology. Humana Press, New York, pp 203–211

20. Heap JT, Pennington OJ, Cartman ST, Carter GP, Minton NP (2007) The ClosTron: a universal gene knock-out system for the genus Clostridium. J Microbiol Methods 70:452–464

21. Heap JT, Kuehne SA, Ehsaan M, Cartman ST, Cooksley CM, Scott JC, Minton NP (2010) The ClosTron: mutagenesis in clostridium refined and streamlined. J Microbiol Methods 80:49–55

22. Heap JT, Cartman ST, Kuehne SA, Cooksley CM, Minton N (2010) In: Mullany P, Roberts AP (eds) Clostridium difficile, vol 1, 1st edn, Methods in molecular biology. Humana Press, New York, pp 165–182

23. Huhulescu S, Sagel U, Fiedler A, Pecavar V, Blaschitz M, Wewalka G, Allerberger F, Indra A (2011) Rifaximin disc diffusion test for in vitro susceptibility testing of Clostridium difficile. J Med Microbiol 60:1206–1212

24. Griffiths D, Fawley W, Kachrimanidou M, Bowden R, Crook DW, Fung R, Golubchik T, Harding RM, Jeffery KJ, Jolley KA, Kirton R, Peto TE, Rees G, Stoesser N, Vaughan A, Walker AS, Young BC, Wilcox M, Dingle KE (2010) Multilocus sequence typing of Clostridium difficile. J Clin Microbiol 48:770–778

25. Goh S, Ong PF, Song KP, Riley TV, Chang BJ (2007) The complete genome sequence of Clostridium difficile phage phiC2 and comparisons to phiCD119 and inducible prophages of CD630. Microbiology 153:676–685

Chapter 17

An In Vitro Model of the Human Colon: Studies of Intestinal Biofilms and *Clostridium difficile* Infection

Grace S. Crowther, Mark H. Wilcox, and Caroline H. Chilton

Abstract

The in vitro gut model is an invaluable research tool to study indigenous gut microbiota communities, the behavior of pathogenic organisms, and the therapeutic and adverse effect of antimicrobial administration on these communities. The model has been validated against the intestinal contents of sudden death victims to reflect the physicochemical and microbiological conditions of the proximal to distal colon, and has been extensively used to investigate the interplay between gut microbiota populations, antibiotic exposure, and *Clostridium difficile* infection. More recently the gut model has been adapted to additionally model intestinal biofilm. Here we describe the structure, assembly, and application of the biofilm gut model.

Key words Chemostat, *Clostridium difficile*, Biofilm, Modeling, Mucosa, Microbiota

1 Introduction

Clostridium difficile infection (CDI) continues to pose a major public health threat and is associated with significant patient morbidity and mortality. Recurrent disease is observed in ~20% of patients [1], which introduces difficulties in treatment management and places further burden on healthcare facilities. The pathophysiological mechanisms of recurrent CDI are not fully understood, but likely involve continued disruption of the host gut microbiota, persistence of *C. difficile* spores, and inadequate host immune response.

The human colon is a highly complex and diverse ecosystem comprising planktonic communities and sessile bacteria within mucosal biofilms. Biofilms are associated with 65% of nosocomial infectious in the USA [2] with treatment costs over $1 billion annually [3, 4]. Studies on intestinal mucosal communities are limited due to the physical inaccessibility of the healthy gut; therefore little is known about intestinal biofilms. Sessile communities differ from

Adam P. Roberts and Peter Mullany (eds.), *Clostridium difficile: Methods and Protocols*, Methods in Molecular Biology, vol. 1476, DOI 10.1007/978-1-4939-6361-4_17, © Springer Science+Business Media New York 2016

their planktonic counterparts, most notably in terms of recalcitrance to therapeutic interventions. The mucosal biofilm and the behavior of *C. difficile* within this biofilm are likely to be of key importance in the disease progression, but are poorly understood.

The importance of investigating the behavior of *C. difficile* within biofilm has recently been recognized by numerous research groups. However, initial studies utilize simple in vitro systems focused on single- or dual-species biofilms, which cannot accurately simulate the complex bacterial communities and environment of the human colon. Investigation of *C. difficile* biofilms is hampered by the same constraints as investigation of *C. difficile* planktonic cultures, namely that behavior in simplified laboratory conditions is markedly different from behavior in the complex, multi-species environment of the colon. Like other areas of *C. difficile* research, investigation of mucosa-associated *C. difficile* communities has utilized a murine model of CDI. However, animal models of CDI, including the hamster and mouse model, are limited by their inability to accurately reflect conditions within humans, and possess an intestinal physiology and microbiome which differs markedly from humans.

We have previously reported the use of an in vitro model of the human colon, which is validated against the intestinal contents of sudden death victims [5]. This model has been successfully utilized to determine the propensity of antimicrobial agents to induce CDI, efficacy of CDI treatment therapies, and the effect of these antimicrobial agents upon *C. difficile* and the indigenous gut microbiota. It is reflective of disease in vivo and correlates well with clinical findings, thus providing an excellent research tool. This model has recently been adapted to study the formation and roles of complex, mixed-species intestinal biofilms, by incorporating 18 removable glass rods into vessel 3 (representing the distal colon and of most physiological relevance to CDI), which promote formation and subsequent sampling and analysis of intestinal biofilm [6]. The biofilm model has been validated for reproducible and consistent formation of mixed-species intestinal biofilms. Optimal biofilm formation and removal techniques have been determined. The biofilm gut model is currently the only in vitro platform enabling analysis of complex, multi-species intestinal biofilm and has previously been utilized to analyze sessile mixed-species communities and investigate the role of biofilms in CDI [7]. We describe here the structure, the assembly, and application of the traditional gut model, and how this model can be adapted to additionally allow the analysis of intestinal biofilm communities.

2   Materials

2.1   Traditional Chemostat Vessel

The triple-stage biofilm gut model consists of three glass fermentation vessels connected in a weir cascade system (Fig. 2). Vessels are maintained at 37 °C via a water-jacketed system connected to a circulating heated water bath. Vessel contents are magnetically stirred and pH values of the vessels are maintained at 5.5 (±0.2), 6.2 (±0.2), and 6.8 (±0.2) for vessels 1, 2, and 3, respectively. The anaerobicity of the system is maintained by the continuous sparging of oxygen-free nitrogen into each vessel. The system is top fed with a complex growth medium at a controlled rate (flow rate 13.2 mL/h) using a peristaltic pump (*see* **Notes 1** and **2**).

1. Chemostat vessels (Soham Scientific, Ely, UK): The working volumes are 280, 300, and 300 mL, for vessels 1, 2, and 3, respectively. The vessel consists of a base, lid, and various attachments (Fig. 1a). The vessel contains a waste outlet port, connected to 6.4 mm bore tubing (Marprene), which attaches to the growth media delivery glassware of the downstream vessel, or waste receptacle (vessel 3—*see* **Note 3**). An O-ring sits on the outer contact surface of the chemostat base where the lid is placed. Ensure that the O-ring and glassware contact surfaces are greased (Glisseal Laboratory grease, Border Chemie). The lid is secured to the base with a metal clamp. A magnetic stirrer bar is placed within the chemostat vessel. The lid unit contains five open ports (B19) housing the attachments outlined below (Fig. 2):

    (a) A glass stopper, which can be removed at any time to allow access to the contents of the vessel for sampling.

    (b) A gas inlet consisting of glass gas delivery tube, which allows the delivery of nitrogen gas into the culture fluid of the vessel.

    (c) A gas outlet to allow gas to escape from the vessel. Both the gas inlet and gas outlet ports are connected to a 0.22 μm vent filter.

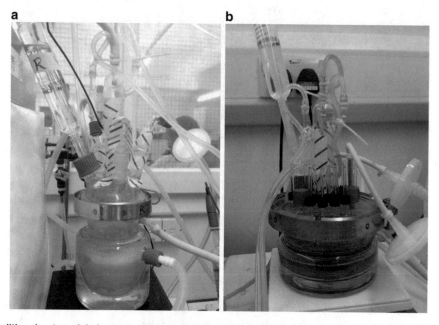

Fig. 1 Traditional gut model chemostat (**a**) and biofilm chemostat (**b**)

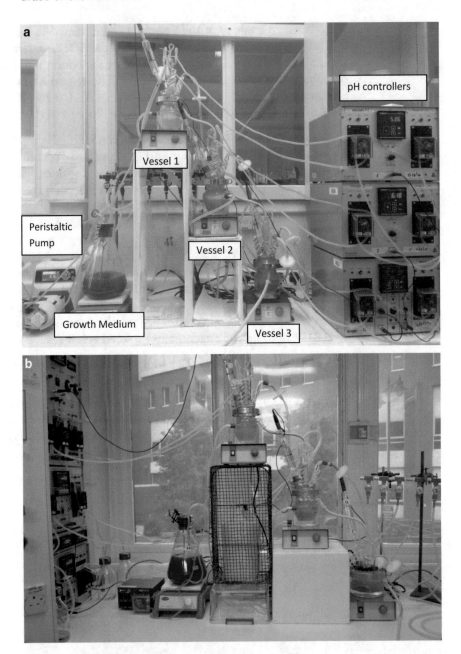

Fig. 2 Traditional triple-stage gut model (**a**) and biofilm gut model (**b**)

(d) A pH probe (attached to a pH control unit) attachment allowing the probe to be inserted into the vessel contents.

(e) A triple-pronged media feeder (central port), which delivers growth media (or the contents from an upstream vessel), acid, or alkali (via autoclaved tubing attached to an automated pH control unit).

2. Stirring: The contents of each vessel and the growth media are constantly stirred magnetically.

3. Nitrogen delivery: Oxygen-free nitrogen is provided via a generator (Parker Hannifin Ltd, UK). A gas manifold connected by silicone tubing allows delivery and control of gas flow to all vessels.

4. pH Control: Each vessel is fitted with a pH probe (P200 Chemotrode, Hamilton, Reno, NV, USA—*see* **Note 4**) connected to a controller controlled by delivering 1 M NaOH/HCl into the vessels using pH controller units (Biosolo 3, Brighton Systems, UK). NaOH is delivered into the vessels by silicone peristaltic tubing. HCl is delivered into the vessels by flexible peristaltic tubing.

5. Temperature control: A circulating water bath (Grant TC120, or similar) able to maintain 37 °C.

6. Growth media: Media constituents are outlined in Subheading 2.3. Media is fed into vessel (via the triple pronged media feeder glassware) using a peristaltic pump (Cole-Parmer Masterflex L/S Digital drive with Masterflex easy load pump head 77800-60 or similar) able to achieve a flow rate of 13.2 mL/h (*see* **Note 5**).

7. Waste: The overflow from vessel 3 flows to an autoclavable waste vessel.

2.2 Biofilm Chemostat Vessel

1. Biofilm chemostat vessel (Soham Scientific, Ely, UK): The biofilm vessel replaces vessel 3 and has a 300 mL working volume, lid, attachments as outlined above (gas inlet changed to a circular pipe, with drilled holes interspersed on the surface to encourage even distribution of gas flow across the rods), and 18 rod attachment ports. The ports for the biofilm vessel attachments are smaller (B14) to allow for rod attachments.

2. Biofilm rods: Ground glass rods (2 mm diameter) are inserted through the lid screwed in place. Upon removal of rods, replacement screw caps are placed onto the lid to maintain the integrity of the system.

2.3 Growth Medium

The model is top fed with a complex growth medium that is prepared in 2 L volumes; constituents are listed in Table 1. Growth medium is prepared in Büchner flasks plugged with a bung adapted to incorporate media delivery ports and magnetically stirred. Sterilization of the growth media is achieved by autoclaving at 123 °C for 15 min after which resazurin (*see* **Note 6**) and glucose are filter sterilized into the medium through a 0.22 μm syringe filter.

2.4 Solid Agar Medium

A list of solid agar medium used during gut model experiments is provided in Table 2.

2.5 Cytotoxin Assay

1. Cells: Vero cells (African Green Monkey Kidney Cells, ECACC 84113001) purchased from NCTT.

Table 1
Growth medium constituents

Constituent	g/L	Supplier
Starch (potato)	3.0	Fisher
Pectin	2.0	Oxoid
Yeast extract	2.0	Oxoid
Peptone water	2.0	Oxoid
Sodium hydrogen carbonate ($NaHCO_3$)	2.0	Sigma
Arabinogalactan	1.0	Sigma
Bile salts no. 3	0.5	Sigma
Cysteine HCl	0.5	Sigma
Tween 80	2.0 mL/L	Sigma
Vitamin K	10 μL/L	Sigma
Sodium chloride	0.1	Sigma
Potassium dihydrogen phosphate (KH_2PO_4)	0.04	Fisher
Di-potassium monohydrogen phosphate (K_2HPO_4)	0.04	AnalR
Magnesium sulfate ($MgSO_4 \cdot 6H_2O$)	0.01	Sigma
Calcium chloride ($CaCl_2$)	0.01	Sigma
Hemin	0.005	Sigma
Glucose	0.4	Sigma

2. Culture medium: Dulbecco's Modified Eagles Medium (Sigma D6546) supplemented with 50 mL newborn calf serum (Invitrogen 16010), 5 mL antibiotic/antimycotic solution (Sigma A5955), and 5 mL L-glutamine (Sigma G7513).

3. Culture vessels: Tissue Culture Flasks (75 mL, Nunc) or Flat Bottom 96 well Trays (Nunc).

3   Methods

3.1   Vessel Assembly

Vessels are assembled individually. The lid connection and all ports and attachments are greased and sealed. Connecting tubing is measured and attached to the upper vessel. All exposed openings are covered with aluminum foil and autoclave tape. Vessels are autoclaved separately. Tubing for media, acid, and alkali is measured and autoclaved. After autoclaving, vessels are connected in

Table 2
Solid medium used in the enumeration of gut microbiota in the gut model

Medium	Target species	Constituents
Fastidious anaerobe agar (FAA)	Total anaerobes and total clostridia	Fastidious anaerobe agar (FAA) supplemented with 5 % horse blood
Bacteroides Bile Aesculin agar (BBE)	*B. fragilis* group	Bacteroides Bile Aesculin agar (BBE) supplemented with 5 mg/L hemin, 10 µL/L vitamin K, 7.5 mg/L vancomycin, 1 mg/L penicillin G, 75 mg/L kanamycin, 10 mg/L colistin
LAMVAB	*Lactobacillus* spp.	LAMVAB agar: 52.5 mg/L MRS broth, 20 mg/L agar technical supplemented with 0.5 g/L cysteine HCl, 20 mg/L vancomycin, adjusted to pH 5
Beerens agar	*Bifidobacterium* spp.	Beerens agar: 42.5 mg/L Columbia agar, 5 mg/L agar technical supplemented with 5 mg/L glucose, 0.5 g/L cysteine HCl, 5 mL propionic acid, adjusted to pH 5 (*see* **Note 10**)
Nutrient agar	Total facultative anaerobes	Nutrient agar
MacConkey agar	Lactose-fermenting Enterobacteriaceae	MacConkey agar
Kanamycin Aesculin Azide agar	*Enterococcus* spp.	Kanamycin Aesculin Azide agar
Brazier's CCEYL agar	*C. difficile* spores	Alcohol shock followed by Brazier's CCEY agar supplemented with 2 % lysed horse blood, 5 mg/L lysozyme, 250 mg/L cycloserine, 8 mg/L cefoxitin
Brazier's CCEYL agar	*C. difficile* total counts	Brazier's CCEYL agar as described above supplemented with 2 mg/L moxifloxacin

situ, tubing is attached, pH probes are calibrated and inserted, the water jacket tubing is connected to the circulating water bath, and gas tubing is connected.

3.2 Preparation of the Gut Model

Each vessel of the gut model is inoculated with approximately 150 mL of pooled fecal emulsion. Vessel 1 is topped up to approximately 280 mL with growth medium and the media pumped started.

3.3 Preparation of Fecal Emulsion

Fecal material is donated by healthy elderly volunteers ($n = 3$–5, ≥ 60 years) with no history of antimicrobial therapy for at least 3 months prior to donation. Fecal samples are stored in a sealed anaerobic zip lock bag for no longer than 12 h during transportation and transfer to an anaerobic cabinet. To ensure the absence of

C. *difficile* populations within the fecal material, samples are plated directly onto CCEYL agar in duplicate and incubated anaerobically at 37 °C for 48 h. Fecal material from any donor testing positive for C. *difficile* should be discarded. Fecal emulsion is prepared by suspending 10% w/v C. *difficile*-negative feces in pre-reduced PBS, and the suspension emulsified in a stomacher until a smooth slurry is formed. Any large particulate matter is removed by filtration through a sterile muslin cloth.

3.4 C. difficile Spore Preparation

C. *difficile* is inoculated onto a single CCEYL plate and incubated anaerobically at 37 °C for 48 h. All growth is removed and subcultured onto ten Columbia blood agar (CBA) plates and incubated anaerobically at 37 °C for 10–14 days. All growth is removed and emulsified into 1 mL of sterile saline, to which 1 mL of 99.6% ethanol is added. The suspension is vortexed for 30 s and stored aerobically at room temperature.

3.5 Planktonic Bacterial Population Sampling and Enumeration

The glass stopper is removed from the vessel and approximately 5 mL culture fluid removed from the vessel via a sterile Pasteur pipette and transferred to a sterile glass tube. One milliliter aliquots are transferred to sterile Eppendorf and stored at 4 °C (cytotoxin assay) or –20 °C (antimicrobial bioassay). The samples are transferred to an anaerobic workstation. Cultures are serially diluted in pre-reduced peptone water to 10^{-7}. Twenty microliters of four appropriate dilutions are inoculated to quarter plates of each culture medium (Table 2) in triplicate and incubated anaerobically (obligate anaerobes) or aerobically (facultative anaerobes) at 37 °C for 48 h. Colonies are identified to genus level on the basis of colony morphology, Gram reaction, and microscopic appearance on selective and non-selective agars.

3.6 Biofilm Analysis

Biofilm-associated bacterial populations are enumerated following careful removal of rods from the biofilm model. Rods are transferred into 5 mL pre-reduced saline, and thoroughly vortexed for 2 min, and the rod discarded. Resuspended biofilm is centrifuged at $16,000 \times g$ for 10 min, the supernatant removed, and pellet resuspended in 2 mL pre-reduced saline. An aliquot (500 μL) is centrifuged and stored at 4 °C for cytotoxin assay. A second aliquot (1 mL) is transferred to a pre-weighed Eppendorf, and centrifuged at $16,000 \times g$ for 15 min, and supernatant discarded. The remaining pellet is weighed and pellet weight calculated by subtracting the Eppendorf weight from the total. The remaining biofilm suspension is enumerated as described for planktonic organisms and units were reported as $\log_{10}$ cfu/g of biofilm.

3.7 Cytotoxin Assay

Vero cell monolayers are cultured to ensure confluent growth upon examination under an inverted microscope. One hundred and sixty microliters of the harvested, trypsinized vero cells are inoculated into the wells to which antitoxin will be added and 180 μL of Vero cells are added to all other wells and incubated in 5 % CO_2 at 37 °C for 2 days or until Vero cell monolayers are confluent upon examination under an inverted microscope. The Vero cells are continuously passaged for the duration of each experiment. One milliliter samples for toxin enumeration are centrifuged at $16,000 \times g$ for 15 min and the supernatant is stored at 4 °C. Sample supernatant and positive cytotoxin controls (48-h culture of *C. difficile* strain 027 210 in brain–heart infusion broth) are serially diluted tenfold in sterile phosphate-buffered saline (PBS-pH7) to 10^{-5}. Serial dilutions are aseptically transferred into microtiter trays containing Vero cell monolayers. Twenty microliters of *C. sordellii* antitoxin is used to neutralize any cytotoxic effect and ensure that cell rounding observed is specific to *C. difficile*. A sample is designated as positive if at least ~80 % of the Vero cell monolayer cells are rounded, and the effect is neutralized by antitoxin. A relative unit is used to quantify the level of cytotoxin present by assigning a titer to the sample based on the greatest dilution of which a positive cytotoxic effect is observed (i.e., if toxin was present in the neat-only dilution this was assigned a titer of 1; if a positive cytotoxin effect was observed in the 10^{-1} dilution then it was assigned a titer of 2).

3.8 Reduced Antimicrobial Susceptibility Surveillance

Breakpoint agars are utilized to monitor for the development and proliferation of antibiotic-resistant or -tolerant organisms. Solid medium specific for the target species is used including an additional supplement of the antimicrobial agent of interest at four times the MIC of that antimicrobial agent for the target species, i.e., surveillance for vancomycin-resistant Enterococci (typical *E. faecalis* vancomycin MIC 1 mg/L)—use kanamycin aesculin azide agar base supplemented with 10 mg/L nalidixic acid, 10 mg/L aztreonam, 20 mg/L kanamycin, plus 4 mg/L vancomycin.

3.9 Antimicrobial Bioassay

The concentration of active antimicrobial agent is determined by an in-house, large-plate bioassay. *See* Table 3 for assay specificities.

Indicator organisms are inoculated onto fresh CBA and incubated aerobically (37 °C) overnight. A 0.5 McFarland suspension (~10^8 cfu/mL) of indicator organism is prepared in sterile saline and 1 mL added to 100 mL molten (50 °C) agar. Inoculated agars are mixed by inversion, poured into 245 mm × 245 mm bioassay plates, and allowed to set. Inoculated agars are dried (37 °C) for 10 min and 25 wells (each 9 mm diameter) removed from the agar using a cork borer. Twenty microliters of target agent calibrator (doubling dilution calibration series) or each filter-sterilized sample from the gut model is randomly assigned to bioassay wells in triplicate. Bioassay plates remain at ambient temperature for 4 h prior to overnight aerobic incubation at 37 °C. Zone diameters are measured using callipers accurate to 0.1 mm. Calibration lines are plotted from squared zone diameters and unknown concentrations from culture

Table 3
Indicator organism and media used for bioassay to determine active concentrations of clindamycin, oritavancin, vancomycin, fidaxomicin, and metronidazole

Target antimicrobial agent	Indicator organism	Agar	Concentration range evaluated
Clindamycin	*K. rhizophila*	Wilkins-Chalgren (Sigma)	4–256 mg/L
Oritavancin	*S. aureus* ATCC 29213	Mueller-Hinton	8–256 mg/L
Vancomycin	*S. aureus* ATCC 29213	Mueller-Hinton	8–512 mg/L
Fidaxomicin	*K. rhizophila*	Wilkins-Chalgren	1–64 mg/L
Metronidazole[a]	*C. sporogenes* (0.5 McFarland in Schaedler's broth)	Wilkins-Chalgren	1–16 mg/L

[a]Assay carried out under anaerobic conditions

supernatants determined. Coefficient of variation values is typically 10% and $R2$ values for calibration lines should be ≥0.9.

Quantification of biofilm-associated antimicrobial activity was determined using the assumption that 1 g of biofilm was equal to 1 mL of planktonic culture fluid.

3.10 Experimental Design

For a typical gut model experiment two triple-stage models are constructed and run in parallel. After the gut models are inoculated with fecal emulsion no further interventions are made for 14 days to allow the system to equilibrate (Fig. 3, period A—*see* **Note 7**). Once steady state is reached (~ day 14) an inoculum of approximately 10^7 cfu *C. difficile* spores (typically ribotype 027, strain 210) is added to vessel 1 of the gut models (period B) and left without intervention for 7 days. This serves as an internal control period whereby the gut flora remain stable and spores quiescent in the absence of antimicrobial exposure. Subsequent interventions are dependant on the aims of the study. Typical examples are listed below.

3.10.1 Induction Gut Model

After the internal control period a further inoculum of approximately 10^7 cfu *C. difficile* PCR ribotype 027 spores is added to vessel 1 of the gut models along with a dosing regimen of antibiotic of interest and dosed to reflect levels present with feces (period C—*see* **Note 8**).

3.10.2 Treatment Gut Model

After the internal control period a further inoculum of approximately 10^7 cfu *C. difficile* PCR ribotype 027 spores is added to vessel 1 of the gut model along with a dosing regimen of clindamycin (33.9 mg/L QD 7 days—period C, Fig. 3). Following

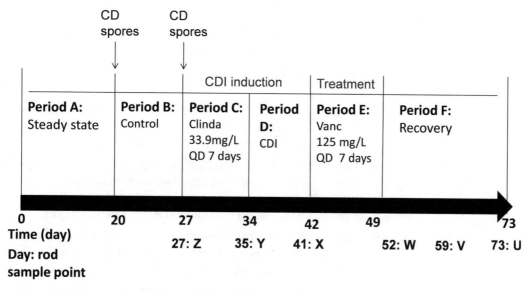

Fig. 3 Typical treatment biofilm gut model experimental timeline

commencement of clindamycin dosing no further intervention is made until *C. difficile* germination, proliferation, and high toxin production are observed (period D), at which point instillation of the therapeutic agent (e.g., vancomycin 125 mg/L, QD, 7 days—*see* **Note 9**) commences. Following cessation of therapeutic instillation the model is left without intervention for 21 days (period F).

Three rod-associated biofilm samples are taken at key stages of the experiment. Due to the finite number of rods ($n = 18$) within the vessel and precautions taken to minimize sessile population bias (i.e., three rod samples per time point), a maximum of six biofilm analysis time points are included in each experiment.

4 Notes

1. Regular observation of gut models is advised to prevent problems. Gas flow, temperature, pH, and fluid levels should be regularly monitored.

2. Excessive frothing of the culture fluid can significantly reduce culture volume. If this cannot be reduced by altering the gas flow, addition of polyethylene glycol (PEG) can help.

3. Blockages of connecting tubing between vessels can occur. This is usually due to buildup of biofilm/cellular matter and can generally be removed by manipulation/massage of the tubing.

4. pH probes must be able to withstand high protein concentrations.

5. Growth media and growth media tubing can become contaminated. The resazurin indicator in the media may cause a color change (red to yellow) if this occurs.

6. Resazurin must be delivered into the medium whilst still warm (≥ 50 °C).

7. Steady state (Period A) can be flexible in length, and should last until microflora populations are stable. Typically this will be ~10–14 days, but can be extended if required.

8. Clindamycin instillation results in consistent CDI induction in the gut model and is therefore the agent of choice for CDI induction during experiments focusing on CDI treatment. Clindamycin is instilled to achieve levels equivalent to those in bile [8].

9. Vancomycin is the first-line treatment agent for CDI and used as a comparator agent to determine superiority/non-inferiority/inferiority of novel anti-CDI agents under investigation.

10. Glucose unstable at excessive temperatures. Medium constituents, including glucose, should be added to cooled, autoclaved distilled water and steamed (100 °C) until molten. Once cooled (approx. 50 °C) propionic acid should be added and pH adjusted using 10 M NaOH and/or 10 M HCl.

Acknowledgements

We acknowledge all the developmental and technical support provided by the Research Team members in Leeds.

References

1. Barbut F, Richard A, Hamadi K, Chomette V, Burghoffer B, Petit JC (2000) Epidemiology of recurrences or reinfections of Clostridium difficile-associated diarrhea. J Clin Microbiol 38:2386–2388

2. Mah TF, O'Toole GA (2001) Mechanisms of biofilm resistance to antimicrobial agents. Trends Microbiol 9:34–39

3. Archibald LK, Gaynes RP (1997) Hospital-acquired infections in the United States. The importance of interhospital comparisons. Infect Dis Clin North Am 11:245–255

4. Costerton JW, Lewandowski Z, Caldwell DE, Korber DR, Lappin-Scott HM (1995) Microbial biofilms. Annu Rev Microbiol 49:711–745

5. Macfarlane GT, Macfarlane S, Gibson GR (1998) Validation of a three-stage compound continuous culture system for investigating the effect of retention time on the ecology and metabolism of bacteria in the human colon. Microb Ecol 35:180–187

6. Crowther GS, Chilton CH, Todhunter SL, Nicholson S, Freeman J, Baines SD, Wilcox MH (2014) Development and validation of a chemostat gut model to study both planktonic and biofilm modes of growth of clostridium difficile and human microbiota. PLoS One 9:e88396

7. Crowther GS, Chilton CH, Todhunter SL, Nicholson S, Freeman J, Baines SD, Wilcox MH (2014) Comparison of planktonic and biofilm-associated communities of *Clostridium difficile* and indigenous gut microbiota in a triple-stage chemostat gut model. J Antimicrob Chemother 69:2137–2147

8. Brown RB, Martyak SN, Barza M, Curtis L, Weinstein L (1976) Penetration of clindamycin phosphate into the abnormal human biliary tract. Ann Intern Med 84:168–170

Chapter 18

MiniBioReactor Arrays (MBRAs) as a Tool for Studying *C. difficile* Physiology in the Presence of a Complex Community

Jennifer M. Auchtung, Catherine D. Robinson, Kylie Farrell, and Robert A. Britton

Abstract

The commensal microbiome plays an important role in the dynamics of *Clostridium difficile* infection. In this chapter, we describe minibioreactor arrays (MBRAs), an in vitro cultivation system that we developed that allows for *C. difficile* physiology to be assayed in the presence of complex fecal microbial communities. The small size of the bioreactors within the MBRAs allows for dozens of reactors to be run simultaneously and therefore several different variables can be tested with limited time and cost. When coupled with experiments in animal models of *C. difficile* infection, MBRAs can provide important insights into *C. difficile* physiology and pathogenesis.

Key words *Clostridium difficile*, Microbiome, Bioreactors, In vitro, Microbial ecology

1 Introduction

Interactions with the commensal microbiome play an important role in the dynamics of *C. difficile* infection. To better interrogate these interactions in a controlled laboratory setting, in vitro cultivation models have been developed to assess *C. difficile* physiology in the presence of the microbiota. Freter and Wilson [1] used single-chamber continuous-flow bioreactors to cultivate hamster cecal communities capable of suppressing *C. difficile* growth in vitro and in *C. difficile* mono-associated mice. Freeman, O'Neill, and Wilcox adapted the three-stage continuous flow cultivation system described by MacFarlane, MacFarlane, and Gibson [2] to study *C. difficile* invasion of human fecal communities [3]. This model has been used extensively to study the impact of (1) different antibiotic regimens on *C. difficile* persistence (e.g., [4–6]), (2) co-infection with different *C. difficile* strains [7, 8], and [3] recurrence of *C. difficile* growth following vancomycin treatment [8].

Adam P. Roberts and Peter Mullany (eds.), *Clostridium difficile: Methods and Protocols*, Methods in Molecular Biology, vol. 1476, DOI 10.1007/978-1-4939-6361-4_18, © Springer Science+Business Media New York 2016

A modified version of this model, incorporating glass rods as a surface for biofilm formation, was also described [9]; this model provides a platform to study physiological differences between planktonic and biofilm-associated populations of *C. difficile*.

Building upon these studies, we developed a simplified, single chamber continuous-flow platform (mini-bioreactor arrays, MBRAs [10]) that allows for cultivation of many different fecal microbial communities in parallel. MBRAs use small volume reactor vessels (25 mL total volume, 15 mL operating volume) fabricated in blocks of six, paired with four 24-channel peristaltic pumps and two 60-spot stir plates to operate 48 reactors in parallel in a single anaerobic chamber. In our initial studies, we seeded MBRA with fecal samples pooled from 12 healthy donors, disrupted a subset of communities with clindamycin-treatment, and challenged treated and untreated communities with *C. difficile*. We found that untreated communities resisted invasion by *C. difficile*, whereas clindamycin-treated communities were susceptible. We used this reactor model to evaluate competition between *C. difficile* clinical isolates of different ribotypes and found that four ribotype 027 clinical isolates exhibited a competitive advantage over clinical isolates of four other ribotypes (ribotypes 001, 002, 014, and 053). These results were validated in a humanized microbiota mouse model of *C. difficile* infection.

Following these initial studies, we have tested the impact of several variations of our previously published MBRA protocol, including changes in fecal donors, composition of medium, retention time, clindamycin-dosage regimen, and *C. difficile* growth status (i.e., challenge with *C. difficile* spores or vegetative cells). In most cases, we have observed that our MBRA model was not impacted by these changes and note these alternative, unpublished protocol modifications throughout the chapter. Because a laboratory setup for the analysis of 48 MBRA communities requires significant capitol investment, we also describe a simplified bioreactor design with less need of specialized equipment.

2 Materials

2.1 Fecal Sample Processing for –80 °C Storage

1. Autoclavable laboratory spatulas.

2. Sterile 1.8–2.0 mL cryogenic tubes.

3. Phosphate buffered saline (PBS): 1 L contains 8 g sodium chloride, 0.2 g potassium chloride, 1.44 g sodium phosphate dibasic, and 0.24 g potassium phosphate monobasic. Adjust pH to 7.4 and filter-sterilize.

4. Portable laboratory scale with sensitivity to 0.1 g.

5. Incubator with capability for 65 °C incubation for 30 min.

6. TCCFA Agar (described in ref. [11]): For 1 L combine, 40 g proteose peptone #3, 5.75 g sodium phosphate monobasic, 2 g potassium phosphate dibasic, 2 g sodium chloride, 200 mg magnesium sulfate heptahydrate, 6 g D-fructose, and 15 g Bacto agar. Autoclave for 20 min, then add a filter-sterilized mix containing 1 g taurocholic acid sodium salt (Sigma), 250 mg D-cycloserine, and 16 mg cefoxitin.

7. Sterile laboratory spreaders, pipetman, and barrier tips.

8. Liquid nitrogen.

9. Low temperature laboratory freezer (−80 °C).

2.2 MBRA Assembly and Operation

1. MBRA are made from DMS Somos Watershed plastic by stereolithography with the previously described dimensions [10]. Our MBRA are manufactured by Proto Labs (www.protolabs.com, formerly FineLine Prototyping), but could be manufactured by other companies with similar capabilities. The CAD file for stereolithography is available upon request. Stereolithography does not produce threads for insertion of fittings within the MBRA; threads can be introduced with a ¼-28 hand tap tool (available from most hardware stores).

2. A 60-position magnetic stir plate is required, such as the MIXDrive60 produced by 2mag, which has inter-magnet spacing that matches the inter-reactor dimensions of the MBRA. One stir plate is needed for every four MBRA strips (24 reactors).

3. Two 24-channel peristaltic pumps with low flow-rate capabilities, such as the series 205S peristaltic pump with 24-channel drive produced by Watson-Marlow, are needed for each set of 24 reactors.

4. A heated anaerobic chamber with a hydrogen sulfide mitigation system and sufficient dimensions to contain the MBRA setup ($90 \times 80 \times 80$ cm ($l \times d \times h$)) is needed. The chamber must also provide an electrical power supply for peristaltic pumps and stir plate. If available, at least one pass-through port with butyl rubber stopper will allow removal of waste from the chamber. The atmosphere in the chamber should contain $\geq 5\%$ H_2, 5% CO_2, and $\leq 90\%$ N_2 (5% CO_2 is needed for adequate buffering of the bioreactor medium, which contains bicarbonate).

5. Tubing, fittings, and source bottle caps are available from Cole-Parmer and Kinesis Inc. and are described in Table 1. This table lists the tubing, fittings, and caps sufficient for a single run of 24 reactors. Although tubing is not reusable, fittings and bottle caps can be reused until noticeable signs of wear are detected.

6. One 500 mL, twenty-four 1 L, and four 2 L glass laboratory bottles with GL45 threaded caps.

Table 1
Tubing, fittings, and caps needed for assembly of 24 reactors

Tubing and fittings from Cole Parmer		
Part number	Description	# packs
EW-45505-82	Adapter, nylon, male luer to 1/4-28 thread, 25/pack	4
EW-45502-56	Female luer tee, Nylon, 25/pack	2
EW-45502-04	Female luer × 1/8″ hose barb adapter, Nylon 25/pack	3
EW-45502-02	Female luer × 3/32″ hose barb adapter, Nylon, 25/pack	1
EW-45505-04	Male luer with lock ring × 1/8″ hose barb adapter, Nylon, 25/pack	8
EW-45502-00	Female luer × 1/16″ hose barb adapter, Nylon, 25/pack	4
EW-96460-26	2-stop Tygon E-Lab, Tubing, 0.89 mm, 12/pack	2
EW-96460-30	2-stop Tygon E-Lab, Tubing, 1.14 mm, 12/pack	2
EW-06424-67	C-Flex Tubing, 1/8″ ID × 1/4″ OD, 25 ft/pack	3
Bottle caps, fittings, and solvent line from Kinesis		
00945Q-2	Omnifit Q-series two hole bottle cap	26
008NB32-KD5L	1/4-28 mm thread to barbed male adaptor (3.2 mm), 5/pack	5
008 T32-150-10	Tubing, PTFE, 1/8″ (3.2 mm) OD × 1.5 mm ID, 10 M	1

7. Holders for MBRA strips can be 3-D printed from ABS or any other suitable plastic. A CAD file for 3D printing that fits the current MBRA design and the 60-spot magnetic stir plate is available upon request.

8. 8 × 3 mm magnetic stir bars (1 per reactor) and 7 mm OD glass tubing precision seal rubber septa (1 per reactor).

9. Sterile 0.22 μm syringe filters.

10. Loctite instant mix epoxy (or equivalent).

2.3 MBRA and C. difficile Cultivation Media (See Note 1)

1. BRM (described in ref. [10]): Original bioreactor medium (Table 2).

2. BRM2 (described in ref. [12]): BRM2 is a modification of BRM with 1 g/L taurocholic acid sodium salt replaced by 0.5 g/L bovine bile (Sigma), which is added prior to autoclaving.

Table 2
Recipe for 1 L of BRM

To 975 mL distilled water, add:	
Quantity	**Reagent**
1 g	Tryptone
2 g	Proteose peptone #3
2 g	Yeast extract
100 mg	Arabinogalactan
150 mg	Maltose
150 mg	D-cellobiose
400 mg	Sodium chloride
10 mg	Magnesium sulfate heptahydrate
10 mg	Calcium chloride dihydrate
40 mg	Potassium phosphate dibasic
40 mg	Potassium phosphate monobasic
5 mg	Hemin
2 mL	Tween 80
Adjust to pH 6.8 and autoclave at 121 °C (≥15 psi) for 45 min Post autoclaving, make a filter-sterilized mix of:	
25 mL	Distilled water
1 g	Taurocholic acid, sodium salt (Sigma-Aldrich)
40 mg	D-glucose
200 mg	Inulin
2 g	Sodium bicarbonate
1 mg	Vitamin K_3

3. BDM: A defined medium with nutrient profile similar to BRM2 (Table 3).

4. BHIS Agar (described in ref. [11]): 37 g/L BBL brain heart infusion, 5 g/L yeast extract, 15 g/L Bacto agar.

5. Clindamycin phosphate and vancomycin hydrochloride.

2.4 MBRA Inoculation and Sampling

1. 1.7–2 mL snap cap tubes.

2. 50 mL screw cap conical tubes.

3. 25 mL sterile serological pipettes.

4. Phosphate buffered saline.

Table 3
1 L recipe for BDM

To 950 mL distilled water, add:

Quantity	Reagent	Quantity	Reagent
600 mg	Ammonium sulfate	170 mg	L-phenylalanine
500 mg	Sodium chloride	180 mg	L-proline
500 mg	Bovine bile	90 mg	L-serine
250 mg	L-alanine	80 mg	L-threonine
190 mg	L-arginine	200 mg	L-valine
210 mg	Glycine	5 mg	Hemin
70 mg	L-histidine	10 mg	Magnesium sulfate heptahydrate
180 mg	L-isoleucine	10 mg	Calcium chloride dihydrate
270 mg	L-leucine	10 mg	Sodium sulfate
240 mg	L-lysine	2 mL	Tween 80
60 mg	L-methionine	1 mL	Trace mineral mix

Autoclave at 121 °C (≥15 psi) for 45 min
Post autoclaving, make a filter-sterilized mix of:

Quantity	Reagent	Quantity	Reagent
30 mL	Distilled water	40 mg	Potassium phosphate monobasic
200 mg	Inulin	40 mg	Potassium phosphate dibasic
574 mg	L-glutamic acid sodium salt	45 mg	L-tyrosine
32 mg	L-asparagine	250 mg	L-aspartic acid
19 mg	L-cysteine	2 g	Sodium bicarbonate
5 mg	L-glutamine	1 mg	Vitamin K_3
24 mg	L-tryptophan	1 mL	Trace Mineral Mix

Also add 20 mL of autoclaved 2 % w/v soluble starch (MP Biomedicals, in distilled water; autoclaved at 121 °C at ≥15 psi for 30 min)

1 L Trace Mineral Mix. In 998.4 mL distilled water, add

Quantity	Reagent	Quantity	Reagent
1.6 mL	Hydrochloric acid	2 mg	Copper(II) chloride dihydrate
2.1 g	Iron sulfate heptahydrate	144 mg	Zinc sulfate heptahydrate
30 mg	Boric acid	36 mg	Sodium molybdate dihydrate
100 mg	Manganese chloride tetrahydrate	25 mg	Sodium metavanadate
190 mg	Cobalt chloride hexahydrate	25 mg	Sodium tungstate dihydrate
24 mg	Nickel(II) chloride hexahydrate	6 mg	Sodium selenite pentahydrate

The stock can be wrapped in foil and stored at 4 °C

(continued)

Table 3
(continued)

To 950 mL distilled water, add:			
Quantity	**Reagent**	**Quantity**	**Reagent**
1 L Trace Vitamin Mix. In 1 L distilled water, add			
900 mg	Potassium phosphate monobasic	1.55 g	Nicotinic acid
15 mg	Folic acid	120 mg	Calcium pantothenate
60 mg	Pyridoxine hydrochloride	1 mg	Vitamin B12
213 mg	Riboflavin-5-phosphate sodium salt hydrate	12 mg	p-aminobenzoic acid
2 mg	Biotin	5 mg	Lipoic acid
58 mg	Thiamine hydrochloride		
Filter-sterilize. The stock can be wrapped in foil and stored at 4 °C			

5. Laboratory wipes (e.g., 4.5×8.5 in Kimwipes).

6. Bleach.

7. 1 and 5 mL syringes.

8. 22 gauge $\times 3''$ hypodermic needles (e.g., Air-Tite Products #N223) and 16 gauge $\times 1.5''$ hypodermic needles.

9. Laboratory centrifuge that can accommodate 50 mL screw cap conical tubes.

2.5 qPCR to Enumerate C. difficile

1. 0.1 mm silica/zirconia beads.

2. 1.7–2 mL screw cap tubes.

3. RNAse, DNAse-free molecular grade water or autoclaved ultrapure water (resistance = 18.2 MΩ cm at 25 °C).

4. qPCR primers were previously described [10] and are listed in Table 4. *tcdA* and broad range bacterial 16S rRNA can be used to determine the ratio of toxigenic *C. difficile* DNA to total DNA present in the population. qPCR primers for *thyA* and *thyX* can be used to distinguish *C. difficile* ribotype 027 strains bearing the *thyA* insertion to strains of other *C. difficile* ribotypes carrying the ancestral *thyX* gene.

5. Power SYBR Green PCR Master Mix (Life Technologies) or equivalent.

6. iCycler iQ PCR plates (Bio-Rad) and microseal "C" optical sealing film (Bio-Rad) or equivalent.

7. Laboratory centrifuge that can accommodate 96-well plates.

8. Real-time PCR machine with capability for detecting SYBR green (e.g., Eppendorf Mastercycler ep realplex2).

Table 4

qPCR primer sequences

Target gene	Primer sequences (Forward and Reverse)	Citation
C. difficile tcdA	F: AGC TTT CGC TTT AGG CAG TG R: ATG GCT GGG TTA AGG TGT TG	[10]
Bacterial 16S *rRNA*	F: ACT CCT ACG GGA GGC AGC AG R: ATT ACC GCG GCT GCT GG	[14]
C. difficile thyA	F: GAT GGC CAG CCT GCT CAT ACA ATA R: TGT TTC ATC AGC CCA GCT ATC CCA	[10]
C. difficile thyX	F: CCA GTT GGG ACA GAC GAA AT R: TGA ACA AGC CCT TGA AAT ACC	[10]

3   Methods

3.1   Fecal Sample Preparation for – 80 °C Storage

1. Prior to receipt of fecal samples, autoclaved laboratory spatulas, PBS, and cryogenic vials should be placed into the anaerobic chamber to pre-reduce for ≥4 h.

2. Upon receipt, fecal samples should be transferred into the anaerobic chamber along with a portable laboratory scale.

3. Each fecal sample should be stirred with a sterile spatula and divided into aliquots in cryogenic vials at a consistent mass (2–3 g depending upon size of cryogenic vial).

4. A 200 mg aliquot should be removed from the fecal sample, resuspended in 1 mL of PBS, heat-killed at 65 °C for 30 min, and 100 µl spread on TCCFA to verify that the sample is *C. difficile* negative.

5. Samples should be labeled, sealed tightly, removed from the anaerobic chamber, flash frozen with liquid nitrogen, and stored at –80 °C. Samples stored in this way can be used for ≥1 year.

3.2   MBRA Assembly for 24 Reactors (Four MBRA Strips)

1. Use the thread-tapping tool to introduce ¼-28 threads into all ports of the MBRA. Rinse with water to remove plastic particulates (Fig. 1a).

2. Cut twenty-four 25 mm segments from the 1/8″ PTFE tubing (Kinesis Inc.).

3. Securely insert each 25 mm segment of PTFE tubing into a male luer to ¼-28 thread fitting (Fig. 1b).

4. Screw the fitting into the top of the MBRA strip.

5. Add 15 mL of water to each reactor chamber and ensure that the bottom of the PTFE tubing is just touching the surface of the water (Fig. 1c, *see* **Note 2**).

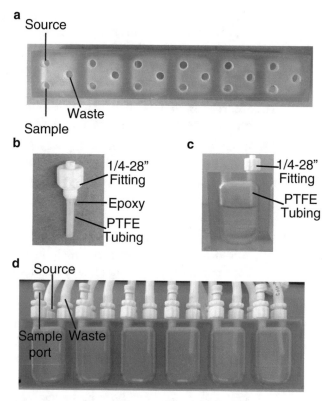

Fig. 1 Initial assembly of MBRA. (**a**) A top-down view of an MBRA strip, indicating the positions at which to secure the source line, waste line, and sample port on one of the reactor chambers. (**b**) An image of a ¼-28″ fitting with inserted PTFE tubing waste line. The position at which epoxy should be applied is also noted. (**c**) Proper length of the PTFE waste line tubing is verified by insertion of a ¼-28″ fitting with inserted waste line into a reactor chamber that is filled with the desired volume of water. (**d**) An assembled MBRA strip, noting the position of the source C-flex tubing, waste C-flex tubing, and sample port with properly folded septum on a single reactor

6. Remove the fittings from the MBRA, maintaining the position of the PTFE tubing.

7. Pour the water out of the MBRA.

8. Using a pipette tip, apply a thin layer of epoxy at the bottom of the ¼-28 thread fitting where it contacts the PTFE tubing to hold in place (Fig. 1b). Take care to avoid excessive addition of epoxy.

9. Allow epoxy to cure, then screw back into the top of the MBRA in the position indicated for the waste line fitting in the MBRA diagram in Fig. 1.

10. Place one 8×3 mm micro stir bar in each reactor within the MBRA.

11. Screw additional male ¼-28 thread fittings in the top of the MBRA at the positions for the source line fittings and sample ports.

12. Screw female luer×1/8″ hose barb adapter fittings into the ¼-28 thread fittings for the waste and source lines.

13. Screw female luer×3/32″ hose barb adapter fittings into the ¼-28 thread fittings for the sample port.

14. Place rubber septa over 3/32″ hose barb adapters and fold top over to make a flat surface (Fig. 1d).

15. Cut eight pieces of C-flex tubing at each of the following lengths: 14, 15.25, 16.5, 17.75, 19, and 20.25 cm for the source and waste lines.

16. Securely fasten the C-flex tubing over the female luer × 1/8″ hose barb adapter fittings for the source and waste lines (*see* **Note 3**).

17. Insert a male luer with lock ring × 1/8″ hose barb adapter fitting into the free end of the C-flex tubing.

18. Insert female luer × 1/16″ hose barb adapter fittings into each end of the 2-stop Tygon E-Lab Tubing (both 0.89 mm and 1.14 mm, *see* **Note 4**).

19. Screw one end of the tubing with the female luer × 1/16″ hose barb adapter fitting into the male luer with lock ring × 1/8″ hose barb adapter fitting already connected to the C-flex tubing on the MBRA. Take care to connect the appropriate, color-coded 2-stop tubing to the appropriate waste and source lines.

20. Cut twenty-four 5 cm pieces of C-flex tubing for connecting the source lines. Insert male luer with lock ring × 1/8″ hose barb adapter fittings into both ends of the tubing.

21. Connect one end of the 5 cm piece of tubing with male luer with lock ring × 1/8″ hose barb adapter fitting to the unoccupied female luer × 1/16″ hose barb adapter fitting at the end of the 0.89 mm 2-stop E-lab tubing. Repeat for the remaining 23 pieces of tubing.

22. Cut sixteen 5 cm pieces of C-flex tubing. For eight of the tubes, insert a male luer with lock ring × 1/8″ hose barb adapter fitting into both ends of the tubing. For the remaining eight pieces of tubing, insert a male luer with lock ring × 1/8″ hose barb adapter fitting into one end of the tubing and a female luer × 1/8″ hose barb adapter fitting into the other end of the tubing.

23. Join the C-flex tubing for the source lines together with female luer tees (Fig. 2a). The C-flex tubing for the reactors on the right-most end of the strip should be connected to opposing sides of the tee by screwing the male luer with lock ring × 1/8″ hose barb adapter fittings onto the tee. A 5 cm piece of C-flex tubing with male luer with lock rings × 1/8″ hose barb adapter fittings on both ends should be connected to the tee that is perpendicular to the remaining two outlets. This newly added tubing should be connected to a second tee junction, with the C-flex tubing for the reactor that is in the third position from the right connected to the opposing side of the tee junction. Another 5 cm piece of tubing, with a male luer with lock ring × 1/8″ hose barb adapter fitting at one end and a female luer × 1/8″ hose barb adapter fitting at the other end should be connected to the perpendicular position of the tee. (During operation, this end will be connected to a

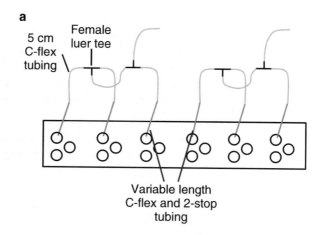

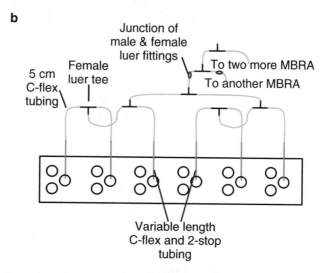

Fig. 2 Connection of source and waste lines. Diagrams of the connections used for the source (**a**) and waste (**b**) lines. More details are described in the text

source bottle for these reactors. During autoclaving, this end should be covered with a piece of aluminum foil to maintain sterility post-autoclaving.) A similar pattern should be used to join the source lines for reactors 4–6 from the right-hand side.

24. Loosely tape the tubing together (grouped in threes) for autoclaving.

25. Begin preparing the waste lines by cutting twenty-four 5 cm pieces of C-flex tubing and inserting the male luer with lock ring×1/8″ hose barb adapter fittings into both ends the tubing.

26. As for the source lines, connect one of the male luers with lock ring×1/8″ hose barb adapter fitting to the unoccupied female luer×1/16″ hose barb adapter fitting at the end of the 1.14 mm 2-stop E-lab tubing. Repeat for remaining 23 pieces of 1.14 mm 2-stop E-lab tubing.

27. Cut twenty 5 cm pieces of C-flex tubing. For 16 pieces of this tubing, insert male luer with lock ring×1/8″ hose barb adapter fittings into both ends of the tubing. For the remaining four pieces of tubing, insert a male luer with lock ring×1/8″ hose barb adapter fitting into one end of the tubing and a female luer×1/8″ hose barb adapter fitting into the opposing end of the tubing.

28. Join the C-flex tubing for the waste lines together with female luer tees (Fig. 2b). This assembly initially proceeds as described for joining the source lines together in **step 23**. However, rather than terminating in a female luer×1/8″ hose barb adapter fitting as described in **step 23**, the joined sets of three waste line tubing will terminate in a male luer with lock ring×1/8″ hose barb adapter fitting and be connected together to opposing ends of a tee junction to make a single waste stream exiting from the MBRA. A 5 cm piece of tubing with a male luer adapter with lock ring×1/8″ hose barb adapter fitting at one end and a female luer×1/8″ hose barb adaptor fitting at the other end should be connected the tee junction. The free end of the female luer×1/8″ hose barb adapter fitting should be capped with foil for autoclaving. Assemble remaining three MBRA reactors in this way.

29. Prior to operation, the waste streams from all four reactors will be connected into a single waste stream. Connecting reactors prior to autoclaving makes manipulation awkward. Therefore, we build and autoclave the waste line connector assembly separately. Build the connector assembly by cutting four 3 cm pieces of C-flex tubing and two 5 cm pieces of C-flex tubing and inserting male luer with lock ring×1/8″ hose barb adapter fittings into both ends of the tubing. Connect two of the 3 cm pieces to opposing ends of a tee junction. Connect one of the 5 cm pieces of C-flex tubing with male luer with lock ring×1/8″ hose barb adapter fittings at both ends to the perpendicular position on the tee junction. Repeat with a second tee junction, the remaining two 3 cm pieces, and a 5 cm piece of tubing. Connect the 5 cm pieces of tubing present on each of the two tee junctions to opposing sides of a new tee junction. Cut a 25–50 cm piece of C-flex tubing (size depends upon configuration in your anaerobic chamber). Place a male luer with lock ring×1/8″ hose barb adapter fitting on one end and a female luer×1/8″ hose barb adapter fitting on the opposing end. Connect the 25–50 cm piece of C-flex tubing to the perpendicular side of the tee junction. The terminal female luer fitting should be covered with foil and the tubing should be grouped together and loosely taped for autoclaving.

30. If your anaerobic chamber setup contains pass-through ports, such as the butyl rubber stoppers present on the Coy Vinyl anaerobic chamber, a ¼″ hole can be drilled through the center

of the butyl stopper. The stopper can be cut to allow insertion of the C-flex tubing, followed by resealing with epoxy, which is reinforced with additional epoxy following autoclaving. If your anaerobic chamber does not have pass-through ports, the waste can be collected within a waste container in the anaerobic chamber and removed daily (*see* **Note 5**).

31. Assemble a waste collection bottle by loosely securing an Omnifit Q-series two-hole bottle cap to the top of a 2 L bottle. Screw male ¼-28 thread fittings into both of the holes of the cap. Screw on female luers with 1/8″ hose barb adapters into both male ¼-28 thread fittings. Cut a 5 cm piece of C-flex tubing and connect to one of the 1/8″ hose barb adapters on the waste collection bottle. Insert a male luer with lock ring 1/8″ hose barb adapter at the opposing end of the 5 cm piece of tubing and cover with foil (This piece of tubing will serve as your air vent; contamination will be prevented by connecting a 0.22 μm syringe filter following autoclaving; *see* **Note 6.**). Cut a 20 cm piece of C-flex tubing and connect to the second 1/8″ hose barb adapter on the waste collection bottle. Place a male luer with lock ring × 1/8″ hose barb adapter in the opposite end of the tubing and cover with foil for autoclaving. This fitting will be connected to the waste line leaving the anaerobic chamber following autoclaving.

32. Autoclave reactors at 121 °C, ≥15 psi for 45 min. Use slow exhaust program typically used for liquids.

33. After reactors cool, tighten fittings and place in anaerobic chamber for at least 72 h prior to use.

3.2.1 MBRA Source Bottle Assembly and Media Preparation

1. Assemble 24 source bottles by placing an Omnifit Q-series two-hole bottle cap on each 1 L media bottle. Opposite the full length piece of PTFE tubing that comes inserted in each cap, insert a ¼-28 mm thread to barbed male adaptor (3.2 mm) and screw in securely. Cut a 20 cm piece of C-flex tubing and place on the ¼-28 mm thread to barbed male adaptor. At the other end of the 20 cm tubing, insert a male luer with lock ring 1/8″ hose barb adaptor fitting. Cover with foil. In the second hole on the Omnifit cap, insert a male luer to ¼-28 thread fitting. Screw a female luer to 1/8″ hose barb adapter fitting on to the male luer fitting. Cut a 5 cm piece of C-flex tubing and place over the 1/8″ hose barb of the female luer fitting. At the other end of the 5 cm tubing, insert a male luer with lock ring 1/8″ hose barb adaptor fitting. Cover with foil. (This will be your vent line during operation and will be coupled to a 0.22 μm syringe filter to prevent contamination.)

2. Media should be prepared as described in the materials section (*see* **Note 7**), with media dispensed into source bottles prior to autoclaving. Caps should be placed loosely on the source bottles

and autoclaved on the slow exhaust cycle for 45 min at 121 °C ($\geq$15 psi). Media should be placed in the anaerobic chamber for at least 72 h prior to use to ensure sterility and anaerobicity.

3. Only eight source bottles are needed at one time for operation of 24 MBRA. We make all 24 L at one time to ensure consistency and place bottles into the chamber $\geq$72 h prior to use. Each liter of medium lasts approximately 1 week with the flow conditions described below.

3.3 MBRA Setup

1. MBRA should be aligned in holders on the magnetic stir plate over the indicated stirring positions. Proper alignment can be verified by setting the stir plate controller to the maximum rpm and verifying that the magnetic stir bars are turning.

2. 2-stop lab tubing for the source and waste should be properly fitted into the clamps on the peristaltic pump. If tubing is placed into the peristaltic pump clamps <24 h prior to intended use, clamps should be locked in place. Otherwise, delay locking clamps until <24 h before use because this reduces the chance of tubing compression.

3. Connect the terminal piece of C-flex tubing on the waste lines from each MBRA strip to the waste line connector assembly by joining male and female luer connections (*see* **Note 8**). Connect tubing to the waste bottle (s).

4. Connect the terminal pieces C-flex tubing on the source lines to the 20 cm piece of tubing on each source bottle.

5. Place a 0.22 μm syringe filter on the 5 cm vent line for each source bottle and on the vent line for the waste bottle.

6. Initiate flow at a modest flow speed (1 mL/min on source pump and 2 mL/min on waste pump) to begin filling the reactors.

7. As reactors begin to fill, check that all reactors reach the same volume and that media exits the reactors into the waste line. If any individual reactors do not fill, tighten any loose fittings and check for problems with individual source lines and replace with prepared extra lines if necessary. If an entire set of three reactors does not fill, check for problems with the source bottle by tightening fittings. If problem is not resolved, replace with a new source bottle, if available. If level of medium rises above the interior waste line in the reactors, check the fittings and exterior waste line for problems and replace if necessary.

8. Once each reactor has filled, reduce the pump settings to your desired flow rate (*see* **Note 9**) and then turn off the pumps.

9. Leave medium in the reactors and waste bottle(s) for 16–24 h prior to inoculation to ensure sterility was maintained.

3.4 MBRA Inoculation

1. Place autoclaved laboratory spatulas, PBS, 50 mL conical tubes, 25 mL sterile serological pipettes, 5 mL syringes, and 16 gauge needles in anaerobic chamber to pre-reduce for ≥4 h.

2. Determine the amount of fecal material that is needed to inoculate the desired number of reactors. Each reactor receives 3.8 mL of supernatant from a 25% m/v fecal slurry. For 24 reactors, a total of 144 mL of 25% m/v fecal slurry should yield sufficient supernatant for inoculation.

3. Transfer frozen fecal samples to the anaerobic chamber and thaw for 15 min.

4. Use a sterile laboratory spatula to transfer fecal material from cryogenic vials to 50 mL conical tubes (12 g total mass). Add 36 mL of anaerobic PBS and seal conical tube tightly. Repeat for two more tubes.

5. Remove conical tubes from chamber, vortex for 5 min, then centrifuge at low speed ($201 \times g$) for 5 min to settle particulates.

6. While samples are centrifuging, sterilize the septa on top of each reactor with a laboratory wipe wetted with 10% bleach. Leave in place for 10 min.

7. Return centrifuged samples to anaerobic chamber.

8. Using sterile serological pipettes, transfer supernatants (~35 mL) to new 50 mL conical tubes.

9. Load 3.8 mL fecal slurry supernatant into 5 mL syringes with 16 gauge 1.5″ needles.

10. Quickly remove laboratory wipe, fully insert the needle through the center of the septum, and inject fecal slurry into the reactor.

11. If desired, save a 1 mL aliquot of fecal slurry for analysis (*see* **Note 10**). Transfer 1 mL to 1.7 mL tube. Centrifuge at $20,000 \times g$ for 1 min. Transfer the supernatant to new 1.7 mL tube and store both tubes at −80 °C.

12. Allow fecal communities to begin growing in batch mode for 16–18 h before initiating flow to reactors. (Ensure that magnetic stir plate control is on and at maximum rpm). If desired, samples can be removed and processed as described in **step 15** prior to initiation of flow.

13. After 16–18, restart peristaltic pumps to initiate flow to reactors.

3.5 MBRA Operation and C. difficile Invasion

1. Once communities have been established with continuous flow for at least 24 h, communities can be disrupted by treatment with antibiotics for 4 days (*see* **Note 11**).

2. Prepare a 25 mg/mL stock of clindamycin phosphate in water and filter-sterilize. Sterilize septa with laboratory wipes and 10% bleach as described above. Inject each reactor to be disrupted with 150 μl of 25 mg/mL clindamycin using a 1 mL syringe and 22 gauge 3″ needle (250 μg/mL final concentration, *see* **Note 12**).

Dose each source bottle with appropriate volume of 25 mg/mL clindamycin to achieve 250 µg/mL final concentration.

3. If you are interested in comparing the composition of your communities before and after treatment (*see* **Note 10**), you should collect a 1 mL sample from each reactor prior to administration of clindamycin. To collect samples, sterilize the septa with bleach and laboratory wipes as described above. Insert a 22 gauge 3″ needle connected to a 1 mL syringe through the septum of each reactor. Carefully remove 1 mL of sample. Transfer to 1.7 mL tube and seal. Remove from the anaerobic chamber and centrifuge at $20,000 \times g$ for 1 min to pellet cells. Transfer supernatants to new tube and store pellets and supernatants at –80 °C.

4. Samples can be removed from reactors daily, if desired, during antibiotic treatment and processed as described above.

5. *C. difficile* will be added to reactors ~24 h following the cessation of antibiotic treatment. Therefore, it is essential to begin preparing *C. difficile* cultures in advance. If spores are to be used, they should be prepared and titered prior to use using appropriate protocols. If vegetative cultures will be used, they should be propagated on BHIS agar two days prior to use. At this time, 5 mL aliquots of BRM2 medium in 15 mL conical tubes should be prepared and pre-reduced. Following propagation on BHIS, *C. difficile* strains should be inoculated into 5 mL aliquots of BRM2 (1 aliquot per strain) and inoculated anaerobically at 37 °C overnight. Following overnight incubation, *C. difficile* strains should be diluted 1:20 in fresh BRM2 and their growth should be monitored periodically until cells reach an optical density at 600 nm of 0.08–0.15. At this point, *C. difficile* cells should be diluted 1:10 into a fresh aliquot of BRM2 and used to inoculate reactors. If you are studying competition between two strains of *C. difficile*, they can be mixed at this dilution step.

6. After 4 days of clindamycin treatment, disconnect old source bottles and replace with fresh source medium lacking antibiotic (*see* **Note 13**).

7. If you will be monitoring *C. difficile* abundance by serial dilution and selective plating, transfer appropriate selective agar (e.g., TCCFA with additional antibiotics), pipette tips, 1.7 mL tubes, and aliquots of BRM2 agar to chamber to pre-reduce (*see* **Note 14**).

8. 16–24 h after replacing clindamycin-containing source medium with fresh medium, sample all reactors. This sample will be used as a community background (negative) control for *C. difficile* in qPCR assays.

9. If using vegetative cells, subculture *C. difficile* as described above in **step 5**. If using spores, *C. difficile* can be added at any time following sampling.

10. Inoculate spores or subcultured *C. difficile* cells into reactors through sterilized septa with 22 gauge 3″ needles and 1 mL syringes. Spores should be added to achieve a final concentration of 10^6 mL in reactors. Addition of 150 μl of *C. difficile* vegetative cells as described above should result in a final density in reactors of 10^4–10^5 cells/mL.

11. After 10–15 min to allow mixing of *C. difficile*, remove 1 mL samples from reactors and transfer to 1.7 mL tubes as described above.

12. If *C. difficile* is to be enumerated by selective plating, remove a 100 μl aliquot for spot plating and transfer to a new tube.

13. Remove remainder of sample in 1.7 mL tube, centrifuge and process as described in **step 3**.

14. If enumerating by selective plating, serially dilute *C. difficile* sample to 10^{-3} and spot plate 10 μl of undiluted, 10^{-1}, 10^{-2} and 10^{-3} dilutions on selective agar. Incubate plates at 37 °C anaerobically for 16–24 h and count colonies.

15. *C. difficile* proliferation can be monitored over time by sampling followed by selective plating as described in **steps 12** and **14** and/or by qPCR with *C. difficile* primers as described below (*see* **Note 15**).

16. Source bottles should be replaced with new source bottles containing fresh medium when remaining volume in the current source bottle is ~100 mL.

17. At the end of the run, the source medium can be replaced with source media bottles containing a 20% bleach solution to sterilize the MBRAs. 20% bleach should be run through the reactors at moderate pump setting (1 mL/min) and left in contact with MBRA for 30–60 min (*see* **Note 16**). Remove reactors from chamber, disassemble, empty, and rinse. Fittings and MBRA strips can be reused until visible signs of wear and tear are detected.

3.6 Alternative Bioreactor Assembly

1. We have made small volume bioreactors using 100–500 mL GL45 thread media bottles fitted with Omnifit Q-series two hole bottle caps. The volume within the reactor is fixed by the length of the PTFE waste tubing. Reactors can be stirred with a standard magnetic stir plate at a low setting and small laboratory magnetic bars (22×8 mm). Media can be delivered and removed with a smaller peristaltic pump. Appropriate pump settings should be determined by measuring the amount of water transferred over a fixed period of time within the setup. Source and waste bottle assembly follow a similar pattern to that described for the MBRAs, with the 2-stop lab tubing connected to C-flex tubing by luer fittings. We have not found a needle of appropriate length to sample these reactors. Therefore, the cap must be removed each time a sample is desired.

2. Other aspects of bioreactor preparation and operation described above can be used with this simplified setup.

3.7 Quantification of C. difficile Levels by qPCR

1. *C. difficile* levels can be quantified directly from bead beaten cell extracts.

2. Prepare tubes for bead beating by adding ~700 mg of 0.1 mm zirconia/silica bead to a 1.7 mL screw cap tube. Add 100 μl of molecular grade water. Leave lid lightly fastened on top. Autoclave for 20 min at 121 °C (≥15 psi). Cool and tighten cap prior to use.

3. Bead beat the cells by resuspending the cell pellet from 1 mL of cells in 500 μl molecular grade water. Transfer to bead beating tube and tighten cap. Homogenize with bead beater at maximum speed for 2 min. Centrifuge at $8000 \times g$ for 1 min to pellet beads. Transfer supernatant to new tube and store at –20 °C until use.

4. For toxigenic *C. difficile*, the toxin A gene (*tcdA*) primers described in Subheading 2 can be used to quantify the levels of *C. difficile*. For absolute quantification, prepare *C. difficile* standards from a known quantity of *C. difficile* cells. To make these standards, grow your *C. difficile* strain overnight in 5 mL of BRM2. Remove a 100 μl aliquot, serially dilute and spot 10 μl of 10^{-3}, 10^{-4}, 10^{-5}, and 10^{-6} dilution on TCCFA, BHIS or BRM2 agar plate. Incubate plate anaerobically at 37 °C overnight to determine CFU/mL. Transfer a 1 mL aliquot from overnight to a 1.7 mL tube, centrifuge at $20,000 \times g$ from 1 min to pellet, remove supernatant, and store pellet at –80 °C until ready for bead beating, which should be performed as described above. Prepare bead beaten extracts from your sample collected before addition of *C. difficile*. Pool 50 μl from each reactor to act as the background community control. Using the CFU/mL data obtained from plating, serially dilute your *C. difficile* standard in to 10^7 CFU equivalents into background community control extract in a total volume of 500 μl. For example, if plating data indicated that *C. difficile* was present at 10^8 CFU/mL (typical concentration for overnight growth in BRM), dilute 50 μl of *C. difficile* bead beaten extract into 450 μl of background community extract. Perform tenfold serial dilutions into background community control DNA (200 μl total volume) to 10^3 CFU/mL. Use 4 μl of each standard, 10^7–10^3, to establish a *C. difficile* standard curve for calibration of qPCR data. Use 4 μl of the background community control as a negative control for *C. difficile*.

5. To perform qPCR on samples, transfer 4 μl of bead beaten cell extract from each sample to the wells of a 96-well optical plate. (All reactions should be done in triplicate.) Transfer 4 μl of each standard as well as negative control to the 96-well optical plate. Prepare qPCR master mix. The 1× concentration for master mix is 12.5 μl Power SYBR Green PCR Master mix, 0.25 μl 5 μM *tcdA* forward primer, 0.25 μl 5 μM *tcdA* reverse primer, and 8 μl molecular grade water. Transfer 21 μl of master mix to each

reaction. Cover plate with optical film and centrifuge briefly at low speed to remove any air bubbles. Amplify in qPCR machine with the following cycle: 95 °C for 10 min, followed by 40 cycles of 95 °C for 15 s, 60 °C for 1 min (fluorescence measured at the end of each 60 °C cycle). A 20-min melting curve can be performed from 60 to 95 °C to ensure that the amplified product is consistent with the *tcdA* product amplified in the standards.

6. Analyze the qPCR data by examining the mean and standard deviations of the cycle thresholds (C_T) values for each replicate. If the standard deviation of the C_T values for any of the replicates are larger than 1.5, consider repeating. Plot a standard curve from the controls, using the log_{10} value of the CFU/mL on the *y*-axis and the average C_T value on the x-axis. Determine the equation and R^2 for the line; it is not necessary to force the line through 0. Use the equation from your standard curve and the C_T values to determine the CFU/mL equivalents from your samples. For samples with C_T values below the range of your standard curve, report the CFU/mL levels as below the limit of detection. If you encounter samples with C_T values above your standard curve, repeat the qPCR on a 1:10 or 1:100 dilution of your sample.

7. As a further normalization for qPCR, the total 16S rRNA gene signal can be determined using the broad-range qPCR primers described in Materials. Because the primers have a broad-range for 16S rRNA genes, care should be taken to avoid contamination with source of bacterial DNA. Use fresh molecular grade water, sterile tubes, and barrier tips for dilutions and qPCR setup. A standard curve can be created from community DNA. In our experience, the MBRA communities in BRM2 support a density of 10^8 cells/mL. However, this can be verified for your specific community by serial dilution and spot plating of MBRA samples on BRM2 agar if desired. Serially dilute community cell extracts from 10^6–10^2 CFU/mL equivalents in molecular grade water in a total volume of 100 μl. Use 4 μl of each standard (10^6–10^2) as well as a molecular grade water as a negative control. Dilute each sample 1:100 in molecular grade water. Transfer 4 μl of each 1:100 dilution, each standard and negative control to qPCR plate. (Set up reactions in triplicate.) Prepare qPCR master mix. 1× concentration for master mix is: 12.5 μl Power SYBR Green PCR Master mix, 0.25 μl 5 μM 16S *rRNA* forward primer, 0.25 μl 5 μM 16S *rRNA* reverse primer, and 8 μl molecular grade water. Transfer 21 μl of master mix to each reaction. Cover plate with optical film and centrifuge briefly at low speed to remove any air bubbles. Amplify in qPCR machine with the cycle described above for *tcdA*. A 20 min melting curve should be performed from 60 to 95 °C to ensure that the amplified product is consistent with the 16S *rRNA* product amplified in the standards.

8. Analyze the qPCR data by examining the mean and standard deviations of the C_T values for each replicate. If the standard deviation of the C_T values for any of the replicates are larger than 1.5, consider repeating. Plot a standard curve from the controls, using the $\log_{10}$ value of the CFU/mL on the y-axis and the average C_T value on the x-axis. Determine the equation and R^2 for the line; it is not necessary to force the line through 0. You will most likely observe a signal from the negative control. As long as this signal is at least 2 C_T units lower than your 10^2 control you should not be concerned. Use the equation from your standard curve and the C_T values to determine the CFU/mL equivalents from your samples. If you encounter samples with C_T values above your standard curve, repeat the qPCR on a 1:1000 or 1:10,000 dilutions of your sample.

9. Normalize your calculated *tcdA* CFU/mL across samples based upon the total bacterial DNA signals. In our experience, C_T values for total bacterial DNA vary by less than two across samples, so the impact is typically modest.

10. If you are using primers to compare levels of two different *C. difficile* populations, such as the *thyA*-containing ribotype 027 strains and strains of other ribotypes that contain the *thyX* gene, use these minor variations to the protocol described below. Previous qPCR experiments with the *thyA* and *thyX* described in Materials have demonstrated that the efficiency of the two primer sets, calculated with the method described by Pfaffl [13] differ by <5%, so direct comparisons of the C_T values detected can be made without comparison to a standard curve. Samples are bead beaten as described above and are diluted 1:10 prior to use of 1 µl as template in qPCR reactions. (Reactions are still performed in triplicate.) The 1× master mix has higher volumes of water (11 µl) to compensate for the decreased template and higher concentrations of primers (100 µM rather than 5 µM). A 1× master mix contains: 12.5 µl Power SYBR Green PCR Master mix, 0.25 µl 100 µM *thyA* or *thyX* forward primer, 0.25 µl 100 µM *thyA* or *thyX* reverse primer, and 11 µl molecular grade water. *thyA* and *thyX* are amplified in separate PCR reactions using the cycling parameters described above.

11. Analyze qPCR results. The ratio of *thyA* to *thyX* is calculated with the equation $2^{(C_T thyX - C_T thyA)}$. The competitive index for a specific day is determined by dividing the ratio on a specific day to the ratio observed on day 0, just after addition of *C. difficile*.

12. Competitions between other strains of *C. difficile* can be monitored by qPCR as long as you have primers that distinguish each strain being competed.

4   Notes

1. Unless otherwise noted, reagent-grade chemicals from any manufacturer can be used in media.

2. The length of the PTFE tubing can be adjusted to change the volume of the reactor vessel. Shortening the line can increase the retention volume whereas lengthening the line can decrease the retention volume. We have used retention volumes as small as 5.2 mL and as large as 20 mL. To avoid contamination of the source medium, leave a headspace volume equivalent to 5 mL of medium.

3. To minimize the amount of source and waste line tubing, C-flex tubing length decreases with the reactors' proximity to the source or waste peristaltic pump. That is, if the peristaltic pump loaded with waste lines is on the right hand side, then the 14 cm C-flex tubing for the waste line will be on the right-most reactor within the MBRA strip. By necessity, this will be the reactor that is most distant from the peristaltic pump loaded with source lines and so the 20.25 cm C-flex tubing for the source line will be on the right-most reactor.

4. The interior diameter of the 2-stop Tygon E-lab tubing is smaller than the 1/16″ female luer fitting hose barb adapter fitting (~1.6 mm). With some effort, both the 0.89 and 1.14 mm tubing can be placed over the hose barb adapter. Placing the fitting over the hose barb adapter is facilitated by heating the ends of the 2-stop Tygon E-lab tubing in hot water (>65 °C) just prior to inserting the fitting into the tubing. During MBRA setup in the anaerobic chamber, you will occasionally encounter problems with a pinched piece of 2-Stop tubing impeding media flow. It is advisable to prepare two extra pieces of 2-stop Tygon E-lab tubing of each size (0.89 and 1.14 mm) with female luer to 1/16″ hose barb adapter fittings on each end. The fittings on the ends of these pieces of tubing can be capped with foil, autoclaved, placed in the anaerobic chamber, and used to replace any damaged tubing discovered during MBRA setup.

5. Many communities cultivated in MBRA produce hydrogen sulfide, which poisons the palladium catalysts used for catalyzing the reaction between atmospheric hydrogen and trace amounts of oxygen. Poisoning of the catalysts with hydrogen sulfide is irreversible and can quickly diminish the life of palladium catalysts, as well as potentially impacting other electronics within the chamber. Further, some oxygen sensors (e.g., Coy Laboratories Anaerobic Monitor Model 12) use palladium to sense oxygen levels and can also be poisoned by hydrogen sulfide in the chamber. Removal of the waste from the chamber through a pass-through port reduces the level of atmospheric hydrogen sulfide that accumulates and works in

conjunction with hydrogen sulfide mitigation systems (e.g., Hydrogen Sulfide Removal Column from Coy Laboratories; Anatox Activated Charcoal from Shel lab) to prolong the life of palladium catalysts and equipment.

6. Depending upon space considerations, multiple waste bottles can be connected in series. In this case, the first waste bottle should be a 1 L bottle with an Omnifit two-hole cap as described above. In place of the vent line, a ¼-28 mm thread to barbed male adaptor (3.2 mm) should be screwed in securely. On the inside of the Omnifit cap opposite this fitting, a ~25 cm piece of 1/8″ PTFE tubing should be inserted. Insertion of this tubing should leave ~100 mL retention volume. A 20–30 cm piece of C-flex tubing can be placed over the ¼-28 mm thread to barbed male adapter fitting and connected to a second 2 L waste bottle. The 2 L waste bottle should have an Omnifit two-hole cap, with male luer to ¼-28 thread adapter fittings and female luer with 1/8″ hose barb adapter fittings screwed into both holes. The 20–30 cm piece of C-flex tubing originating from the first waste bottle can be connected directly to the hose barb of one of the female luers. The second female luer can be connected to a 5 cm piece of C-flex tubing and male luer with lock ring 1/8″ hose barb adapter fitting to create a vent line. The tubing for the waste bottles should be adjusted in length to ensure that there are no kinks or curls in the line that would impede the flow of media.

7. BRM2 medium is appropriate for most *C. difficile* MBRA experiments and is the most cost-effective medium. BRM contains taurocholate rather than the bovine bile found in BRM2, making this medium more expensive as well as leading to communities with abundant *Bilophila* species that are not observed in BRM2 [10, 12]. BDM attempts to simulate the nutrient composition of BRM2 using defined media. Although microbial communities cultivated in BDM are different than those cultivated in BRM2 (Auchtung and Britton, unpublished results), *C. difficile* is still capable of proliferating in these communities following disruption with clindamycin.

8. As long as connections are made quickly after removal of foil and are not touched against gloves or surfaces, there is a minimal chance for contamination. If fittings become dislodged or touch surfaces, soak them in 10% bleach for 10 min prior to reconnection.

9. For the Watson-Marlowe pumps described above, a flow setting of 1 on the source pump will give a flow rate of 1.875 mL/h, resulting in an 8 h retention time. This setting is what we have typically used for our *C. difficile* invasion experiments. However, we have also successfully implemented this model with a pump setting of 0.5 (0.94 mL/h; 16 h retention time), although *C. difficile* titers are ~1 log lower in these communities (Auchtung

and Britton, unpublished results). We typically use a flow setting on the waste pump that is 2× the flow setting on the source pump to prevent clogging in the waste lines.

10. Microbial communities can be analyzed by amplification of the 16S rRNA gene as previously described [10, 12]. An alternative protocol for microbial community characterization by selective plating has been previously described [3]. Metabolites present in supernatants can be analyzed using protocols appropriate for the metabolite of interest.

11. We typically wait for 24–48 h before disrupting communities with clindamycin treatment, although we have also had success disrupting communities that have been established for 14 days prior to antibiotic treatment and challenge with *C. difficile* (Auchtung and Britton, unpublished results). Previously, we published a regimen of twice daily dosing of reactors with clindamycin (final concentration 500 μg/mL) for 4 days [10]. However, we have found that adding clindamycin directly to reactors once (final concentration 250 μg/mL) followed by addition to the source medium (250 μg/mL) for 3 or 4 days also leads to community disruption and *C. difficile* invasion (Auchtung and Britton, unpublished results). Because this less invasive approach to antibiotic administration successfully disrupts communities, it is now the approach that we use in our experiments.

12. We would recommend leaving a subset of reactors untreated as a control while initially establishing your MBRA model. Once MBRA operation conditions have been robustly established, then all reactor communities could be disrupted with clindamycin if the purpose of your experiment is to study *C. difficile* physiology when proliferating in a disrupted community.

13. When switching source media bottles, disconnect the fitting on the old source bottle from the source line on the reactors and quickly connect the fitting on the new source bottle. Take care to avoid contaminating any of the fittings. Transfer the 0.22 μm filter from the vent line on the old source bottle to the new source bottle. Pulse the source peristaltic pump for 2–3 s at maximum speed to ensure that source medium is being drawn up the interior PTFE tubing line within the source bottle.

14. With a large number of reactors, it is easier to sample reactors into deep well 96-well plates rather than individual 1.7 mL tubes. We also perform serial dilutions in 96-well assay plates using a multichannel pipettor.

15. In our invaded communities, *C. difficile* typically persist at 10^5–10^6 cells/mL (e.g., [10]). In untreated communities, *C. difficile* normally washes out to undetectable levels by days 2–4 following inoculation (e.g., [10]). If desired, *C. difficile* proliferation within a community can be disrupted by treatment

with vancomycin. Vancomycin treatment (5 μg/mL final concentration) for 3 days (administered as described for clindamycin treatment) is sufficient to kill all vegetative cells and will also lead to a slight decrease in *C. difficile* spores due to washout of reactors. Cessation of vancomycin treatment can lead to germination of remaining spores, thereby simulating some aspects of a recurrent *C. difficile* infection (Auchtung and Britton, unpublished results).

16. 20% bleach contact times longer than 1 h lead to discoloration of MBRA.

Acknowledgements

The authors acknowledge Robert Stedtfeld for his work designing the MBRAs. This work was supported by award 5U19AI090872-02 from the National Institutes of Allergy and Infectious Diseases to R.A.B.

References

1. Wilson KH, Freter R (1986) Interaction of *Clostridium difficile* and *Escherichia coli* with microfloras in continuous-flow cultures and gnotobiotic mice. Infect Immun 54:354–358

2. Macfarlane GT, Macfarlane S, Gibson GR (1998) Validation of a three-stage compound continuous culture system for investigating the effect of retention time on the ecology and metabolism of bacteria in the human colon. Microb Ecol 35:180–187

3. Freeman J, O'Neill FJ, Wilcox MH (2003) Effects of cefotaxime and desacetylcefotaxime upon *Clostridium difficile* proliferation and toxin production in a triple-stage chemostat model of the human gut. J Antimicrob Chemother 52:96–102

4. Freeman J, Baines SD, Jabes D et al (2005) Comparison of the efficacy of ramoplanin and vancomycin in both in vitro and in vivo models of clindamycin-induced *Clostridium difficile* infection. J Antimicrob Chemother 56:717–725

5. Baines S, O'Connor R, Saxton K et al (2008) Comparison of oritavancin versus vancomycin as treatments for clindamycin-induced *Clostridium difficile* PCR ribotype 027 infection in a human gut model. J Antimicrob Chemother 62:1078–1085

6. Baines SD, Crowther GS, Freeman J et al (2014) SMT19969 as a treatment for *Clostridium difficile* infection: an assessment of antimicrobial activity using conventional susceptibility testing and an in vitro gut model. J Antimicrob Chemother 70:182–189

7. Baines SD, Crowther GS, Todhunter SL et al (2013) Mixed infection by *Clostridium difficile* in an in vitro model of the human gut. J Antimicrob Chemother 68:1139–1143

8. Crowther GS, Chilton CH, Todhunter SL et al (2015) Recurrence of dual-strain *Clostridium difficile* infection in an in vitro human gut model. J Antimicrob Chemother 70:2316–2321

9. Crowther GS, Chilton CH, Todhunter SL et al (2014) Comparison of planktonic and biofilm-associated communities of *Clostridium difficile* and indigenous gut microbiota in a triple-stage chemostat gut model. J Antimicrob Chemother 69:2137–2147

10. Robinson CD, Auchtung JM, Collins J et al (2014) Epidemic *Clostridium difficile* strains demonstrate increased competitive fitness compared to nonepidemic isolates. Infect Immun 82:2815–2825

11. Sorg JA, Dineen SS (2005) Laboratory maintenance of *Clostridium difficile*. Wiley, Hoboken, NJ

12. Auchtung JM, Robinson CD, Britton RA (2015) Cultivation of stable, reproducible microbial communities from different fecal donors using minibioreactor arrays (MBRA). Microbiome 3:42

13. Pfaffl MW (2001) A new mathematical model for relative quantification in real-time RT–PCR. Nucleic Acids Res 29:e45

14. Fierer N, Jackson JA, Vilgalys R et al (2005) Assessment of soil microbial community structure by use of taxon-specific quantitative PCR assays. Appl Environ Microbiol 71:4117–4120

Chapter 19

A Practical Method for Preparation of Fecal Microbiota Transplantation

Elizabeth Perez, Christine H. Lee, and Elaine O. Petrof

Abstract

Clostridium difficile is a challenging infection that can be difficult to treat with antibiotic therapy. This chapter outlines the processing material for fecal microbiota transplantation (FMT), also known as stool transplant. Fecal transplantations are effective in treating recurrent *C. difficile* infection (CDI). FMT uses a stool sample collected from a healthy, screened donor to restore healthy microbiota in the colon of a patient with CDI for symptom resolution. Here, we describe a rapid method for FMT preparation that uses inexpensive and disposable materials.

Key words Human biotherapy, FMT, Fecal microbial transplantation, Stool transplant, *C. difficile* infection, Specimen preparation, Microbiota

1 Introduction

Clostridium difficile infection (CDI) is becoming more prevalent in both hospitals and in the community, particularly in patients who receive antibiotics, which predispose them to developing the disease. Antibiotics eradicate the normal intestinal microbiota, which leads to the loss of resistance against this opportunistic pathogen. CDI can often be difficult to treat, and can result in significant morbidity and mortality [1]. The management of recurrent CDI (defined as recurrence of CDI symptoms for ≥48 h within 8 weeks following the completion of a course of CDI treatment lasting at least 10 days [2]) poses a significant challenge, as it is becoming more common and there are limited treatment options for achieving cure. In such cases, fecal microbiota transplantation (FMT) has proven to be highly successful in case series and case reports, with success rates of approximately 90 % [3–9]. FMT involves a process in which a healthy donor's stool is diluted and filtered, and the liquid portion of the specimen is administered to an affected patient

Adam P. Roberts and Peter Mullany (eds.), *Clostridium difficile: Methods and Protocols*, Methods in Molecular Biology, vol. 1476, DOI 10.1007/978-1-4939-6361-4_19, © Springer Science+Business Media New York 2016

either rectally or via nasogastric/duodenal tube. FMT serves to reconstitute the altered colonic microbiota, in contrast to antibiotics, which further disrupts the microbiota. However, wide variability exists in the methods involved in preparation of FMT and the selection of the donors, which is a concern for clinicians, hospital laboratories, and regulatory bodies alike [3]. Despite its potential, the inconvenience and cumbersome use of blender or stomacher methods (which involve sharp blades or moving parts) and the lack of standardized protocols have made it difficult for hospital and clinical laboratories to embrace and offer this treatment [3].

Here we detail a rapid "blender/Stomacher-free," inexpensive method that strictly uses disposable materials for preparing the specimen for FMT. This methodology, which can be used for both clinical and research purposes, has been approved by Health Canada for preparing donor stool for FMT. Furthermore, clinical and research laboratories at several hospitals have adopted this procedure. This protocol was developed to provide a standardized, readily adaptable, and affordable method of processing stool for FMT that could be performed in any standard microbiology laboratory without the use of highly specialized equipment. It should be noted that before proceeding with human studies, each center should notify the appropriate regulatory body (e.g., Health Canada) prior to proceeding with FMT, according to regulatory guidance and requirements [10].

2   Materials

Prepare all solutions using commercially available bottled water. Store fecal matter at the indicated temperature. Adhere to the institutional waste disposal regulations when disposing of biologic waste materials.

The materials needed are shown (Fig. 1).

2.1 Patient and Donor Selection

1. Collection container (*see* **Note 1**).
2. Plastic biohazard bag.
3. Styrofoam box.
4. Ice pack.

2.2 Processing of Feces

1. Bleach.
2. Plastic or wooden spatula.
3. 300 mL of commercial bottled drinking water.
4. 4×4 gauze (*see* **Note 2**).
5. Tongue depressors.
6. BD 2 oz (60 mL) syringe.
7. 15 mL Conical tube.

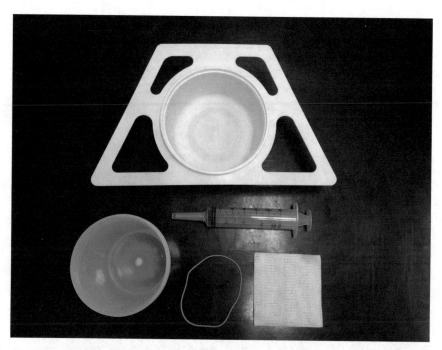

Fig. 1 Some materials required for the processing and collection of fecal material are shown. Fecal collection hat with detachable brim (*top center*). The tight-fitting snap-on lid (that comes with the collection hat) is not shown here. Immediately below is shown the 60 mL collection syringe. *Bottom left* shows the disposable plastic collection container. Any sterile clean plastic container can be used for this purpose, provided that the gauze (shown on *bottom right*) can be secured to the lip of the container for filtration purposes

3 Methods

3.1 Donor Selection and Screening

First, the donor must complete a donor questionnaire to assess the suitability of donating stool for FMT (Table 1). Then, a donor must undergo a comprehensive blood and stool screening for potentially transmissible pathogens (Table 2). Provide the collection instructions and kits to the fully qualified, healthy donors. As this chapter is focused on the preparation of the donor material, only the donor selection is reviewed here (*see* **Note 3**).

1. Instruct the donor not to take any medications, such as laxatives and anti-diarrheal drugs, a minimum of 3 days prior to or during the specimen collection (*see* **Note 4**). For a minimum of 3 months prior to collection, the donor must not have received any oral or intravenous antibiotics.

2. Instruct the donor to collect the feces specimen into the clean, dry collection hat provided (*see* Fig. 2) and follow the stool collection and transportation standard operating procedure (*see* below). The donor should avoid urine, paper, or other waste materials coming into contact with the specimen. Following the collection of stool into the collection hat, the donor should remove the detachable "brim" of the hat and tightly seal the container with its lid.

Table 1
Example of questions for donor screening questionnaire

Question type	Question details
Are you:	1. Feeling healthy and well today? 2. Currently taking an antibiotic? 3. Currently taking any other medication for an infection? 4. Currently taking any immunosuppressant medication by mouth or injection?
Do you have:	1. History of chronic diarrhea persisting >10 days? 2. History of blood in stool not related to hemorrhoid? 3. History of change in bowel habit, alternating from constipation to diarrhea? 4. Any type of active cancer that is not cured? 5. Any active autoimmune diseases?
Have you:	1. Had any vaccinations in the past 12 weeks? If yes, please indicate which one(s) 2. Had contact with someone who had a smallpox vaccination? 3. Lived with a person who has hepatitis A? 4. If yes, have you received vaccine against hepatitis A? 5. Had a blood transfusion? 6. Had a transplant such as organ, tissue, or bone marrow? 7. Had a graft such as bone or skin? 8. Come into contact with someone else's blood? 9. Had an accidental needle stick? 10. Had sexual contact with anyone who has HIV/AIDS or has had a positive test for the HIV/AIDS virus? 11. Had sexual contact with a prostitute or anyone else who takes money or drugs or other payment for sex? 12. Had sexual contact with a prostitute or anyone else who takes money or drugs or other payment for sex? 13. Had sexual contact with anyone who has hemophilia or has used clotting factor concentrates? 14. Female donors: Had unprotected sexual contact with a male who has had sexual contact with another male? 15. Had sexual contact with a person who has hepatitis? 16. Had a tattoo? 17. Had ear or body piercing? 18. Had or been treated for syphilis, gonorrhea, or chlamydia? 19. Been in juvenile detention, lockup, jail, or prison? 20. Been outside the USA or Canada? If yes, list the places(s) 21. Receive a blood transfusion in the UK or France? (review list of countries in the EU) 22. Receive money, drugs, or other payment for sex? 23. Male donors: had unprotected sexual contact with another male? 24. Had a positive test for the HIV/AIDS virus? 25. Used needles to take drugs, steroids, or anything not prescribed by your doctor? 26. Used clotting factor concentrates? 27. Had hepatitis? 28. Had malaria? 29. Had Chagas' disease? 30. Had babesiosis? 31. Received a dura mater (or brain covering) graft? 32. Had sexual contact with anyone who was born in or lived in Africa? 33. Have any of your relatives had Creutzfeldt-Jakob disease?

Table 2

Examples of basic donor screening tests

Serologies	Hepatitis Bs antigen (HBsAg); hepatitis C antibody; syphilis serology; human immunodeficiency virus (HIV) 1/2; human T-lymphotropic virus (HTLV) I/II
Stool	*C. difficile* toxin; enteric pathogens; ova and parasites, polymerase chain reaction (PCR) for norovirus, adenovirus, and rotavirus

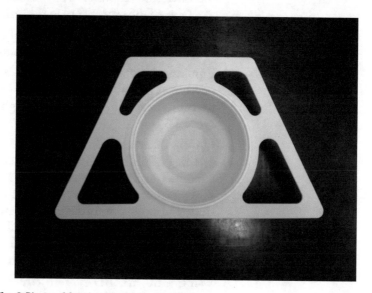

Fig. 2 Photo of fecal collection hat is shown

3. Have the donor place the container in the plastic bag provided, seal tightly, and deliver to the collector.

4. Label the bag (*see* **Note 5**) with the date, time of collection, and the donor's designated letter (*see* **Note 6**).

5. When this is completed, wash hands thoroughly with soap and water.

6. Maintain the stool sample at 2–8 °C until it can be transported to the laboratory. Stool sample should be kept in a Styrofoam™ box with a frozen ice pack inside and the lid tightly closed (*see* **Note 7**). Transportation should occur within 5 hours of collection.

3.2 Processing of Feces

This protocol may be used in any facility that possesses a Level 2 BSC (Biological Safety Cabinet), but should not be attempted elsewhere due to risk of production of aerosols from the sample, contamination, or infection of the patient or those processing the sample (*see* **Notes 8, 11**).

1. Visually inspect the stool for visible blood, mucus, and/or urine contamination in the sealed container. If the sample is contaminated, it must be discarded.

2. Disinfect the surface of the Level 2 BSC using bleach (*see* **Note 9**). The remainder of the steps will take place in the BSC.

3. Weigh an empty container equal to the one that the specimen was collected in, and "tare" the scale. Then weigh the specimen and container. Record this weight, which gives approximate weight of stool since the containers all weigh roughly the same.

4. Remove excess stool into the empty container until only 50 g of specimen remains with a clean disposable plastic or wooden spatula. Discard the excess stool in the sealed container (*see* **Note 10**).

5. Add 300 mL of commercial bottled drinking water to the 50 g of stool. Record exact volume of water used.

6. Emulsify the mixture for 3–5 min by hand using two tongue depressors as spatulas (*see* **Notes 11** and **12**). Allow the mixture to settle for 5 min. Record the weight of the stool mixture (*see* **Note 13**).

7. On top of a clean container, spread one 4×4 gauze across the opening of the container and attach it securely to the top of the container using a rubber band (*see* Fig. 3). Push down slightly in the center of the gauze, to make a small "crater" or depression, and pour the mixture slowly but steadily into the center of the gauze. The supernatant should seep through, which will be collected in the next step, and particulate matter should remain trapped in the gauze (which will be discarded).

8. Using a 60 mL BD syringe (*see* Fig. 4), draw up 50 mL of supernatant from the disposable container (*see* **Note 14**). Repeat with a new syringe for a total volume of up to 100 mL.

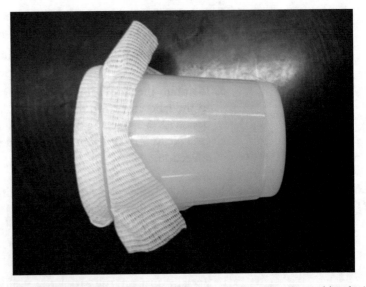

Fig. 3 Photo illustrating how to secure the gauze to the disposable plastic container for filtration of the fecal material

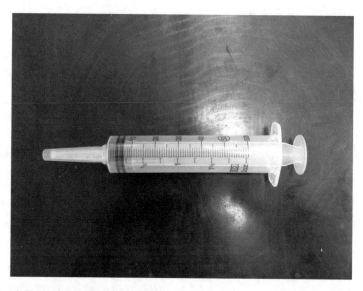

Fig. 4 Photo illustrating the type of syringe used for collection of the fecal material. It is important to use a wide-bore syringe so that the syringe does not "jam." Although the vast majority of large particulate matter is filtered out with the gauze, some of the fecal sediment that goes through the gauze can still cause the syringe to occlude if a wide-bore syringe is not used

Do not expel the filtrate from the syringes—it will be stored in the syringe until it is administered to the patient.

9. Draw up 10 mL of filtrate and place it in a 15 mL conical tube with a tight-fitting screw cap. This sample should be preserved at −20 °C or colder for quality control purposes.

10. Check that the filtrate has preserved its typical brown color of stool. Particulate matter will require re-filtration. Abnormal color (e.g., presence of blood) may indicate an inappropriate sample that will need to be discarded.

11. Label the syringes and the 15 mL tube with a unique identifying number or label that will allow for the future identification of the sample, and ensure that it is administered to the correct patient, and can be traced back to the donor.

12. The syringes with supernatant can be refrigerated at 2–8 °C for up to 24 h, or frozen at −20 °C for up to 30 days. The quality assurance sample will be stored at −20 °C or colder indefinitely.

13. Discard all of the waste from the hood, including the original sample container, the excess stool, the plastic or wooden spatula, and gauze into a tightly sealed double-bagged plastic bag. Disinfect the surface of the bag with bleach before removing it from the biological safety cabinet. The bag should then be autoclaved and discarded as biohazardous waste according to local protocols.

14. Using bleach, wipe down the surface of the BSC (*see* **Note 9** on using bleach in the BSC).

4   Notes

1. Using collection containers with a lid that snaps shut makes it easier to shake the contents and achieve a more homogenous mixture.

2. Usually only one 4×4 gauze, secured on top of a clean container using a rubber band, is sufficient to strain the particulate matter.

3. If the material is intended for human use, it is important to obtain the appropriate clinical expertise and to review patient data to ensure that the patient is appropriate for the therapy. For example, for recurrent *C. difficile* infection treatment in adults, we require that the patient must be at least 18 years of age, and has had multiple (2+) episodes of CDI or is refractory to standard therapy (antibiotic therapy). The treatment should be discussed with the patient by a qualified health care professional and informed consent for the procedure should be obtained. It is important to make sure to discuss the possible benefits of the therapy as well as the potential harm it may cause.

4. The donor should not be on any medications for 72 h at the time of collection.

5. If biohazard bags are not available, most institutions require that the bag be marked with a biologic waste tag, to indicate that the material is of human origin.

6. The date and the designated donor's letter will serve as the lot number for the FMT. For example, when the sample is collected on February 31, 2015, and the designated donor letter is "B" then the lot number will be 310215B.

7. Most institutions require double-enclosed transport of human samples—by virtue of being in the plastic stool hat with a sealable lid, then in a plastic bag that is sealed, and then in a tightly closed styrofoam container, the sample easily meets these stringent requirements for transport.

8. Several limitations to this protocol should be noted. This protocol is developed for preparation of donor stool only. Its use in patients with recurrent *C. difficile* infection or any other medical application requires close appropriate clinical supervision and is beyond the scope of this protocol.

9. Leave the bleach on for no more than 20 min, and be sure to wash off completely by rinsing with water or it will corrode and stain the metal surface of the BSC.

10. Alternatively, if more precise weight is needed, take the empty container, tare the scale, and weigh 50 g of stool directly into that container to use and discard excess.

11. Wear appropriate safety gear for this step (labcoat, gloves, goggles/droplet face shield).

12. The homogenization should be conducted until the consistency of the sample approaches that of a "milk shake," which may take more or less time than specified, depending on the firmness of the stool sample.

13. A systematic review of fecal bacteriotherapy by Gough et al. has shown that FMT is not as effective if less than 50 g of stool is used during the preparation step [11]. Therefore, careful attention should be accorded to ensure that 50 g of sample is collected and homogenized.

14. Adequate homogenization of the sample is necessary. If the filtrate is not homogenous, it will become jammed in the syringe. Inspect the filtrate for clumps and mix it further if needed before drawing it up into the syringe.

References

1. Mitchell BG, Gardner A (2012) Mortality and *Clostridium difficile* infection: a review. Antimicrob Resist Infect Control 1(1):20

2. Cohen SH et al (2010) Clinical practice guidelines for *Clostridium difficile* infection in adults: 2010 update by the Society for Healthcare Epidemiology of America (SHEA) and the Infectious Diseases Society of America (IDSA). Infect Control Hosp Epidemiol 31:431–455

3. Allen-Vercoe E et al (2012) A Canadian Working Group Report on fecal microbial therapy: microbial ecosystems therapeutics. Can J Gastroenterol 26(7):457–462

4. Hamilton MJ, Weingarden AR, Sadowsky MJ, Khoruts A. (2012) Standardized frozen preparation for transplantation of fecal microbiota for recurrent *Clostridium difficile* infection. Am J Gastroenterol 107(5):761–7

5. Kassam Z et al (2012) Fecal transplant via retention enema for refractory/recurrent *C. difficile* infection. Arch Intern Med 172(2): 191–193

6. Mattila E et al (2012) Fecal transplantation, through colonoscopy, is effective therapy for recurrent *C. difficile* infection. Gastroenterology 142:490–496

7. Kelly C et al (2012) Fecal microbiota transplantation for relapsing *C. difficile* infection in 26 patients. Methodology and results. J Clin Gastroenterol 46:145–149

8. Guo B et al (2012) Systematic review: faecal transplantation for the treatment of *C. difficile*-associated disease. Aliment Pharmacol Ther 35:865–875

9. Garborg K et al (2010) Results of faecal donor instillation therapy for recurrent *C. difficile*-associated diarrhea. Scand J Infect Dis 42:857–861

10. Minister of Health (2015) Guidance document of fecal microbiota therapy for the treatment of C. diffcile infections. Health Canada. http://www.hc-sc.gc.ca/dhp-mps/consultation/biolog/fecal_microbiota-bacterio_fecale-eng.php.

11. Gough E, Shaikh H, Manges AR (2011) Systematic review of intestinal microbiota transplantation (fecal bacteriotherapy) for recurrent *Clostridium difficile* infection. Clin Infect Dis 53(10):994–1002

Chapter 20

Ion-Exchange Chromatography to Analyze Components of a *Clostridium difficile* Vaccine

Richard R. Rustandi, Feng Wang, Catherine Lancaster, Adam Kristopeit, David S. Thiriot, and Jon H. Heinrichs

Abstract

Ion-exchange (IEX) chromatography is one of many separation techniques that can be employed to analyze proteins. The separation mechanism is based on a reversible interaction between charged amino acids of a protein to the charged ligands attached to a column at a given pH. This interaction depends on both the pI and conformation of the protein being analyzed. The proteins are eluted by increasing the salt concentration or pH gradient. Here we describe the use of this technique to characterize the charge variant heterogeneities and to monitor stability of four protein antigen components of a *Clostridium difficile* vaccine. Furthermore, the IEX technique can be used to monitor reversion to toxicity for formaldehyde-treated *Clostridium difficile* toxins.

Key words Ion-exchange chromatography, HPLC, 5mTcdA, 5mTcdB, Binary toxins, *C. difficile*, Vaccine

1 Introduction

Ion-exchange chromatography (IEX) is a useful analytical tool for characterization of protein charge variant heterogeneities. IEX separation relies on surface charge-charge interactions between a protein and the resin of the column. There are two types of IEX chromatography: anion-exchange chromatography (AEX) and cation-exchange chromatography (CEX). With AEX negatively charged ions exposed on the protein surface bind to positively charged functional groups on a column and with CEX positively charged ions exposed on the protein surface bind to negatively charged functional groups on a column. In practice, proteins bind to the IEX column in the absence of high salt and can be eluted by increasing either the salt (typically NaCl) concentration or pH gradient (*see* **Note 1**) [1–3].

Clostridium difficile infection (CDI) is the leading cause of nosocomial diarrhea in the Western world. The main toxigenic virulence factors are two large glucosyltransferase proteins, toxin A (TcdA) and

Adam P. Roberts and Peter Mullany (eds.), *Clostridium difficile: Methods and Protocols*, Methods in Molecular Biology, vol. 1476, DOI 10.1007/978-1-4939-6361-4_20, © Springer Science+Business Media New York 2016

toxin B (TcdB), which are proposed to be the primary factors responsible for the symptoms of CDI [4]. Recent CDI outbreaks have been linked to hypervirulent strains which secrete an additional toxin, referred to as binary toxin, CDTa and CDTb, in addition to producing TcdA and TcdB. These hypervirulent strains have been associated with an increase of morbidity and mortality [5, 6]. Vaccination against these toxins is desirable to combat CDI. We have developed a novel tetravalent *C. difficile* vaccine containing all four toxins produced from an insect cell expression system. Data for this novel tetravalent vaccine composed of TcdA, TcdB, and binary toxin components CDTa and proCDTb for the prevention of CDI were presented previously [7, 8]. There are five amino acid mutations each for TcdA (5mTcdA) and TcdB (5mTcdB). Four of the mutations are in the enzymatic domains, and are designed to reduce toxicity, while one is located in the cysteine protease domain to minimize proteolysis of the vaccine components. In addition, 5mTcdA and 5mTcdB required formaldehyde treatment to fully eliminate any residual toxicity. Similarly, three amino acid residues in enzymatic domain of CDTa were mutated to eliminate toxicity and one cysteine residue was mutated to remove aggregation, to generate a molecule referred to as 4mCDTa [9, 10]. The current tetravalent *C. difficile* vaccine consists of 5mTcdA, 5mTcdB, 4mCDTa, and proCDTb in which each has a p*I* of 5.9, 4.8, 8.7, and 4.5, respectively. The broad range of p*I*s across the four vaccine components from acidic to basic necessitated the use of both AEX and CEX chromatography.

In this chapter, we describe details of the AEX and CEX chromatography methods used to analyze charge heterogeneity of each *C. difficile* vaccine antigen. In addition, we demonstrate the utility of these methods for observing changes in charge distribution profiles during stability studies. Lastly, we show how we have applied these methods to detect reversion of formaldehyde-treated 5mTcdA and 5mTcdB samples.

2   Materials

2.1   Chemical Reagents

1. Mobile Phase A (MPA): 10 mM Sodium phosphate, pH 7.2.
2. Mobile Phase B (MPB): 10 mM Sodium phosphate and 1 M NaCl, pH 7.2.
3. Storage solution: 10 mM Sodium phosphate with 0.1 % NaN_3, pH 7.2.
4. Wash solution: MilliQ water.

2.2   Equipment

1. HPLC system (Agilent) (*see* **Note 2**).
2. Anion-exchange column, Propac WAX-10; 4.6 mm ID × 250 mm length, 5 μm particle size, 300 Å pore size (Thermo) for 5mTcdA, 5mTcdB, proCDTb antigens (*see* **Note 3**).

3. Cation-exchange column, Propac WCX-10; 4.6 mm ID×250 mm length, 5 μm particle size, 300 Å pore size (Thermo) for 4mCDTa antigen (*see* **Note 3**).

4. Pre-column filter, 0.5 μm (MacMod) (*see* **Note 4**).

5. Mobile phase filtration unit with 0.22 μm filter (*see* **Note 5**).

---

3 Methods

3.1 Solution Preparation

3.1.1 Mobile Phase A (2 L)

Use 1 M sodium phosphate pH 6.5 solution from Teknova (*see* **Note 5**) and add 20 mL of 1 M sodium phosphate pH 6.5 solution. Add 1930 mL of MilliQ water and adjust pH to 7.2 with 50% NaOH and 1 N NaOH. Make up to a final volume of 2 L MilliQ water. Filter through 0.22 μm filtration unit (*see* **Note 5**).

3.1.2 Mobile Phase B (2 L)

Use 20 mL of 1 M sodium phosphate pH 6.5 solution and add 400 mL 5 M NaCl from Teknova (*see* **Note 5**) Add 1530 mL of MilliQ water and adjust pH to 7.2 with 50% NaOH and 1 N NaOH. Make up to a final volume of 2 L with MilliQ water. Filter through 0.22 μm filtration unit (*see* **Note 5**).

3.1.3 Storage Solution (1 L)

Use 10 mL of 1 M sodium phosphate pH 6.5 solution and add 900 mL MilliQ water and 1 g NaN_3. Adjust pH to 7.2 with 50% NaOH and 1 N NaOH. Adjust to a final volume of 1 L with MilliQ water. Filter through 0.22 μm filtration unit (*see* **Note 5**).

3.2 Sample Preparation

All *C. difficile* vaccine antigens were produced in an insect cell/baculovirus expression system and purified using multistep chromatography techniques with purities of 95% or above. Formaldehyde treatment procedures for 5mTcdA and 5mTcdB have been described previously [11]. Samples were diluted to 0.1 mg/mL in Mobile Phase A for IEX HPLC. Heat-stressed *C. difficile* vaccine antigens were prepared by incubation at 37 °C for various time points.

3.3 IEX HPLC

1. Assemble the HPLC system by connecting the pre-column filter (0.5 μm) and IEX column to the solvent delivery system.

2. The system is equilibrated by the following condition:

   Column equilibration: Mobile Phase A for 30 min at 0.5 mL/min.

   Detection: Fluorescence mode ($\lambda_{ex} = 280$ nm, $\lambda_{em} = 350$ nm) (*see* **Note 6**).

   Flow rate: 1 mL/min.

   Temperature: Ambient (21–25 °C).

3. After above step is completed (flat baseline), inject buffer blanks and perform gradient run. It is highly recommended that this step is repeated twice to establish a flat baseline using

the intended gradient. Initial separation can be performed using a linear gradient from 0 to 100% mobile phase B for 20 min and then continue at 100% mobile phase B for 5 min. At this condition, tetravalent *C. difficile* vaccine antigens are eluted. The separation resolution can be adjusted by changing the gradient condition. The optimal separation conditions for each of the tetravalent *C. difficile* vaccine antigens are shown:

5mTcdA (pI=5.9) and proCDTb (pI=4.6) AEX gradient

(a)   MPA: 80% for 20 min.
(b)   MPB: 20–28% linear gradient for 15 min.
(c)   MPB: 28–100% linear gradient for 5 min.
(d)   MPB: 100% for 3 min.

5mTcdB (pI=4.9) AEX gradient

(a)   MPA: 55% for 7 min.
(b)   MPB: 55–80% linear gradient for 20 min.
(c)   MPB: 100% for 2 min.

4mCDTa (pI=8.7) CEX gradient

(a)   MPA: 96% for 10 min.
(b)   MPB: 4–9% linear gradient for 20 min.
(c)   MPB: 100% for 2 min.

4. The IEX chromatogram profiles for 5mTcdA, 5mTcdB, 4mCDTa, and proCDTb are shown in Fig. 1. The 5mTcdA preparation has at least four additional acidic variants (to the right of the main peak), and one basic peak (to the left of the main peak). The 5mTcdB preparation contains at least one acidic (at 13 min) and one basic variant (at 9 min near the shoulder of the main peak). The 4mCDTa preparation (the one analyzed

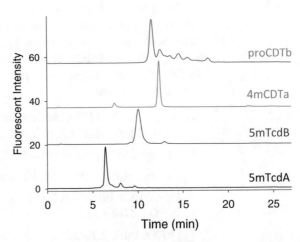

Fig. 1 Chromatograms of four different *C. difficile* vaccine antigens (run under the gradient conditions described in Subheading 3) demonstrating their charge heterogeneities. The three antigens, 5mTcdA (pI=5.9; MW=307 kDa), 5mTcdB (pI=4.8; MW=270 kDa), and proCDTb (pI=4.5; MW=95 kDa), are acidic proteins while CDTa (pI=8.7; MW=48 kDa) is a basic protein

Table 1 Charge Heterogeneities of *C. difficile* Vaccine Antigens

Sample	% Main	% Acidic	% Basic
5mTcdA	85.5	13.0	1.5
5mTcdB	96.5	2.2	1.3
4mCDTa	86.5	13.5	ND
proCDTb	43.3	56.7	ND

ND not detected

with a CEX column) has only one acidic variant (to the left of main peak). Finally, proCDTb contains multiple peaks of acidic variants (at least six different acidic heterogeneities to the right of the main peak). Table 1 lists the % main, % acidic, and % basic components for all four antigens (*see* **Note 7**).

5. The IEX method is also used to analyze the individual antigen stability profiles upon heat stress at 37 °C. The four *C. difficile* antigens, 5mTcdA, 5mTcdB, 4mCDTa, and proCDTb, were heat-stressed at 37 °C for up to 6 months. Figure 2 illustrates IEX profiles for the four antigens upon such heat stress. The acidic peaks increase significantly in 5mTcdA after 1 week, while for 5mTcdB the main peak broadens and a new acidic peak appears at 23-min retention time. In 4mCDTa, two new acidic peaks appear at 8.2 and 11 min after 6-month incubation, while for proCDTb all the acidic peaks have, in general, increased after 3 months (*see* **Note 8**).

6. Residual toxicity is still observed even after four amino acid mutations were introduced in the enzymatic domains for 5mTcdA and 5mTcdB. Hence, additional treatment using formaldehyde is performed to completely remove toxicity. Treatment of 5mTcdA and 5mTcdB with formaldehyde (specifically, without added lysine) results in loss of positive charges from reacted protein lysine residues. Formaldehyde-treated protein becomes more acidic and appears at later retention times by AEX. Furthermore, the AEX peaks for formaldehyde-treated 5mTcdA and 5mTcdB broaden due to heterogeneous populations of various reaction adducts of lysines with formaldehyde. Figure 3a and b shows AEX data on formaldehyde-treated 5mTcdA and 5mTcdB, respectively. The black chromatogram traces represent the proteins before formaldehyde treatment while the red traces are after treatment. When the formaldehyde-treated samples are incubated at 25 °C for 2 weeks, the AEX peaks shift back toward the less acidic region (from the red traces to the blue traces) indicating that a chemi-

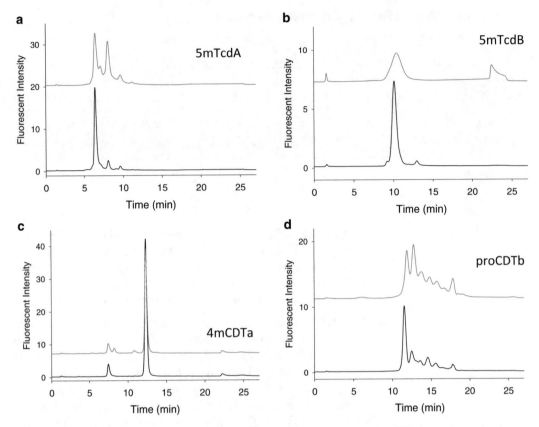

Fig. 2 Heat-stress (37 °C) study of the four *C. difficile* vaccine antigens using IEX chromatography demonstrates an increase in acidic variants (*red traces*) compared to proteins frozen at −70 °C (*black traces*); (**a**) 5mTcdA at 1 week; (**b**) 5mTcdB at 3 months; (**c**) 4mCDTa at 6 months; (**d**) proCDTb at 1 month

cal reversal or reversion is occurring. Wang et al. have clearly demonstrated that this AEX shift back (from red trace to blue trace) correlates with reversion to toxicity in mice for 5mTcdB [11] (*see* **Note 9**).

4   Notes

1. Although IEX elution can be performed using either salt or pH gradients, the former method is preferred due to its simplicity and improved robustness. Elution using a pH gradient requires proper pH-controlled mobile phase preparations which is a common source of error in pH gradient methods. In addition, the HPLC system temperature must be properly controlled since pH may change with temperature.

2. Any HPLC system with a binary pump can be used but a quaternary pump is preferred since wash and storage solutions

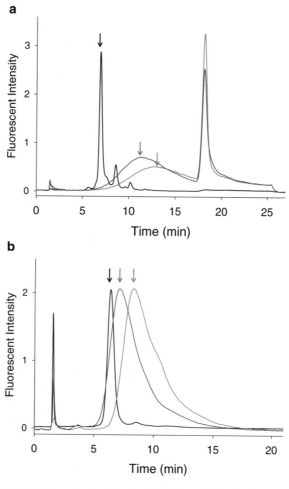

Fig. 3 Chromatograms showing the impact of formaldehyde treatment on AEX profiles and reversion back toward non-treated forms upon stress for 5mTcdA (**a**) and 5mTcdB (**b**). In both overlays the *black trace* shows the untreated profile, the *red trace* shows the formaldehyde-treated profile, and the *blue trace* shows formaldehyde treated with stress at 25 °C for 2 weeks

can be pumped into the column directly without the need to change bottle solutions. It is very important that the column is flushed and stored with storage solution at the end of the run. Subsequently, the HPLC system needs to be flushed thoroughly with wash solution to remove salt and to prevent crystal formation and then flushed with storage solutions to guard against microbacterial growth inside the HPLC machine.

3. Various IEX columns from different vendors have been evaluated but these particular weak AEX and CEX columns provide the best protein recovery and good resolution for all four *C. difficile* antigens.

4. Use of a pre-column filter is highly recommended as a substitute for a guard column. The particular pre-column filter described here is hand tightened and inexpensive compared to a guard column.

5. The filtration of mobile phases is important for running IEX since solid salts from sodium phosphate, sodium chloride, and sodium azide may contain particles that could clog the HPLC system lines, column, and detector. For this reason we recommend the use of 1 M sodium phosphate and 5 M NaCl stock solutions from Teknova to reduce possible particulates from solid salts.

6. Detection can be performed either by using UV absorbance at 280 nm and/or 220 nm or fluorescence mode ($\lambda_{ex} = 280$ nm, $\lambda_{em} = 350$ nm). Because of the high salt concentration used with gradient separation, a higher background may be seen, especially at 220 nm, and there is also baseline drift observed during gradient runs. All of these issues can be overcome by performing fluorescence mode detection, which also provides better sensitivity. *Caution:* UV detection at 280 nm or fluorescence may not give accurate % peak area composition for impurities and fragments due to different numbers of tryptophan and tyrosine residues.

7. The identification of basic and acidic peaks in 5mTcdA and 5mTcdB is still under investigation. Initial mass spectrometry characterization indicates that the acidic peak in 4mCDTa (to the left of the main peak on a CEX column) is the N-terminal-acetylated form of 4mCDTa. Also initial data from mass spectrometry indicate that some of the acidic peaks observed in proCDTb contain phosphorylation sites.

8. In general, heat-stress caused all antigens to increase in acidic variants except for 5mTcdB which demonstrated a broadening of the main peak and a new, relatively broad, acidic peak at 23 min. Furthermore, 5mTcdB is known to aggregate upon heat-stress and the acidic peak at 23 min could be due to the aggregate species. Similarly, 5mTcdA also aggregates very rapidly at 37 ° C and, after 1 month, 5mTcdA precipitates out of solution. Although the actual mechanism of charged variants increases in each of these *C. difficile* vaccine antigens is not known currently, however, in general, common chemical modifications from asparagine to isoaspartate or aspartate (deamidation) are the most likely route of acidic variants in proteins [3, 12].

9. The reversion phenomena described is common for various inactivated toxoid vaccines treated with formaldehyde [13–16]. To date, the reversion is typically confirmed by performing an expensive in vivo animal toxicity study [17], but here we demonstrate that a simple AEX method could be used as a surrogate marker for reversion to toxicity (at least in the case of *C. difficile* 5mTcdB vaccine antigen).

Acknowledgments

The author would like to thank our colleagues in purification and formulation Bioprocess R&D for providing us with material and technical support. We gratefully thank our management, Drs. Sha Ha, Richard Peluso, Jeff Blue, and Sangeetha Sagar, for support of this work.

References

1. Himmelhoch SR (1971) Chromatography of proteins on ion-exchange adsorbents. Methods Enzymol 22:273–286

2. Wang F, Peklansky B, Anderson C, Wang Y, Rustandi RR (2012) Improved ion-exchanged HPLC method in mAb using pH gradient and its comparison with cIEF. J Liq Chromatogr Relat Technol 35:1259–1269

3. Vlasak J, Ionescu R (2008) Heterogeneity of monoclonal antibodies revealed by charge-sensitive methods. Curr Pharm Biotechnol 9:468–481

4. Pruitt RN, Chambers MG, Ng KK, Ohi MD, Lacy DB (2010) Structural organization of the functional domains of *Clostridium difficile* toxins A and B. Proc Natl Acad Sci U S A 107:13467–13472

5. Warny M, Pepin J, Fang A, Killgore G, Thompson A et al (2005) Toxin production by an emerging strain of *Clostridium difficile* associated with outbreaks of severe disease in North America and Europe. Lancet 366:1079–1084

6. Gerding D, Johnson S, Rupnik M, Aktories K (2014) *Clostridium difficile* binary toxin CDT: mechanism, epidemiology, and potential clinical importance. Gut Microbes 5:1–13

7. Heinrichs J, Wang S, Miezeiewski M, Secore S, Xie A, Zorman J et al (2012) Design, production and pre-clinical evaluation of a novel toxin-based vaccine for the prevention of *Clostridium difficile* disease. In: Fourth international *Clostridium difficile* symposium, 20–22nd Sept, Bled, Slovenia

8. Heinrichs JH (2013) Evaluation of a novel vaccine for the prevention of *Clostridium difficile* disease. In: *Third annual vaccine congress*, London

9. Heinrichs JH, Bodmer JL, Secore SL, Goerke AR, Caro-Aguilar I, Gentile MP, Horton MS, Miezeiewski MR, Skinner JM, Sondermeijer PJA, Subramanian S, van der Heijden-Liefkens KHA, Wang S, Xie J, Xoconostle RF, Zorman JK (2013) Vaccine against *Clostridium difficile* comprising recombinant toxins. Patent WO2013112867, August

10. Xie J, Horton M, Zorman J, Antonello JM, Zhang Y, Arnold BA, Secore S, Xoconostle R, Miezeiewski M, Wang S, Colleen PE, Thiriot D, Goerke AR, Gentile M-P, Skinner JM, Heinrichs JH (2014) Development and optimization of high-throughput assay to measure neutralizing antibodies against *Clostridium Difficile* binary toxin. Clin Vaccine Immunol 21:689–697

11. Wang B, Wang S, Rustandi RR, Wang F, Mensch CD, Hong L, Kristopeit A, Secore S, Dornadula G, Kanavage A, Heinrichs JH, Mach H, Blue JT, Thiriot DS (2015) Detecting and preventing reversion to toxicity for a formaldehyde-treated *C. difficile* toxin B mutant. Vaccine 33:252–259

12. Robinson NE, Robinson AB (2001) Molecular clocks. Proc Natl Acad Sci U S A 98:944–949

13. Quentin-Millet MJ, Arminjon F, Danve B, Cadoz M, Armand J (1988) Acellular pertussis vaccines: evaluation of reversion in a nude mouse model. J Biol Stand 16:99–108

14. Holmgren J, Svennerholm A, Lonnroth I, Fall-Persson M, Markman B, Lundbeck H (1977) Development of improved cholera vaccine based on subunit toxoid. Nature 269:602–604

15. Akama K, Kameyama S, Otani S, Sadahiro S, Murata R (1971) Reversion of toxicity of diphtheria toxoid. Jpn J Med Sci Biol 24:183

16. Akama K, Ito A, Yamamoto A, Sadahiro S (1971) Reversion of toxicity of tetanus toxoid. Jpn J Med Sci Biol 24:181

17. Wang S, Rustandi RR, Lancaster C, Hong LG, Thiriot DS, Xie J, Secore S, Kristopeit A, Wang SC, Heinrichs JH (2016) Toxicity assessment of Clostridium difficile toxins in rodent models and protection of vaccination. Vaccine 34:1319

Chapter 21

A Size-Exclusion Chromatography Method for Analysis of *Clostridium difficile* Vaccine Toxins

Catherine Lancaster, Richard R. Rustandi, Paola Pannizzo, and Sha Ha

Abstract

High-performance size-exclusion chromatography (HPSEC or SEC) is a method that can be applied to measure size distribution of proteins, including aggregates, monomers, and fragments. In the biopharmaceutical industry the quantitation of aggregates contained in biotherapeutics and protein-based vaccines is critical given the potential impact on safety, immunogenicity, and efficacy. Hence, aggregation analysis of therapeutic proteins or protein-based vaccine products is almost always a requirement of regulatory agencies. SEC, also referred to as gel-filtration chromatography, separates molecules by size through a porous resin stationary phase. Under isocratic flow small molecules are retained on the column longer than large molecules. Here we describe the use of this SEC technique to characterize aggregation levels for four different protein antigens for a *Clostridium difficile* vaccine.

Key words Size-exclusion chromatography, HPLC, TcdA, TcdB, Binary toxin, *C. difficile*, Vaccine

1 Introduction

SEC is a useful method for size separation of protein monomers from aggregated forms (dimers, trimers, and oligomers). In the biopharmaceutical setting, SEC is a standard technique for characterization of protein aggregates. SEC offers many advantages over other sizing methods, primarily that mild elution conditions allow minimal impact on the protein structure. SEC columns contain stationary phase consisting of spherical beads with pores whereby proteins can be eluted isocratically in the presence of buffer (mobile phase). While the buffer moves through the column, small molecules diffuse in and out of the matrix pores (partitioning). The smallest molecules move furthest into the matrix pores and hence stay longer in the column. The largest molecules are unable to diffuse into the pores and travel through the column at the fastest rate. Therefore, using SEC, separation of biomolecules can occur based on their hydrodynamic radius and molecular size. Aqueous mobile phase often containing salt (added to reduce nonspecific binding of analyte to the stationary phase) is typically utilized in an isocratic

Adam P. Roberts and Peter Mullany (eds.), *Clostridium difficile: Methods and Protocols*, Methods in Molecular Biology, vol. 1476,
DOI 10.1007/978-1-4939-6361-4_21, © Springer Science+Business Media New York 2016

flow. Ultraviolet (UV) detection is most often used for measuring protein by SEC, but fluorescence detection can also be utilized to increase sensitivity. In addition, a more complex combination of detectors employing multi-angle light scattering (MALS), refractive index (RI), and UV is often utilized for measuring the radius and molecular size of each species [1, 2].

Clostridium difficile infection (CDI) is a frequent cause of nosocomial and community-acquired diarrhea and a major health care problem. Strains associated with CDI are known to produce two large toxins, TcdA and TcdB, which are both glucosyltransferase enzymes of similar size, 308 kDa and 270 kDa, respectively [3]. In addition, recent outbreaks associated with more severe morbidity and mortality are known to be caused by hypervirulent strains also containing binary toxin (CDTa and CDTb). CDTa is a 48 kDa protein with ADP-ribosylation activity that binds to CDTb to form binary toxin [4]. ProCDTb is an approximately 95 kDa precursor and non-active form of CDTb. Merck has developed a tetravalent recombinant-based vaccine candidate targeting four toxins of *Clostridium difficile* designed to prevent CDI. Three components of the vaccine (TcdA, TcdB, and CDTa) are mutated at their enzymatic domains to remove toxicity and hence they are called 5mTcdA, 5mTcdB, and 4mCDTa, respectively [5]. Further reduction of toxicity is necessary for 5mTcdA and 5mTcdB by formaldehyde treatment to make 5mTxdA and 5mTxdB [6]. The components of this Merck *C. difficile* vaccine include 5mTxdA, 5mTxdB, as well as 4mCDTa and proCDTb. For this vaccine, the antigens are manufactured by infecting SF+ insect cells with recombinant baculovirus expressing *C. difficile* vaccine components. The process used for purification of these antigens yields drug substance products with >95% purity.

Here we describe an SEC method that is used to characterize 5mTxdA, 5mTxdB, 4mCDTa, and proCDTb protein vaccine components. With this method, percent of monomer and aggregated forms of each of these proteins is monitored. In addition to the four drug substance components of the Merck *C. difficile* vaccine candidate, this method has been applied to 5mTcdA and 5mTcdB, pre-formaldehyde-inactivated intermediates. This method is also used to support process and formulation development of the vaccine components and to ensure acceptable levels of monomer and aggregate in drug substance lots.

2   Materials

2.1   Chemicals and Reagents

1. Mobile phase: 25 mM Sodium phosphate, 300 mM NaCl, 0.05% sodium azide, pH 6.8 prepared from stock solutions of (*see* **Note 1**) 1 M sodium phosphate pH 6.5 (Teknova), 5 M NaCl (Teknova), 10% sodium azide (Teknova), and 50% NaOH (Fisher).

2. Storage buffer (0.05 % sodium azide) (made from 10 % sodium azide).

3. Bovine serum albumin (BSA) (2 mg/mL) (Thermo).

2.2   Equipment

1. HPLC system (Waters Alliance with Waters Dual Absorbance UV detector) (*see* **Note 2**).

2. SEC column, TSKGel Super SW3000 Silica 4 μm 250 Å column (4.6 mm × 30 cm) (Tosoh) (*see* **Note 3**).

3. Pre-column filter, 0.5 μm (MacMod) (*see* **Note 4**).

3   Methods

3.1   Solution Preparation

1. Mobile phase A: 25 mM Sodium phosphate, 300 mM NaCl, 0.05 % sodium azide, pH 6.8 (4 L).

   To approximately 3.5 L ultrapure water add 100 mL of 1 M sodium phosphate pH 6.5, 240 mL of 5 M NaCl, 20 mL of 10 % sodium azide. Add 50 % NaOH, dropwise, to pH 6.8. Adjust the volume to 4 L using ultrapure water (*see* **Note 1**).

2. Storage buffer: 0.05 % Sodium azide.

   To 1990 mL ultrapure water, add 10 mL of 10 % sodium azide.

3.2   Sample Preparation

1. Samples are diluted to 2 mg/mL in mobile phase. No sample preparation is needed if the starting concentration is less than 2 mg/mL.

3.3   SEC HPLC

Assemble the HPLC system by connecting the pre-column filter (0.5 μm) and SEC column to the solvent delivery system. The system is equilibrated by the following condition:

Column equilibration: 100 % Mobile phase A for 1 h at 0.2 mL/min (*see* **Note 5**).

Detection: UV mode at 280 nm (*see* **Note 6**).

Flow rate: 0.2 mL/min.

Temperature: Ambient (21–25 °C).

After equilibration is complete, one or several blank water or mobile phase injections can be made. The recommended run time for this method is 35 min, where all *C. difficile* protein samples elute prior to 20 min. The last ~10 min will ensure complete wash prior to the next injection (*see* **Note 7**). A total of 10 μg of *C. difficile* protein samples should be injected for each run. The volume of injection will vary depending on protein concentration (*see* **Note 8**). BSA can also be injected as a system control at 10–20 μg to ensure the separation of monomer and aggregate forms.

The SEC chromatogram profiles using this method for 5mTcdA, 5mTcdB, 5mTxdA, 5mTxdB, 4mCDTa, and proCDTb are shown in Fig. 1. In all cases, the main peak represents the monomer of the given protein. Large toxins (5mTcdA/5mTxdA and 5mTcdB/5mTxdB) elute the earliest followed by proCDTb and finally 4mCDTa, the smallest of the *C. difficile* vaccine components. The method is not capable of resolving proteins of 308 kDa (5mTcdA/5mTxdA) and 270 kDa (5mTcdB/5mTxdB) sizes and hence is not suitable for drug product characterization. However this method can be applied to monitoring the amount of aggregate, monomer, and fragment in drug substance and intermediates. Table 1 shows the percent of aggregate, monomer, and fragment in the samples which are displayed in Fig. 1.

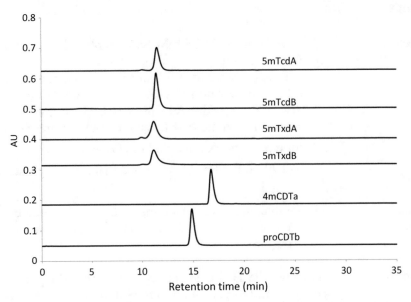

Fig. 1 SEC chromatograms from four *C. difficile* vaccine components (5mTxdA, 5mTxdB, proCDTb, 4mCDTa) as well as intermediates 5mTcdA and 5mTcdB. Ten micrograms of each protein was injected on a TSKGel Super SW3000 column, under isocratic flow at 0.2 mL/min. UV 280 nm signal is shown

Table 1

Relative distribution of monomer, aggregate, and fragment forms of *C. difficile* vaccine components

Sample	% Aggregate	% Monomer	% Fragment
5mTcdA	0.2	99.8	N/D
5mTcdB	1.2	98.8	N/D
5mTxdA	3.2	96.8	N/D
5mTxdB	5.8	94.2	N/D
4mCDTa	0.5	98.2	1.2
proCDTb	0.2	99.8	N/D

This method has been applied for screening and selecting conditions for formaldehyde inactivation, minimizing the amount of aggregate formed during the inactivation process. It should be noted that the formaldehyde treatment of these toxins under the given conditions did not result in a main peak product of increased size which was confirmed by HPSEC MALS/RI/UV showing a monomer molecular weight for the main peak (data not shown). Therefore, the cross-linking that occurs via formaldehyde is thought to be mostly an intra-molecular cross-linking rather than an inter-molecular cross-linking.

This method has also been applied for monitoring stability of *C. difficile* vaccine components. Figure 2 shows the SEC profiles for 5mTcdB before and after a stress at 37 °C for 6 months. As displayed, aggregate is significantly increased upon stress and fragments also increase. Similarly, proCDTb was monitored before and after 6 month 37 °C stress and showed increased aggregate and fragment, but to a lesser extent than for 5mTcdB (see Fig. 3). In this case, several proCdtB aggregate peaks are observed suggesting presence of a dimer as well as a higher order aggregate after such stress. 5mTcdA was not evaluated at the 6 month 37 °C condition since this protein precipitates out of solution after just 1 week at 37 °C. Results for 5mTcdA 1 week stress at 37 °C are shown (Fig. 4) and the loss of protein due to precipitation is seen by decreased peak area in this method. Additionally, 4mCDTa, 5mTxdA, and 5mTxdB were not formally monitored in such a stability study, but the same method could be applied to these antigens to evaluate the impact of stress or long-term stability on aggregation of these proteins.

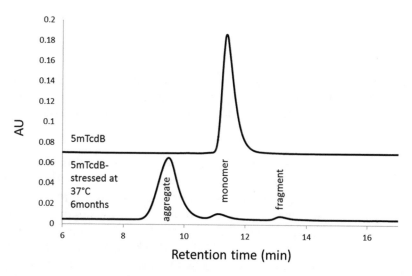

Fig. 2 Chromatogram overlays for 5mTcdB stressed at 37 °C for 6 months compared to a control. The chromatograms illustrate the ability to monitor increase in aggregate and fragment of 5mTcdB using this method

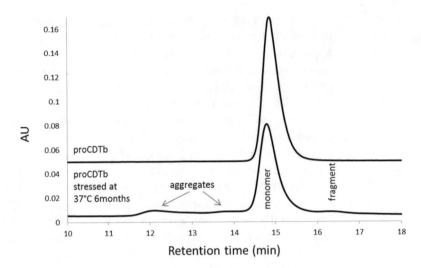

Fig. 3 ProCDTb chromatogram overlay for control material and that stressed at 37 °C for 6 months. The overlay shows an increase in aggregate forms (both dimer and high-order aggregate) as well as an increase in fragment

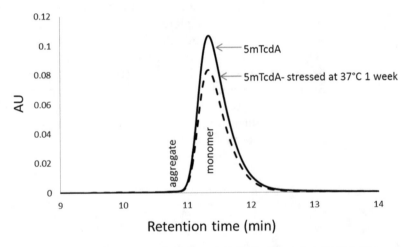

Fig. 4 Chromatograms of 5mTcdA control (*solid line*) and 5mTcdA stressed at 37 °C for 1 week (*dashed line*) which show a loss in total peak area of monomer, consistent with visual precipitate observed for this protein upon stress at this condition. The 37 °C stress study was terminated for this antigen early since it precipitates out of solution

For this vaccine program, a variety of expression systems were originally evaluated for production of these antigens and baculovirus expression was chosen based on many parameters including yield and quality of the four vaccine components. However, for CDTa, the product using the 3mCDTa mutant was heavily aggregated as seen by SEC (Fig. 5). This aggregation was due to a single cysteine residue in the N-terminus and therefore a fourth mutation was introduced by replacing cysteine with alanine to avoid aggregation in the baculovirus system [5]. This SEC method was applied

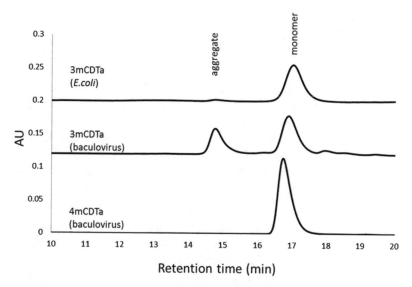

Fig. 5 CDTa chromatograms comparing 3mCDTa from *E. coli* expression system, 3mCDTa from baculovirus expression (prone to aggregation), and 4mCDTa from baculovirus expression. The fourth mutation was introduced to reduce aggregation in the baculovirus-expressed product

for process engineering and optimization in order to produce monomeric CDTa, which turned out to be 4mCDTa (Fig. 5) in the expression system which was chosen for this product.

SEC is an important tool for monitoring size variants of proteins. It has been applied in the method described to *C. difficile* vaccine development to support formulation and process development and to ensure product consistency and stability.

4   Notes

1. The preparation of mobile phase may vary from that listed, but a recommended preparation procedure is described. Sodium phosphate and sodium chloride concentrations are critical to reproduce the method as listed; sodium azide is added to prevent contaminating fungal or bacterial growth and is not required for the method to perform as shown. Additional filtration and degassing of mobile phase can be performed but may not be needed.

2. Any HPLC or UPLC system with UV detector can be used.

3. Various SEC columns have been evaluated for these toxins. TcdB specifically showed some non-specific protein column interactions with several columns tested. Carryover and elution in the inclusion volume were observed for TcdB with several columns tested. This antigen in particular has made the identification of a suitable column for all four proteins most difficult. The given SEC column provides the best resolution and recovery of those tested.

4. Use of a pre-column filter is recommended but not required.

5. The column equilibration shown here is for previously used columns. For a new column, a further equilibration should be performed in order to coat and pacify the column prior to use. Several water or mobile phase injections followed by approximately 5–10 BSA injections should be performed to prepare the column for use. BSA can be injected at 10–20 µg per injection. The baseline and peak area from injection to injection should be monitored and once two BSA injections overlay well and baseline flattens, test sample injections can be made on the column.

6. UV detection at 280 nm wavelength is used for this SEC method to monitor the protein. Lower wavelength such as 220 nm is sometimes used to increase signal of proteins and can be done only if sodium azide is removed from the mobile phase. Sodium azide has significant absorbance at wavelengths closer to 200 nm but this is not an issue at 280 nm. Fluorescence detection ($\lambda_{ex} = 280$ nm, $\lambda_{em} = 350$ nm) may also be utilized to increase sensitivity if needed. Note that the linear range has been evaluated using UV 280 nm only, and the 10 µg injection is within the linear range for this detection method but should be evaluated if using alternate methods. MALS/RI/UV may also be applied to measure molecular size of these proteins.

7. The run time can be adjusted to 30 min if desired.

8. Linearity has been evaluated for 5mTcdA, 5mTcdB, 4mCDTa, and proCDTb. The linear range varied slightly for each of the antigens, but all are linear between approximately 5 and 20 µg. The mass of 10 µg was chosen as appropriate for all antigens.

Acknowledgments

The authors would like to thank the many contributors and colleagues in Bioprocess Research and Development for providing us with material and technical support. We gratefully thank Assunta Ng and Paola Pannizzo for their critical contributions to this method development, optimization, and qualification and John Loughney for the thorough review of this work. We also would like to thank our managers, Drs. Richard Peluso and Sangeetha Sagar, for the support of this work.

References

1. Hong P, Koza S, Bouvier E (2012) Size-exclusion chromatography for the analysis of protein biotherapeutics and their aggregates. J Liq Chromatogr Relat Technol 35(20):2923–2950

2. Fekete S, Beck A, Veuthey JL, Guillarme D (2014) Theory and practice of size exclusion chromatography for the analytics of protein aggregates. J Pharm Biomed Anal 101:161–173

3. Pruitt RN, Chambers MG, Ng KK, Ohi MD, Lacy DB (2010) Structural organization of the functional domains of Clostridium difficile toxins A and B. Proc Natl Acad Sci U S A 107:13467–13472

4. Gerding D, Johnson S, Rupnik M, Aktories K (2014) Clostridium difficile binary toxin CDT: mechanism, epidemiology, and potential clinical importance. Gut Microbes 5:1–13

5. Heinrichs JH, Bodmer JL, Secore SL, Goerke AR, Caro-Aguilar I, Gentile MP, Horton MS, Miezeiewski MR, Skinner JM, Sondermeijer PJA, Subramanian S, van der Heijden-Liefkens KHA, Wang S, Xie J, Xoconostle RF, Zorman JK (2013) Vaccine against Clostridium difficile comprising recombinant toxins. Patent WO2013112867, August

6. Wang B, Wang S, Rustandi RR, Wang F, Mensch CD, Hong L, Kristopeit A, Secore S, Dornadula G, Kanavage A, Heinrichs JH, Mach H, Blue JT, Thiriot DS (2015) Detecting and preventing reversion to toxicity for a formaldehyde-treated *C. difficile* toxin B mutant. Vaccine 33:252–259

INDEX

Adam P. Roberts and Peter Mullany (eds.), *Clostridium difficile: Methods and Protocols*, Methods in Molecular Biology, vol. 1476, DOI 10.1007/978-1-4939-6361-4, © Springer Science+Business Media New York 2016

Printed in the United States
By Bookmasters